Changing Emotion
with Emotion

Changing Emotion *with* Emotion

A PRACTITIONER'S GUIDE

Leslie S. Greenberg

 AMERICAN PSYCHOLOGICAL ASSOCIATION

Published by
American Psychological Association
750 First Street, NE
Washington, DC 20002
https://www.apa.org

Order Department
https://www.apa.org/pubs/books
order@apa.org

In the U.K., Europe, Africa, and the Middle East, copies may be ordered from Eurospan
https://www.eurospanbookstore.com/apa
info@eurospangroup.com

Typeset in Charter and Interstate by Circle Graphics, Inc., Reisterstown, MD

Printer: Sheridan Books, Chelsea, MI
Cover Designer: Beth Schlenoff Design, Bethesda, MD

Library of Congress Cataloging-in-Publication Data

Names: Greenberg, Leslie S., author.
Title: Changing emotion with emotion : a practitioner's guide / by Leslie S. Greenberg.
Description: Washington, DC : American Psychological Association, [2021] |
    Includes bibliographical references and index.
Identifiers: LCCN 2020048842 (print) | LCCN 2020048843 (ebook) |
    ISBN 9781433834691 (paperback) | ISBN 9781433836060 (ebook)
Subjects: LCSH: Emotions. | Psychotherapy.
Classification: LCC RC489.E45 G73 2021 (print) | LCC RC489.E45 (ebook) |
    DDC 616.89/14—dc23
LC record available at https://lccn.loc.gov/2020048842
LC ebook record available at https://lccn.loc.gov/2020048843

https://doi.org/10.1037/0000248-000

Printed in the United States of America

10 9 8 7 6 5 4 3 2

Contents

Changing Emotion
with Emotion

INTRODUCTION
Working With Emotion in Psychotherapy

There is a burgeoning interest in how to work with emotion in psycho-therapy. Different schools offer distinct perspectives and have developed different methods, which were compared in a recent book (Greenberg et al., 2019). I take a further step in the present book by offering a transdiagnostic, transtheoretical perspective to working with emotion. This perspective is based on three main ideas: (a) emotion is central in many forms of psychological dysfunction, (b) both acceptance and change of emotions are important to curing suffering regardless of type of emotional disorder, and (c) work on transforming the underlying emotional cause of psychological dis-ease is important for enduring change and differs from modification of symptoms and provision of coping skills.

The intended audience for this book includes mental health clinicians of all schools and students in all helping disciplines. Other professionals who work with people suffering from emotional difficulties also should find the views expressed here informative. How to work with emotions in therapy has not been explicitly taught in psychology, psychiatry, or social work graduate programs even though clinicians working on the front lines meet people's emotional suffering day in and day out. This book is designed to help you

https://doi.org/10.1037/0000248-001
Changing Emotion With Emotion: A Practitioner's Guide, by L. S. Greenberg

think clearly about how to work with emotion and to provide you with methods to do so.

Along with explanations in each chapter of the key steps and skills involved with emotion change, I provide descriptions of clients and transcripts excerpted from actual therapy sessions. I have omitted personal details and changed names to protect all individuals' privacy. I also have embedded brief commentary within brackets in the clinical dialogues. These comments are the result of task analyses I performed on each session to pinpoint the specific moments when one can perceive—whether through words, silence, tone, gesture, facial expression, or tears—that a change is occurring or is being facilitated or acknowledged. By providing analyses of these microevents within each therapy dialogue, my aim is to help you recognize the processes described; these analyses may also serve as group discussion topics or as models for either supervision or deliberate practice.

Until recently, a specific disorder approach has governed diagnosis and treatment. Growing evidence, however, indicates that similar processes underlie depressive and anxiety disorders (Kendler, 1996; Kessler et al., 2005) as well as other disorders. In addition, evidence points to high rates of comorbidity of up to 40% to 80% in clinical and also in epidemiological studies (T. A. Brown, Campbell, et al., 2001; Kessler et al., 2005). A major problem in the field is that interventions that are specific to a disorder pay relatively limited attention to the aspects of the comorbid disorder. Given these concerns, clinicians are increasingly in agreement that we need a new way to classify, and treat, disorders (Barlow et al., 2004). A transdiagnostic approach needs to identify core, common, maladaptive processes and target them in treatment (Barlow et al., 2004) as well as delineate where and how these treatments need to be adjusted depending on the client or diagnostic groups. People with schizophrenia, for example, may need additional processes.

Different models of psychotherapy think about—and work with—emotion in distinct ways, but a goal of all treatment approaches is to help people alleviate emotional suffering. Many features of these diverse approaches are similar, but they may often be viewed as more different than they really are because of their various language systems (Abbass, 2015; Fonagy et al., 2002; Fosha, 2004; Greenberg, 2011; Greenberg & Safran, 1987; Jurist, 2019; McCullough, 1999; Perls et al., 1951; Rogers, 1957). In this book, I hope to present a coherent view of emotion to inform an agreed on approach to the treatment of peoples' underlying emotional problems. I also hope to propose a transdiagnostic perspective that specifies underlying principles and methods for working with deeper emotional pain. I believe that, in the long run, this proposed approach will improve the treatment of people who suffer from different disorders. This approach is for working with implicit body-based emotional states that function beneath levels of awareness and are more related to right-hemispheric implicit processes than to left-hemispheric linguistically processed explicit knowledge.

WHY TARGET EMOTION TO CURE SUFFERING?

Early on, Alexander and French (1946) introduced the notion of the corrective emotional experience and claimed that reexperiencing the old difficulties with a new ending was the secret of all therapeutic change. The proposal was that actual lived experience of a new solution to old problematic patterns convinces people that new solutions are possible, thus inducing them to change their old patterns. With repeated novel experience, the corrected reactions become, over time, automatic and transform into new, higher level forms of functioning.

Goldfried (1980) suggested that the corrective experience occupies a central role in the therapy change process across orientations. He proposed providing the client with new, corrective experiences as a common clinical strategy. I highlight the importance of corrective experience as a concept that originated in psychoanalytic circles but has clear relevance to all orientations and perhaps represents a core principle of change (Goldfried, 1980). In this book, I suggest that the best way to achieve a corrective emotional experience is to transform one emotion by activating another one; I discuss how to facilitate this process.

Most people come to therapy because they are in emotional pain. They may present with symptoms of depression, anxiety, eating disorders, addiction, or personality or interpersonal problems, but they need help dealing with the underlying sadness, shame, anger, fear, and sometimes even unrestrained manic pleasure. Several pathologies described in the fifth edition of the *Diagnostic and Statistical Manual of Mental Disorders* (*DSM-5*; American Psychiatric Association, 2013) can be considered as having originated from emotional difficulties. Individuals with mood disorders, such as depression, feel trapped in a complex web involving sadness, shame, and guilt; those with anxiety disorders are taken by dread and fear; and those with borderline personality disorders experience different alternating emotions that are always highly intense.

Despite recognizing some differences in varied diagnostic groups, a number of therapeutic approaches have always treated people, regardless of diagnosis, in the same fashion (Goldfried & Davison, 1976). Many that focus on emotion from the start have proposed the curative value of the therapeutic relationship, specifically the clinician's empathic responding to feeling and the use of interventions to access emotion regardless of type of disorder (Fosha, 2000; Greenberg, Rice, & Elliott, 1993; Perls et al., 1951; Rogers, 1957). From this perspective, the clinician who can master empathy and emotion eliciting interventions does not need to rely on learning different protocols for different disorders. Treatment is basically the same, whether the *DSM-5* defines the client's clinical issue as anxiety, a mood disorder, posttraumatic stress disorder, addiction, or a personality disorder. This transdiagnostic feature of many current emotion-oriented treatments and of both early, humanistic, and behavioral approaches has been present since the development of those treatments because they relied more on problem or process specification as well as on case formulation than on diagnosis (Fosha, 2000; Greenberg, 2011; Greenberg & Safran, 1987; McCullough, 1999; Perls et al., 1951; Rogers, 1957). So, in some fashion, a transdiagnostic approach is going back to the fundamental principles of these approaches.

Growing evidence shows that activating and working with emotion in therapy predicts outcome regardless of diagnostic grouping. Recently, the results of a meta-analysis (Peluso & Freund, 2018) indicated that client expression of emotion evidences a medium effect size with psychotherapy outcomes. The results of this meta-analysis generally replicated conclusions of other systematic reviews and meta-analyses. The magnitude of the effect sizes observed in the recent analysis ($d = .85$) was similar to findings in both the Diener et al. (2007) and A. Pascual-Leone and Yeryomenko (2016) reviews of the relationship between emotional experience and expression and outcome. Thus, there is evidence that emotional expression in therapy relates to outcome—and that it is not diagnosis specific.

Some theoretical views caution against the idea that expressing emotions is desirable; instead, they champion the value of restraint or suggest different stages of readiness for change and, by implication, for emotion work (Miller & Rollnick, 2013; Prochaska & DiClemente, 1983). Others suggest that emotion work with borderline or traumatized clients and the exploration of childhood memories can be disorganizing and countertherapeutic. For example, both transference-focused psychotherapy and mentalization-based therapy (Bateman & Fonagy, 2004; Yeomans et al., 2015), two psychodynamic evidence-based approaches for severe personality disorders, question the activation of childhood memories for certain clients. I agree that clinicians should exercise some caution about when to activate and when to regulate emotions, as well as what emotions should be regulated or activated and when clients should be invited to go back to childhood or to traumatic experiences. I discuss these caveats throughout the book.

HOW DOES EMOTION TRANSFORMATION WORK?

This book focuses on methods that facilitate the transformation of emotion by helping clients with all types of disorders arrive at painful maladaptive emotions and then leave these emotions by accessing new, adaptive emotions. I suggest that you cannot leave a place until you arrive at it, so one has to feel an emotion to change an emotion. The focus is on methods for both accessing emotion and changing emotion. I discuss generic methods of accessing emotion, including empathically attuning to affect, focusing on bodily felt experience, and processing episodic memories to help people reexperience the past in the present. The importance of new, corrective, emotional experiences and of memory reconsolidation processes is stressed, as well as how it is the having of new adaptive emotional experiences, in the presence of the activated old painful experience, that is crucial in transformation. In addition to generic methods of working with affect, I also discuss more structured methods for arriving and leaving emotion, such as chair work and imaginal reentry to past situations.

A key transdiagnostic principle of emotion transformation is that the best way to change an emotion is with another emotion. To quote Spinoza's (1967) *Ethics (Part IV)*: "An emotion cannot be restrained nor removed unless by an opposed and stronger emotion" (p. 195). This is a fundamental psychological process that all clinicians need to understand. This form of emotion transformation differs from *emotion regulation*, which is itself a rapidly developing transdiagnostic principle developed mainly within modificational traditions (Gross, 2013; Linehan, 1993). Emotion regulation involves the control of emotion—managing unwanted emotions, meaning it is a second-level process that helps with coping and symptom treatment. Jurist (2019) pointed to a difference between "emotion regulation" and "emotion modulation": *Emotion modulation* involves the transformation of emotion at the level of emotion generation so that emotion is experienced in a modulated fashion. *Emotion transformation*, which produces modulated emotion, occurs at the basic, first, or primary, level—the level at which the emotion is generated before it has to be managed. Achieving change at this primary level makes for change in the underlying dis-ease and is a prerequisite for the later higher level, more deliberate regulation processes needed for the complexities of managing emotion in one's social world. In the therapeutic context, emotion regulation acts—after the fact—on the primary process of emotion generation as an aid to coping and symptom. This will be discussed more fully in Chapter 11 on emotion regulation.

I argue that the royal road to managing emotion is by transforming emotion at the level of its generation rather than by controlling already generated dysfunctional emotion. For example, in people who have anger problems, rage is a reaction to, and a way of protecting themselves from, the hurt and disorganizing effects of their underlying shame or fear. The best way to manage or regulate dysregulated anger is not by anger management but by modulation of the anger via transformation of the more primary underlying shame or fear to which the dysregulated anger is a reaction. When the person no longer feels ashamed or no longer is afraid, they do not rage, and their emotion is more modulated (Greenberg, 2015; Jurist, 2019).

In working with emotion, therapists first need to help people arrive at emotions, which involves staying in contact with their feelings. Doing so allows feelings to serve their adaptive purpose. However, some painful feelings are maladaptive; they are responses to past experiences of abandonment, neglect, or trauma. Once one has accepted these emotions, the emotions need to be transformed. This is the *leaving stage*, which is the key therapeutic process of changing emotion with emotion. Consider, for example, how the withdrawal tendencies in shame—of wanting to sink into the ground and disappear—cannot coexist with the opposing approach tendencies of assertive anger to thrust forward to protect one's boundaries. Or, consider how the withdrawal tendency in fear—to run away—can be transformed by the approach tendency in sadness of reaching out to receive comfort.

Therapists who work with emotion, thus, first facilitate acceptance of emotion by helping people sit with their difficult feelings in a session. When a client expresses an emotion, the therapist responds by empathizing compassionately with the painful aspect of the experience and facilitates the client's acceptance and articulation of the meaning of the emotion. In so doing, therapists pay attention to the client's moment-by-moment experience and help the client to not judge their emotions but really accept them. Therapists at this time also help clients put their emotions into words because putting feeling into words in and of itself has adaptive and regulating value (Kircanski et al., 2012). But in addition to acceptance, they also help clients experience new emotions to change the old emotions (Fredrickson et al., 2000; Greenberg, 2015; Lane et al., 2015).

Therapists work to help people effectively process their emotions by getting them to approach, accept, express, regulate, tolerate, understand and reflect on, and maybe, most importantly, to transform their emotions (Greenberg, 2002, 2015). These are all important processes, and each is a basis for a different form of intervention. To help process emotion in this way, therapists first need to offer a relationship in which the therapist is present, is empathically attuned to affect moment by moment, and creates a working alliance. This is a strongly process-oriented approach.

Therapists need to keep their finger on the client's emotional pulse moment by moment and follow the client's shifts and need to respond differentially to these shifting states. This means, for example, that the therapist may sense change through the following: a client's voice as it rises in pitch or volume, disconnected eye gaze, body postures, or tight facial expressions that reveal the client is not feeling safe. Doing so helps therapists sense that they may have said something that led the client to not feel heard; they therefore can adjust accordingly. Therapists are reading both the client's and their own bodily felt sense and action tendencies moment by moment to guide intervention, to intercede to correct any misattunement, or both. They then watch to see the effect of their intervention: if their responses cause a client's facial expression to soften or their breathing to deepen, or, if there had been a misattunement, to see if the client is again feeling safe in the relationship and that any break in the alliance has been repaired.

A process-oriented approach, central to working with emotion, is fundamentally a phenomenological approach that works with a client's subjective experience of the world as it emerges for them (Heidegger, 1953/2000; Merleau-Ponty, 1964, 1968). Working phenomenologically in this way, the therapist pays attention to the client's subjective experience and to shifts in the client's experience. The therapist views people as dynamic, self-organizing, emotion-processing systems that change moment by moment, and a crucial therapist skill involves following and facilitating a next step in emotion processing. Close attention to the present emotional experience of clients is central. Perceptual skills of observing what clients are doing and when are as or more important than intervention skills, which are only as good as their appropriate timing. From a process orientation, it is not so much what therapists do but when they do it that is important.

OVERVIEW OF THE BOOK

The book is broken into three parts: Part I, Understanding the Fundamentals (Chapters 1–4), Part II, Arriving at Emotion (Chapters 5–8), and Part III, Leaving Emotion (Chapters 9–12). Part I provides the conceptual and research scaffolding for the emotion-based approach as a transtheoretical, transdiagnostic, and transcultural way to conduct therapy.

Chapter 1 covers the theory of emotion and emotional change. It presents the basic theory of emotion and emotion schematic processing; it also makes the case for having new emotional experience to change old emotional experience. The chapter presents the significance of implicit emotional experience, the role of the body and action tendency, and the basics of memory reconsolidation.

Chapter 2 discusses research on using emotion to change emotion. The chapter reviews emotion activation and other emotion change processes, indicating the transdiagnostic nature of these processes.

Chapter 3 elaborates the basic principle of change being proposed in this book—changing emotion with emotion—and discusses memory reconsolidation in greater depth as a key process in emotional change. It provides clinical examples of the process of changing emotion with emotion.

Chapter 4 discusses why it is important for therapists to deal with their own emotions and their fears of emotion. Many therapists and trainees have some form of fear of both their own and their clients' emotions; therefore, learning to become comfortable with their own and their clients' emotions is necessary in working with emotion. The chapter moves on to discuss how different views of self and rules of expression affect emotions across cultures as well as inform the clinical decisions therapists need to make both in terms of respecting these differences and of making their proactive choices to educate about and dismantle systemic racism.

Part II begins with Chapter 5, which introduces the foundational skill for arriving at and processing emotion: empathic attunement to affect. Flowing from this skill comes *moment-by-moment attunement to affect*, a process of keeping one's finger on the client's emotional pulse. The chapter discusses and demonstrates attunement as well as the importance of responding in the landscape of feeling rather than in the landscape of action or meaning, and how focusing internally on feeling influences the client's next moment. The chapter also discusses the important differential effects of empathic understanding, empathic exploration, and empathic conjecture in helping clients gain access to their feelings.

Chapter 6 presents the skill of focusing on bodily felt feelings to access and process emotion. It offers examples of different forms of guiding awareness to bodily felt experience and emphasizes the importance of putting words to experience. The chapter discusses the difference between emotional arousal and depth of experience; it also discusses and demonstrates the differential importance of each in therapeutic change.

Chapter 7 looks at clients' experience and process of blocking emotion in sessions, and it highlights the self-protective function of blocking and interrupting emotion. Avoidance and defense are revisioned as self-interruptive coping strategies coming out of a person's attempts to protect the self—to prevent disintegrating or falling apart. It is not that clients are avoiding the pain of the emotion; rather, it is the fear that they will be overwhelmed, will drown or fall apart, and will no longer be able to function that they are protecting against. The chapter presents results of research studies that used both grounded theory and a task analytic approach to the self-interruption or blocking of emotion.

Chapter 8 looks at a task analytic study of the unblocking of emotion and discusses the skills for undoing the blocks to emotion. Highlighted in this chapter is the importance of key steps in helping people approach dreaded emotions: validating clients' fear of emotion and facilitating the realization of client agency in the blocking process. The chapter presents the use of a particular form of two-chair dialogue for helping clients experience that they are agents in their process of self-interruption of emotion.

Part III focuses on the leaving of emotions. The chapters in this part discuss the processes and skills needed to facilitate transformation.

Chapter 9 discusses the importance of reclaiming previously disclaimed feelings and mobilizing unmet needs. This chapter highlights not only how to help clients access previously disallowed needs but also how to facilitate the feeling of having deserved to get the need met. Once a client feels deserving, this leads to the automatic emergence of new feelings. Transcripts in this chapter demonstrate the methods of mobilizing heartfelt needs to generate new emotions to change old emotions.

Chapter 10 deals with reexperiencing the past in the present through the activation of episodic memories, and it presents different methods of accessing episodic memories. The chapter also outlines age regression by either speaking to the imagined child or going back to become the wounded child and speaking as if one is the child; it demonstrates this method with transcripts. The chapter presents other methods, such as going back by means of an affect bridge, tracking a current feeling to its origins, or using somatic experience to arouse memories. Going back to the past helps mobilize clients' unprocessed emotions and unmet needs to make them amenable to transformation by the activation of new feelings to change old feelings. For example, the fear or shame of abuse is changed by the experience of empowering anger, which comes from the healthy feeling of entitlement to the need for protection. Likewise, the fear and sadness of lonely abandonment is changed through grieving what was missed and the internalization of both self and other compassion.

Chapter 11 focuses on emotion regulation. It looks at deliberate regulation to enhance coping and at implicit regulation through automatic processes to enhance transformation at the level of emotion generation. The difference between emotion regulation (coping and self-soothing of dysregulated symptomatic feelings) and emotion transformation (transformation of the client's core painful emotions by bringing in compassionate soothing) is discussed. The chapter also addresses the use of different types of imaginal transformation and a variety of chair dialogues that have been developed for working with transforming emotions.

Chapter 12 focuses on narrative and emotion, specifically, the consolidation of emotional change into new narratives. Stories are our primary way of making meaning, and we make sense of what we feel not only by labeling what we feel in words but by the way we organize our emotional experience into narratives. The chapter discusses how an emotion-oriented therapy facilitates clients' coming to know and understand their own lived experience, articulate them as told stories, and create new stories based on new emotion. It also describes markers of different types of problem-based stories and change stories.

Following Part III is "Looking Ahead: A Unified Approach to Psychotherapy" in which I offer concluding thoughts about how adopting an emotion-centric therapy framework that is transdiagnostic, transtheoretical, and transcultural will help many more people who need therapy to actually get it. Rather than providing only symptom reduction, this framework will provide a transformation of the underlying dis-ease, thus resulting in more enduring change.

WHAT ARE THE ESSENTIALS FOR LEARNING TO WORK WITH EMOTION IN PSYCHOTHERAPY?

When working with emotion in therapy it is essential to develop clarity about whether the clinical focus is on having people experience their emotions in relation to the object or context which activates the emotions, or on helping the client manage their own emotions more generally. Therapeutic work can be seen as belonging in one of these two domains, working on emotions in relation to their objects—say fear of father, or shame about body—or working on one's relationship to one's emotions, such as difficulty in accessing emotion or being overwhelmed by emotions. Understanding which of these forms is the focus of the therapeutic work and when the focus is shifting helps the therapist and client better formulate what they are doing at any point in therapy in the treatment. Looking at whether one is focusing on changing emotion or on changing one's relationship to the emotion is an overarching frame that will help readers as they work through the different chapters of this book. It will be apparent that Chapter 9 on needs, and Chapter 10 on experiencing the past in the present, are more centrally focused on changing emotion, whereas Chapters 7 and 8 on interrupting and unblocking emotion respectively, and Chapter 11 on regulating emotion are most centrally about helping people change how they relate to their emotions.

With either of the above clinical goals as the focus of the emotion work, the therapist will need to develop skills and knowledge in a few key areas. As I elaborate in Chapter 4, therapists first need to develop an emotion-friendly attitude; this primarily means being friendly to their own emotions, which in the long run will help them to be friendly to others' emotions. Probably the best way to do this is for therapists to work on their own emotions in personal therapy or engage in some form of self-experience as part of their training. The ethic of "know thyself" is better stated as "be aware of and accept one's own emotions." This is a process of paying attention to what one feels in everyday living and using this information for daily decision making as well as for transformation. Therapists cannot guide people through terrain that is totally foreign to them; they need to be able to deal with their own emotions to help others deal with their emotions.

Therapists also need some knowledge of the nature and function of emotion at a theoretical level to help clients understand why it is important to focus on emotion, how feeling bad can lead to feeling good, and how it is worthwhile to delve into the memory of past experiences rather than bury them. Clinicians also need to know what research has shown about working with emotions to know that there is evidence on which to base their work.

Therapists need skills to facilitate both awareness and acceptance of emotion and emotional change. Four core skills in the arriving phase are (a) moment-by-moment empathic attunement and the ability to (b) help people focus on bodily feelings, (c) to focus on the present experience of emotion, and (d) to overcome blocks to emotion. Leaving emotion by transforming it, as indicated by the preceding chapter summaries, takes place when clients are able to access their needs, reexperience the past in the present, regulate emotions, and consolidate their experiences into a new narrative.

I have practiced and supervised now for nearly more than 50 years, and this book presents my updated, ever-developing learnings on how best to work with emotion in psychotherapy. Many of the microskills I describe in this book have developed out of my supervising clinicians from around the world over the past decade and from task analyses of work on emotion. My hope for you, the reader, is that this book helps you gain sharper awareness and focus for staying with others as they plunge into painful emotions. I also hope that the many demonstrations of empathy in action I share in this book strike a chord and that you learn both the confidence and humility you need to make your clients feel safe. Finally, it is my sincere hope that you are able to share in your clients' joy and help them overcome any trepidation they have as they create new stories for themselves that are grounded in emotion transformation.

PART I UNDERSTANDING THE FUNDAMENTALS

1 EMOTION THEORY

Emotion, in my view, is the basic datum of human experience. However, we need to bring cognition to emotion to help us make sense of it and to translate its action tendencies into decisions, behavior, and meaning. Emotion is not a single category of phenomena but, rather, a complex domain of human experience. In this chapter, I look at the nature and function of emotion and describe the role of both emotion schemes and needs in therapeutic change.

Defining "emotion"—and the words used to describe it—is somewhat controversial because different views exist (Barrett, 2017; Panksepp, 1998; Panksepp & Biven, 2012; Russell, 2003). Theorists generally agree that *emotion* is a complex reaction pattern involving physiological, experiential, and behavioral and elements (Ekman & Davidson, 1994) and that emotions help people evaluate the significance of situations for their well-being. In this book, I use the terms "affect" and "feeling" as well as "emotion" when discussing emotional processes in therapy. As Damasio (1999) suggested, a useful way of thinking about these terms is to imagine a tree with a trunk and roots, major branches, and leafy minor branches.

Affect can be thought of as the physiologically based roots and trunk of the tree, such as excited or calm; emotions, as the major branches, such as

https://doi.org/10.1037/0000248-002
Changing Emotion With Emotion: A Practitioner's Guide, by L. S. Greenberg

categorically labeled emotions like anger, sadness, and fear; and feelings are the small leafy branches, which are the much more socially and cognitively influenced, like annoyed, disappointed, or suspicious. I use these three terms throughout the book somewhat interchangeably and according to which word seems to best fit the context. I do so, though, with the sense that "affect" emphasizes the more implicit physiological aspects; "emotion," the more basic categorical labels; and "feelings," the more finely differentiated social and cognitive aspects. In addition, to work therapeutically with emotion, I show that it also is clinically important to discriminate different types, sequences, and levels of emotion as well as the degree of adaptiveness and maladaptiveness of emotion.

Emotion serves a number of important evolutionarily derived functions to aid survival. First and foremost, emotion rapidly provides an action tendency to help us survive. Second, it simultaneously provides us with information about what is going on in the situation in relation to our needs, and it communicates our intentions to others (Greenberg, 2015). Third, emotion is our primary signaling system. It is embodied; that is, by our bodily expression of emotion, we communicate our states nonverbally to others. For example, when fear is activated, it provides us with an action tendency: to flee. When we feel fear, it tells us that we are in danger, and our expression or our physical action communicates our state to others. The appraisal of danger and the fear that is felt is not in words; it is presymbolic. It is a basic meaning based on an apprehension of an experienced meaningful pattern that is relevant to our well-being. This fear is not produced by a thought in language but is a sensing, an orientation, and an inclination that needs further processing to make sense of it.

ACTION TENDENCY, INFORMATION, AND EXPRESSION

As Frijda (2016) argued, what is most basic in human functioning are not feelings but modes of action readiness that aim to establish, modify, maintain, or terminate a given self-object relationship. Action tendencies prepare us for adaptive action. The action tendency in fear, as mentioned earlier, is to move away from the dangerous stimulus. Fear motivates us to seek protection and safety. When the goal is achieved, the emotion cycle ends: The relationship with the environment changes, and emotion is deactivated. What is universal across cultures are not emotions as feelings but, rather, emotions as dispositions for various forms of action readiness. Our feelings in this view, then, are reflections in consciousness that accompany action inclinations. Action tendencies have an aim. If the current situation lends itself to it, the state of readiness will activate an action or action sequence from the individual's repertoire that appears capable of achieving the aim of modifying or maintaining relationships. Actual actions appear when these subthreshold activations turn into full-blown action.

Emotion is best understood as fundamentally an action readiness, and it also is a motive state. Action readiness and the action itself are more basic than feelings because feelings largely are conscious reflections of states of action readiness. LeDoux (2012) suggested that, at a neurological level, what is most basic are survival circuits that mediate a coordinated set of adaptive brain and behavioral responses. Emotions do not exist in the brain as neurological entities with specific locations. Instead, what probably are hard-wired are the brain circuits for survival tendencies, such as defense against harm, which develop into basic emotions like anger and fear. It is these brain circuits and their adaptive functions that are conserved across mammals and that, rather than subjective emotional experience, are universal. In working with emotion, how we name them and how they feel may vary; however, it is the action tendencies that are most basic and universal.

Emotions are also our primary meaning system (Forgas, 1995). Evidence clearly points to the neurological primacy of affect. LeDoux's (1996) research on the emotional brain demonstrated that it is possible for our brains to register the emotional meaning of a stimulus before the perceptual system has fully processed that stimulus. Thus, the automatic emotional response has already occurred before one can stop it—be it jumping back from a snake, snapping at an inconsiderate spouse, or yelling at a disobedient child. The neocortex, however, also has been found to have fibers leading back to the amygdala and provides a path for cognitive feedback to the emotion systems. This is the path by which deliberate conscious cognitive processes can be used to help regulate emotion. An important consequence of this method of functioning is that people can respond emotionally without thought because a situation is perceived to fit a category it activates. The activation of the amygdala occurs quickly and can be achieved without the intervention of cortical areas, although only for approximately 12 milliseconds (Markowitsch, 1998).

In addition to action tendency and information, emotional expression, the third major component of emotion, provides people with their primary means of communication. An infant's cry signals to the mother the type of distress the child is in, and the scowl of the angry father signals disapproval or danger. Emotional expression qualifies what is expressed verbally, and it often is more salient than the cognitive content of the communication.

The semantic meaning of the words one expresses frequently is not the most important part of a message. Facial expression, eye and lip expression, direction of gaze, frown, and tone of voice all are registered by the recipient's brain; this plus the context helps interpret what the expresser means and feels. Bodily expression is an important part of communication. Emotion, therefore, is not just a feeling but an action tendency, information, and expression.

IMPLICATIONS FOR THERAPY

Research in affective neuroscience suggests that the processing of ecologically important stimuli (i.e., emotional and social) is conducted by dedicated, modular systems that operate rapidly and automatically, and are largely independent of our conscious awareness (Adolphs & Anderson, 2018; Tamietto & de Gelder, 2010). It has been shown that interference in the naturally occurring process of emotion activation and completion underlies development of many major disorders. Disclaiming the action tendency in emotion, not acknowledging how one feels, and suppressing emotion are major forms of dysfunctional emotion processing (Foa & Kozak, 1986; Greenberg & Safran, 1987). When activated by a provoking stimulus, an emotion follows a natural five-phase sequence: (1) emergence, (2) entry into awareness, (3) ownership by the individual, (4) expression through action, and (5) completion after which a new emotion emerges and the cycle begins again. It is only when this process is repeatedly interfered with, such as when awareness or ownership is prevented, when expression is interrupted, or when action and completion are blocked, that we become stuck in chronic, painful emotions (Greenberg, 2002; Gross & Levenson, 1997; Pennebaker, 1990). As a result of this interference, potentially meaningful implicit information that is necessary for meeting our needs through adaptive action is kept out of awareness. Accordingly, an important task for therapists is to facilitate the experience and expression of previously disallowed emotional experiences in clients.

Emotions give people feedback about their reaction to situations, so it is important to help clients pay attention to what their emotions are telling them and to use this information to guide their behaviors and get their needs met (Damasio, 1994). Consciously feeling the emotion in connection with the object evoking it gives people control over their reactions; they become agents who are having an emotion rather than passive victims of emotion. The process of arriving at, allowing, and accepting emotions, however, is not enough to deal therapeutically with painful emotion. In addition to arriving at emotions, therapists also need to help clients leave certain painful emotions by activating new adaptive emotions that help change the old emotions. Clients need to consolidate their experiential change in new narratives consisting of new views of self and world (Greenberg, 2011). This process of accepting emotion and changing emotion with emotion as well as creating new narratives involves understanding different types of emotions and principles of emotional change. The best way to change an emotion is with an opposing emotion.

Needs

Emotions are embodied connections to our most essential needs (Frijda, 1986). They rapidly alert us to situations important to our well-being. They tell us if things are going our way and organize us to react adaptively. Emotion is generated psychologically by the automatic appraisal of situations in relation to needs, and, therefore, emotions can be seen as carrying needs within them. As part of the process of providing goal-directed action tendencies, emotion evaluates whether something is good or bad for us; it must be distinguished from reason, which evaluates if something is true or false. What is good or bad for us is essentially determined by need or goal attainment. This means the brain is constantly evaluating the state of the organism and whether, in its interaction with the environment, things are going the organism's way—whether its needs are being met.

Emotions and needs are intimately intertwined. Does this mean needs precede emotion? The answer is no. Needs, rather than being inborn, develop from basic organismic biases and preferences, such as a preference for light over dark, soft over hard, warm over cold, maybe even smiles over growls (Greenberg, 2019). Neonates and all organisms are not born with motivations, such as attachment, achievement, and control; rather, they are born with an emotion system designed to aid survival: The infant is an affect-regulating being designed to move toward those emotions that promote survival and move away from those that do not. Closeness, tenderness, soothing, hunger satiation, and so on are sought after because they produce emotions that feel good, and evolution designed organisms to evaluate whether the environment is good or bad for them and to move accordingly. Amoebas, single-cell organisms, taste the environment, and if it tastes good, they move forward; if it tastes bad, they spin away. The thing that meets emotions' goal of survival and growth becomes experienced as good and develops into desires and needs, which are sought after. The infant, thus, is guided by an automatic affect-regulation system that is constantly trying to have the feelings they want and not have feelings they do not want. Emotion and need now exist in an interdependent relationship, both implying the other.

For therapy, this means that empathic understanding of emotion requires an understanding and articulation of needs. Empathic responses do not simply offer words for feelings; they include the need embedded in the emotion. A therapist's response is not just, "So, this left you feeling sad," which often could drop like a lead balloon when the client says, "Yes," but that is enhanced by including the unmet need, "So sad. You needed her comfort, and not getting anything left you so empty and lonely." This elaborated response of feeling and need provides a sense of direction and helps clients differentiate and deepen their experience. The client may respond by saying, "Yes, I really need her comfort, and I sort felt hung out to dry— almost like I didn't exist."

The Self

Working with emotion from a process-oriented perspective, it is important to think of the self as a dynamic self-organizing system. The self in this view is a constant process in which embodied experience, once felt, can be reflected on and symbolized by the processes of consciousness and language. Hence, there is a constant dialectic between experiential and reflective processes that produces the sensation of who we are and allows for the creation of narratives by which we live. A lot has been written about the self. William James (1890) distinguished the self as "Me" and as the self as "I." Daniel Stern (1985) described four interrelated senses of "self": the emergent self, core self, intersubjective self, and verbal self. Hofmann and Doan (2018) in a contemporary treatment of emotion and the self also distinguished between a core self and a social self. In working with emotion in therapy, a person's reflective self is seen to be constantly interacting with all emerging affect so that when people articulate their experience of what they feel and who they are, it is as much created as discovered. What people feel always involves how they explain their experience to themselves. People create their final emotional experience by putting their felt sense, itself a synthesis of more basic elements, into words.

The self is a process of self-organization constantly being created to take particular forms. It is a temporal process unfolding in the present in interaction with the environment. The self is seen as arising in the moment in contact with the environment (Perls et al., 1951). It is formed in relation to others; it is decentralized and unfolds in time, and is organized moment by moment into different forms, such as happy, self-critical, worthless, cautious, or bold. The self is more like a constantly flowing river than a structure in that it is much more constituted by integrating experiences and reflections over time than by integrating spatial locations and a situational knowledge. It is a dynamic self-organizing process that creates the person we are about to become. It is forming and informing forms of being. The person is constantly putting the self together in the situation. Like touch only exists in touching, so the self only exists in experiencing something within a situation. Thus, in therapy, we are concerned with self-organizing processes and the flexibility of this process rather than with finding a true self.

People organize in different ways at different times, and they develop some characteristic ways of organizing emotionally, giving a certain stability to the way personality and character structure are being constructed. People have certain experiential or reflective patterned sequences and ways of being that are more likely to occur than others. These more frequently organized states could be thought of as "self parts." We all have different self-states associated with different emotions. We switch states depending on context and activated emotion. When fear is threatened, a protective self-organization is triggered automatically. When the threat ceases, the person switches into another self-state. There is some stability in the dynamic process of self-formation with different parts that are repeatedly organized; a person may organize repeatedly as humorous, as timid, as self-critical, or as assertive. Some therapeutic work involves facilitating how these parts interact. Therapists need to be aware of the constructive process involved in self-experience: that people may have many self-organizations, and even these maintain a constant process of dialectical construction.

EMOTION TYPES

Emotions, their action tendencies, their information processing, and their expression aspects all developed evolutionarily to help humans survive and thrive. Emotions and their functions are fundamentally adaptive, but, to aid clinical work, it is important to make clinical distinctions between different types of emotion. I have found it most helpful to first distinguish between "adaptive" and "maladaptive" emotion and between "primary," "secondary," and "instrumental" emotion. Each of these categories implies different generation processes and calls for differential intervention. In addition, in discussing working with emotion, it is helpful to distinguish between different degrees of arousal of too much emotion (dysregulated) and too little emotion (blocked or intellectualized).

Emotions can be seen as healthy (*adaptive*), or unhealthy (*maladaptive*), and as primary or not primary. *Primary emotions* are the very first emotions people have in response to internal or external stimuli, that is, their gut feelings. *Secondary emotions* are those that come as reactions to primary emotions. They are more self-protective or defensive, are not adaptive, and obscure the primary emotions. *Instrumental emotions* are experienced or expressed primarily to achieve an aim and often are more manipulative in nature. Primary emotions can be adaptive, in which case they help us adapt to the situation by giving us good orientation to the environment and good information. Or they can be maladaptive and, as a function perhaps of past trauma or attachment problems, are not responses that help us cope adaptively with situations. They are reactions in the present to the past and do not directly seek the attainment of need satisfaction.

Emotional dysregulation refers to poorly modulated emotion responses that do not lie within the normal range of responding. Dysregulation involves the inability to control or regulate emotional responses to provocative stimuli. Primary maladaptive or secondary emotions can become dysregulated. Primary maladaptive emotions like fear of danger, shame of unworthiness, or sadness of lonely abandonment can become so intense that they are intolerably painful. Dysregulated emotions, however, are, more often than not, secondary symptomatic emotions. These are emotional overreactions or exaggerated ways of responding to environmental and interpersonal challenges (e.g., bursts of anger, crying), and may lead to accusing or passive-aggressive behaviors, or create chaos or conflict.

Primary adaptive emotions, such as sadness at loss, anger at violation, or fear at threat, are people's immediate gut response to a situation. They give people good information about what is important to them. Primary emotions are not the same as *evolutionary basic emotions*, which are fundamental and universal, and have different action tendencies. "Primary" means whatever is triggered first in response to a stimulus. So, for example, anger, sadness, and fear are basic emotions, and could be primary because they were triggered first, whereas envy, enchantment, admiration, or weariness are not basic emotions but could be the first complex feelings a person may have. In addition, we must distinguish between shorter emotion episodes (like crying at a loss) versus the long-lasting sadness at the loss, which is better referred to as a mood.

Secondary emotions, such as depressed hopelessness covering shame at not being good enough, rage covering shame at loss of self-esteem, however, are responses to preceding emotional reactions, and, as mentioned earlier, often obscure or interrupt more primary emotional reactions. For example, an individual who feels fear at the possibility of danger may subsequently experience the secondary emotion of anger at the threatening stimulus or shame about their fear. These can also be emotions that are secondary to more cognitive processes (e.g., anxiety in response to catastrophic thinking). Most secondary emotions are symptomatic feelings, such as panic and anxiety, or feelings of depletion and hopelessness in depression. For example, a depressed client with tears running down their face and a complaining tone to their voice says, "I just can't take this anymore. Why do I have to suffer so much?" There is a hopeless quality as well as a tone of protest in the client's voice and expression. This is secondary hopelessness or resignation. In responding to this utterance, the therapist needs to acknowledge the secondary emotion but then needs to guide the client to the underlying primary vulnerable emotion—in this case, perhaps a feeling of shame and worthlessness.

Other-directed blaming or rejecting anger is generally a secondary emotion that needs to be validated and explored to get at the underlying painful (probably maladaptive) emotion. In people who have a history of domestic violence, other-directed secondary rage often covers shame. Rage was needed in their childhood as self-protection against pain. Frequently, this rage can become an automatic response to any kind of vulnerability or perceived threat; so, it appears primary but is generally secondary protection against underlying vulnerability.

Emotions are generated both by top-down and bottom-up processes. People have *automatic emotions* generated bottom up, whereas *cognitively derived emotions* generated by top-down deliberative processes are based on such things as beliefs; an idealized view of the self; and socially derived expectations, moral standards, and values. Those emotions that are more influenced by cognition and social factors, are, in my view, generally secondary emotions, such as when catastrophic thoughts lead to anxiety (McGilchrist, 2009). Catastrophic thoughts are driven by core emotion schemes of fear and by the resulting frightened or insecure self-organization.

An additional nonprimary emotional response category is instrumental emotion, which has been termed *manipulative emotion*, seen as an expression used to get what one wants or for secondary gain. Typical examples are the expression of anger to control or to dominate, or crocodile tears to evoke sympathy. Instrumental emotion can be generated with different degrees of awareness of conscious intent. Here, therapists need to help people become aware of the aim of their emotional expression and explore more direct ways to communicate their emotions.

Although secondary emotions are generally not adaptive responses to the environment in that they do not help the person get what they need, primary emotions can be either adaptive or maladaptive. Primary adaptive emotions are those automatic emotions in which the implicit evaluation, verbal or nonverbal emotional expression, action tendency, and degree of emotion regulation fit the stimulus situation and are appropriate to it (e.g., sadness at loss that reaches out for comfort, fear at threat that prepares the individual to escape). These automatic emotions prepare the individual for adaptive action and help them get their needs met. In therapy, to guide problem solving, the client attends to and expresses these emotions to access the emotions' adaptive information and action tendency. Because they are core and irreducible responses, they therefore are not explored to unpack their cognitive–affective components. For example, anger at maltreatment is a primary, irreducible, and core emotional response that needs to be evoked and symbolized in therapy in order to access the adaptive action tendency to push the offender away and establish appropriate boundaries.

On the other hand, primary maladaptive emotions are enduring painful feelings that initially were adaptive responses to bad situations but are now misplaced. These are feelings such as fear at one's boss's raised voice resulting from having had an aggressive father or fear of one's partner's warm embrace because of past sexual abuse. These feelings produce responses that are disproportionate or inappropriate to the situation and need to be accessed to make them available to new experiences.

How does one help access primary feeling? First, therapists need to stay with whatever feeling the client is experiencing and ask the client to pay attention to it and explore it. Then, by understanding and empathizing with their clients, therapists get to more primary feelings by focusing on whatever else the client may be feeling. The therapist might ask, "What else were you feeling? Were you feeling anything else at the time? Right now, are there any feelings underneath the feelings you're talking about?" It is important to understand that there is customarily more than is being articulated at anyone moment.

EMOTION SCHEMATIC PROCESSING

In addition to the aforementioned distinctions about different types of emotions, an important concept is that of *emotions' schematic memory*, or emotion schemes and the self-organizations they produce. *Schemes*, or internal models, are an increasingly common theoretical notion to explain human functioning. They are networks in the brain that are dynamic organizations through which the world and interactions with it are coded; they operate by forming and influencing people's current views. Schemes are internal mental structures that are initially innate but develop through interactions of lived emotional experiences (J. Pascual-Leone, 1987, 1991; J. Pascual-Leone & Johnson, 1991, 2011). One can imagine that, initially, there are affective, motivational, cognitive, and behavioral predispositions; these biases and preferences are often original inborn schemes that are active and seek application. For instance, a scheme for faces seeks or searches faces, and a scheme for being soothed or rocked seeks these experiences and "feels satisfied" (scheme successfully applied) when they arrive.

The basic psychological units (generating mechanism) of emotional meaning are the *emotion schemes*, which are action- and experience-producing structures. As such, they differ from cognitive schemas, which produce beliefs and inform (inject form into) and assign truth values to experiential, conceptual, and language productions (Greenberg, 2011; J. Pascual-Leone, 1991; J. Pascual-Leone & Johnson, 1991, 2011). We come into the world with rudimentary psychoaffective motor programs to aid survival, and from these programs (in combination with other inborn biases and preferences), we begin to build our experience of the world. We do not learn how to be angry or how to be sad—these are hardwired feelings—but what we become angry at or what we become sad about is a function of learning formed into, and, later on, activated through, emotion schemes. The presence of emotion in any given moment indicates than an emotion scheme or, more accurately, a set of emotion schemes, has been cue activated and is currently guiding the processing; that is, it is now up and running, and thus is accessible to change. Activated emotion schemes are synthesized into higher level self-organizations, such as feeling worthless or feeling insecure, and are a target of therapy.

Emotion Schemes and Self-Organization

Although emotion schemes generate emotional responses, self-organizations are higher level patterns of experience and behavior formed by a synthesis of emotions schemes and other processes, such as complex cognitive and personal (i.e., affective and cognitive) schemes. Whereas shame is an emotion generated by emotion schemes, a self-organization might be feeling worthless or feeling insecure. Self-organizations are based on combinations of a variety of emotions and ways of coping with the emotion, such as fear, sadness and shame, and constitute one's way of managing feelings like withdrawing or clinging. A group of schemes are coactivated by some set of cueing stimuli, and this synthesis of schemes plus any already activated schemes generate different ways of responding and different conscious states. These events can trigger responses that lead an individual to shift rapidly from one state to another, like shifting from rage to sadness, fear to humor, and so on. In addition, different self-organizations are related to trying to satisfy different basic needs.

Basic affects or emotions are innate, yet emotion schemes are learned and arise from our past experiences. They are memory structures that synthesize affective, cognitive, and behavioral elements in a quick and automatic way and are related to implicit, unconscious, and idiosyncratic mechanisms, thus forming the basis for organization of the self. Emotion schemes are formed over our life history through memory process and experiences of the whole organism. Thus, emotion schematic memories are networks of representations built from lived experience, including emotions, images, sensations, evaluations, meanings, cognitions, learned experiences, behaviors, and scripts of how to act. Once something happens that is important to the organism, an emotion scheme with specific meanings is likely to be constructed. When needs are not met, maladaptive emotion schematic memories of the painful feelings of unmet need are formed. When present stimuli, situations, or meanings are close to the ones that happened in the past, our emotion schemes get activated and generate emotions, producing an *experiential state*. Often, when we talk about "accessing emotion," we mean activating the output of a complex network of emotion-laden schematic memories. When we say, "accessing fear, sadness, or anger," we often mean accessing an unprocessed complex, a set of feelings or affects intertwined with cognitions and related to situations (contextualized) that bear on early attachment and identity-related experiences.

In this view, memories and feelings do not reside, fully formed, in the unconscious, waiting to be unveiled when the forces of repression are overcome, as Freud (1915/1955) originally proposed. Rather than seeing the unconscious as a cauldron of forbidden impulses and wishes, the *adaptive unconscious* (Gazzaniga, 1998) is conceptualized as involving an extensive set of processing (schemes of all sorts) that executes complex evaluations and computations that interrelate and generate responses without requiring intention or effort. Much of this processing may be unavailable to conscious awareness, or, at least, awareness is unnecessary for such processing to occur. It is important to understand that emotions are a function of implicit rather than explicit processes. A therapy of emotion will need to work with implicit processes; emotion schemes are the implicit prime generators of emotional experience and the tacit or explicit targets of therapeutic change.

Appraisals have become central in the understanding of emotion generation, which results from appraisal of a situation in relation to need. How are appraisals made? *Appraisals,* in my view, are judgments or evaluations that result from application and synthesis of a number of activated schemes (J. Pascual-Leone, personal communication, August 6, 2020). A number of schemes are tacitly activated, and once synthesized, the schemes result in the formation of an evaluation, such as danger, loss, or comfort. Highly activated schemes are dynamically synthesized, thus leading to a judgment or evaluation. Appraisals can be seen as a higher level construct dependent on a complex set of processing and scheme activation at a more fundamental level.

To demonstrate the functioning of emotion schemes, imagine a situation in which a person felt fear when meeting a new boss in an apparently harmless situation. This person has fear schemes that, to differing degrees, constantly scan the environment for danger, and when stimulated to a certain level by environmental triggers (cues)—even when there is no real threat in the situation—activate the appraisal of danger in relation to a need for safety and produce the emotion of fear. Previous experiences related to vulnerability or failure, or both, if needs for validation or protection were not met contribute to creating emotion schemes that are now activated in this situation. Consequently, the sound of the boss's voice, a look on their face, or an environmental aspect of light, sound, or experiences similar to those of the original situation may raise the fear schemes' activation level and cause a fear response.

Emotion schemes are responsible for the great majority of people's emotional experience. Essentially, emotion schemes provide an integrated and automatic response, which includes emotions, cognitions, and action tendencies, in a kind of package or preprogrammed operation (Greenberg, 2011). Maladaptive emotion schemes are the main reason people look for psychotherapy. In addition, people's emotional experience based on their emotion schemes is highly subjective. The internal emotional state and experience differ from one person to another, or from one time to another, in the same person. The feeling, cause, context, degree of regulation, and intensity all depend on each person's past experience. For example, when "Shelley" is sad, her feeling differs from what "Rhonda" feels when she is sad; however, we understand there is some similarity between these experiences. As different as each person's sadness may be, when a person is sad, there is something of the same flavor to sadness across people. It would be confusing if what one person called "sadness," another called "joy." There is some essence to similarity. Experience is totally personal and contextual, but something is common to enable us to mutually understand that it is sadness and not joy or fear.

Dynamic Nature of Emotional Response

The emotion process is dynamic. Human beings are dynamic self-organizing systems that change moment by moment (Greenberg & Pascual-Leone, 1995). You may be walking along, feeling slightly anxious as you anticipate a business meeting, and you suddenly come across a familiar spot with an old tree that reminds you of your first kiss under that tree. Immediately, the sight of the tree brings back a past; you smile as the memory becomes more vivid, and you may even blush while your heart beats faster. This same tree may evoke a different emotional reaction from someone else who fell out of that tree as a child. While savoring your memory of your first kiss, a person with a vicious-looking dog walks by, and you draw back in fear because you were once been bitten by a similar type of dog. As you walk past the dog cautiously and reach a safe distance, you see another person approaching, and as he gets closer, you recognize him as a close friend you haven't seen for a while. You feel surprised and happy, and greet him in joy. All this took less than a minute. People are dynamic self-organizing emotion systems always in process with their feelings and thoughts fluctuating moment by moment and adapting to the environment. In addition, the different emotional states may be activated by a real-world stimulus (the tree), a memory (the kiss), or a mixture of both (the dog and the past attack).

To be human is to continually oscillate between different emotional states, and such fluctuations are not under our voluntary control. The seat of emotion is the limbic system, which comprises four main parts: the hypothalamus, amygdala, thalamus, and hippocampus. Several other structures may be involved in the limbic system, but unanimous consensus on them has not been reached. The amygdala, which has direct connections with many other parts of the brain and body in combination with other parts of the limbic system, is predominantly responsible for the speed and dynamic nature of our emotional responses. It bypasses the thinking brain (cerebral cortex) because there is no time to think when we face life-threatening dangers or threats, and the amygdala has to "sound the alarm." Even when it is memories that are evoked and the reaction may be more subtle, feelings are rapid and automatic. Memories of violation and feelings of anger or of unrequited love or loss come to mind unbidden. We do not want to feel them and we do not want to think about a given situation, but our emotion system persists. Our efforts to stop feelings and thoughts often are in vain. In a nutshell, emotion schemes are processed automatically and unconsciously, emerging from the interaction between innate emotional responses and personal experiences. They consist largely of preverbal and affective elements as bodily sensations that produce higher order organizations at the corner-stone of the self. They become the basic structure for our meaning creation. The felt experience of who we are comes from the synthesis of these schemes (Greenberg & Pascual-Leone, 1995; Oatley et al., 2006; J. Pascual-Leone, 1991).

Many complex emotional states exist, and names for emotional states are unlimited. Terms for emotions that go beyond basic emotion are quite diverse: words like "astonished," "ecstatic," "bashful," and "wary." Mixed or complex emotional states are formed by a synthesis of activated schemes in the internal world. People rarely feel pure, basic emotions. Children and adults (at times) may feel pure anger or pure joy, but as people move from childhood to adulthood, these pure emotions that came so naturally get intermixed and lose their purity. Adults rarely function with pure emotions but have complex schematically based emotional experiences that are tinged with interpretation, idiosyncratic meanings, and syntheses of a variety of basic emotions. These emotion schemes, however, have their roots in basic emotions.

The deafening sound of a thunderbolt will frighten any human being or animal by activating fear just as it would have frightened an ancient ancestor walking the African plains. This is a species-natural response. Emotions, however, predominantly do not appear in this kind of universal response but, rather, in particular and idiosyncratic ones. Most adult experi-ences involve complex mixed emotions instead of basic ones. For example, one person's irritation may be mixed with fear, whereas another's anger may be mixed with sadness. In addition, complex emotional states like jealousy may be a combination of anger, fear, and sadness. Also, different situations and roles require complex blends of feeling. For example, a parent needs a certain mixture of emotions to be a good parent. A certain degree of anger and pride is needed to maintain authority, but softness and warmth are also needed to provide nurture, and joy and playfulness to provide fun. All these different emotional states are then synthesized into a being a firm, loving parent who provides the responses a parent needs to give.

Activation of Emotion Schemes

Basic emotions form the foundation of emotion schemes. But each scheme, on its own, as it develops over time and when synthesized with a number of other schemes, produces increasingly complex emotional states. It is unusual for many clients to feel purely sad or angry; rather, they feel highly refined and complex emotional states like "being thrown on the dump heap" when rejected or "adrift at sea in a rudderless boat" when having lost a sense of direction. The following excerpt illustrates the activation of complex emotion schemes in the context of a client's current life.

CLIENT: What happens with Michael is, when I see him enter the room, I feel emotion towards him . . . [shift to emotional differentiation] just like different emotions, but up until about a week ago, like friendship.

THERAPIST: Is that kind of like . . . a feeling of warmth? [empathic conjecture, differentiating emotional experience and symbolizing it]

CLIENT: Exactly! I was about to say a trust, a warmth . . . just this complete contentment. [symbolizing the synthesized bodily felt sense]

THERAPIST: That feels really good inside.

CLIENT: Exactly, and, um, it's followed by this gut-wrenching, sick feeling of dread [symbolizes, then shifts to reflexive mode and explains the experience] because the only other person in the last 4 years that has made me feel that way was Simon, and it turned out to be exactly opposite to everything that was really going on . . . like when I thought he most liked me and most accepted me for who I was. It was a huge act.

Therapy involves working with complex emotional states, such as the ones in the preceding dialogue, to help people unpack them and get back to some of the experience of the basic emotions involved. It can be clarifying and liberating for adults to be able to feel their basic anger or sadness uncontaminated by the guilt, fear, or disgust that usually attend them and to experience these emotions without the complexity of having to manage them in socially appropriate ways. The more people are disconnected from their basic emotions, the more complicated they become, and they lose touch with an internal emotional compass that tells them if something is good or bad for them; they also lose touch with what they actually feel in their bodies and become disoriented.

To anticipate what lies ahead, I briefly describe how to work therapeutically with these core painful emotion schemes once activated. A therapy to change emotion follows a two-stage approach of arriving at and then leaving emotional experience (Greenberg, 2002). In the first stage, the therapist listens and lets the story and its emotional significance emerge. So, in the preceding excerpt, the therapist is working with the emotion schemes of dread and distrust to ensure that the client fully arrives at the experience by focusing back on the activated maladaptive emotional experience of dread. To further attend to, welcome, symbolize, and explore it, the therapist might say, "Let's stay with this feeling of sickness and dread that just hits you in the gut when you are reminded of Michael. Can you stay with it and breathe?" This draws the client's attention to the trauma-based emotion memory schemes and the responses associated with them. The client, articulating a belief that helps narrate the experience, might now say, "It's like I can't open up. I'll just be hurt again."

Having arrived at a core maladaptive feeling and an articulated sense of its personal meaning, the goal in therapy is to shift to having the client access a more adaptive emotional resource as an antidote to the maladaptive feeling. This shift heralds the movement to the second stage of the emotion-based approach. Focusing on the alternate feeling already present in the room—the feeling of "trust, a warmth . . . just this complete contentment"—might do this. If this were not present as the source of an alternate voice, the therapist could access a more adaptive emotional response by helping the client articulate a need. The therapist might ask, "What do you need in this deep feeling of hurt and distrust?" The client might respond with, "I just need to be held and comforted. I do so want some of the warmth." The therapist would then put this more adaptive voice in a dialectical interaction with the voice of dread by saying, "So, what are you saying to the dread and to the voice that says, 'I can't open up'?" The client might say, "I know I need to go slow to protect myself, but I also need to recognize what is different in this relationship."

PRINCIPLES OF EMOTIONAL CHANGE

Six principles of how to work with emotions have been gleaned from the psychology literature. They are (a) emotion *awareness*: symbolizing core emotional experience in words; (b) *expression*: saying or showing what one feels using words or action; (c) *regulation*: soothing or reducing emotional arousal; (d) *reflection*: making narrative sense of their experience; (e) *transformation*: undoing a maladaptive emotion with another adaptive emotion; and (f) *corrective emotional experience*: a new lived experience with another person. These principles are seen as best brought about in the context of an empathic therapeutic relationship that facilitates these processes. The first three can be thought of as serving emotion utilization in which the client is helped to use emotion to cope effectively with situations; the next three can be viewed as serving emotional development. These principles have been described in detail elsewhere (Greenberg, 2011, 2017; Greenberg & Watson, 2006), and the one central and most novel principle—transformation by changing emotion with emotion—is elaborated on later in this chapter. I discuss these six principles of emotional change throughout this book in the context of methods that implement them; this discussion can also be found in other sources (Greenberg, 2011; Watson & Greenberg, 2017).

TWO PHASES OF WORKING WITH EMOTION

Working with emotion can be conceptualized as having two phases: *arriving* and *leaving*. The first phase, arriving at one's emotions, involves helping people become aware of their emotions, accept them, and put their feelings into words. The second phase is one of leaving the place at which the client arrived and involves moving on and transforming core painful, maladaptive feelings. This transformation involves identifying the negative self or other views associated with these emotions; identify the need in the core painful emotion; and then generate new, more agentic emotions and self-organizations, which will implicitly or explicitly destructure (i.e., destroy the structure of something) any negative beliefs about self, world, or other. The person is then helped to access, experience, and rely on alternate, healthy emotional responses and needs. Change is consolidated in a new narrative.

Feel It to Heal It

As painful as some feelings may be, people need to feel their emotions before they can change them. You have to feel it to heal it. It is important to help people understand that they cannot leave a place until they have arrived there first and that the only way out of painful emotion is to go through it. In the early phase of therapy, it is helpful to provide clients with a rationale as to how working with emotion will help. Doing so supports clients' collaboration with the aim to work on emotions expressed within salient personal stories. For example, the therapist might say, "Your emotions are important; they are telling you that this is important to you. Let's work on allowing them and getting their message." The therapist also helps the client start approaching, valuing, and regulating their emotional experience. The focus of treatment begins to be established in this early stage. Therapists and clients collaboratively develop an understanding of the person's core painful narrative and work toward agreement on the underlying determinants of presenting symptoms.

Accordingly, helping clients to disclose, subjectively enter, and situate their most emotionally vulnerable and painful stories needs to be a central focus. The therapist works with clients to help them disclose emotionally salient lived experiences so they can tolerate, accept, and story their most vulnerable emotions of pain, hurt, anger, and rage for further reflection, regulation, and new meaning-making. Acceptance of these emotions and the important meanings they convey about the intentions, goals, and beliefs of the self and other is the first step in awareness work.

In this first step, gaining awareness involves helping clients pay attention to, and make contact with, sensations. This is a nonverbal form of knowing what one is feeling. This type of awareness of feelings is not an intellectual understanding of feeling. Clients should not feel that they are on the outside looking in at themselves; rather, they should have a bodily sensed awareness of what is felt from the inside—like the sensing of the throbbing of a toothache. Clients should be encouraged to welcome their emotions, dwell on them, breathe, and let them come. They need to accept their feelings as information. It is helpful for people to become aware of how they interfere with, or interrupt, their emotions rather than allow themselves to experience the emotions. Inquiring as to how clients are avoiding their feelings helps accomplish this.

Various theories of psychotherapy propose that the inhibition—or what is often called "interruption"—of emotional experience and its expression is a central phenomenon underlying psychopathology and, as such, is an important focus in therapy (Fosha, 2000; Greenberg, Rice, & Elliott, 1993; Linehan, 1993; McCullough, 1999). On a rudimentary level, most approaches agree that emotions signal to people which situations to avoid and which to approach, and that we are conditioned to avoid situations in our environment that are associated with unpleasant experiences. Because of the aversive nature of certain affective experiences, such as shame and fear, these emotions themselves can become what we avoid. *Emotional suppression*, the avoidance of affective responses, has been related to poor psychological and health outcomes (Gross, 1998, 2002; Gross & John, 2003). What has come to be called *experiential avoidance* in cognitive behavior therapy to describe the chronic avoidance of unwanted internal experiences has been linked to many different mental health problems and to the dampening of positive emotions (Gross, 1998, 2002; Gross & John, 2003; Kashdan et al., 2006; Roemer et al., 2005) Thus, long-term reliance on emotion avoidance for coping is detrimental to physical and emotional well-being. Although people can attempt to control the occurrence of emotion by avoiding internal and external stimuli (e.g., blocking thoughts, engaging in distraction, keeping away from certain environmental cues), the activation of emotion is often out of their control. The blocking of emotion in therapy becomes an important target of treatment, as I discuss in Chapters 7 and 8.

Clients also need to be taught that emotions are not reasoned, final conclusions on which they must act. Emotions provide valuable information but not reliable conclusions. Clients need to look at their feelings not as truth but as something to be explored. And no bad feelings are one's last feeling. They will change. Emotions do not come into awareness in the form of factual information; looking at emotions in their context transforms them into clues that can be interpreted and are amenable to understanding. People, therefore, can afford to feel emotions without fear of dire consequences. Emotion is neither an action nor a conclusion. People may need to control their actions, but they should not try to control their primary internal experience. For people whose emotions are overwhelming, the task, at first, is not so much one of allowing the emotions and welcoming them as it is learning how to regulate them. After helping people pay attention to and welcome their emotions, therapists need to help clients describe their emotions in words. Describing a feeling in words makes emotional experience more available for reflection. Naming emotion also is a first step in regulating emotions.

Once people have arrived at a particular place, they need to decide whether that place is good for them. If, however, they decide that being in this place will not enhance them or their intimate bonds with others, then this is not the place to stay, and clients have to find the means of leaving. Therapists and clients together need to ask, "Is this feeling adaptive, or is it a maladaptive feeling possibly based on a wound of some kind?" If the person's core feelings are healthy, they should use those feelings as guides to action. If those core feelings are unhealthy, the person needs to process those feelings further to promote change.

Build a Sense of Agency in the Self

People can only recognize that a feeling is not helpful to them once they have fully accepted it. The paradox is that if the feeling is judged as unacceptable—as "not me"—it cannot be changed because the person has not accepted it. Only when a feeling has been accepted can it be evaluated and changed, if necessary. People's core maladaptive feelings are mainly related to three major, basic emotions: fear–anxiety, shame, and sadness (Greenberg, 2015; Timulak, 2015). They also related to three basic views of the self: (a) feeling fragile and insecure, and viewing the self as being unable to hold together without support—a "weak me" sense of self; (b) feelings of worthlessness and a view of the self as a failure—a "bad me" sense of self; or (c) a feeling of lonely abandonment—a "sad me" sense of self. To change the core vulnerability that leads them to so much fear, sadness, and shame, people first have to access it. Next, they need to identify the wound that resulted in their basic negative view of themselves. Then, they need to heal the basic vulnerability and begin to build a stronger sense of self. These maladaptive feelings are almost always accompanied by negative views of self, others, or the world. People often experience these feelings as a negative voice in their heads—a harsh, internal voice that has been learned, often through previous maltreatment by others, and is destructive to the healthy self. Once articulated, these core feelings and views of self, world, and others can be changed by accessing alternate experiences to undo them. Accessing maladaptive feelings and identifying destructive beliefs paradoxically facilitates change, first by accessing the state that needs to be exposed to new experience and, second, by stimulating the mobilization of a healthier side of oneself by a type of opponent process mechanism.

New, more agentic emotions and self-organizations destructure any negative beliefs about self, world, or other. This step is at the core of the leaving phase and involves changing emotion with emotion. Helping people focus on their healthy needs for protection, comfort, and affection in response to being maltreated as well as on their needs for autonomy and competence aims to free them from the oppression of their desperate need for approval. In therapy, I have observed that people's healthier life-giving emotions are often activated in response to their own experienced emotional distress. People are tremendously resilient, especially when they are in a supportive environment. Everyone has the capacity to bounce back. Ultimately, their ability to take care of and support themselves allows them to face distress in a healthy way. When people are suffering or experiencing pain, they generally know what they need. They know they need comfort when they are hurt. They know they need to master situations in which they feel out of control. They know they need safety when they are afraid. Knowing what they need helps them to get in touch with their resources to cope. Helping people to stay with their experiences of their distressing feelings thus helps them get what they need, and this motivates change. The major healthy emotions appear to be empowering anger, the sadness of grief, and self-compassion all with approach tendencies that activate the organism to act to get what is needed. Having accessed adaptive emotions and needs, and having developed a healthier, internal voice, people create a new narrative using their new emotion to change their old narratives (Angus & Greenberg, 2011).

It is only through the experience of healthy emotion that emotional distress can truly be cured. Therapists cannot rationally argue clients into healthier emotional processes or reframe to develop new narratives. They can, however, assist clients in overcoming their unhealthy feelings by helping them to identify their painful maladaptive feelings, access their emotional resources, combat their negative voices with their healthier voices, and develop a new narrative to consolidate their transformation. The therapist's job is to bring people to face their dreaded emotions and find their alternate, healthy feelings, and then use those alternate feelings to transform their unhealthy feelings.

CONCLUSION

Emotion is the basic datum of human experience to which we bring cognition to help us make sense of it and translate its action tendencies into decisions, behavior, and meaning. This chapter discussed how important it is clinically to discriminate different types, sequences, and levels of emotions when working with them in therapy. In addition to discriminating levels of primary or secondary emotion, it is important to identify degrees of adaptiveness. Are the emotions on the surface or are they underlying, and are the emotions adaptive or maladaptive? All these variations make a difference in how the emotions are to be dealt with clinically. Emotion schematic processing also needs to be discriminated from inborn basic emotion programs because they are the source of most adult emotional experience.

This chapter also outlined a set of principles for working with emotion and argued that arriving at, allowing, and accepting emotions—although important—is not enough for dealing therapeutically with painful emotion. Therapists need to help clients leave certain painful emotions by activating new adaptive emotions that help change the old emotions and ultimately lead to generation of new narratives about the self.

The chapters in Parts II and III illustrate in more detail the clinical phases of working with emotion that are described briefly in this chapter. First, however, let's turn to Chapter 2 for the empirical base for emotion work in psychotherapy and then on to Chapter 3 for an in-depth clinical example demonstrating the principle of changing emotion with emotion.

2 RESEARCH ON EMOTIONAL CHANGE

In this chapter, I review several lines of research that, taken together, help make the case for a unified transdiagnostic theory of working with emotion in psychotherapy that is aimed at changing clients' painful emotions with adaptive emotions. This discussion of studies demonstrates that similar emotion activation and other emotion change processes occur across different forms of treatment, different diagnostic groups, and varied clinical presentations, indicating the transdiagnostic nature of these processes. I also describe various measures used to quantify depth of emotional experiencing in sessions and therapeutic gain from emotion work. I also look at how the therapist process of facilitating emotional processing has been studied so far and relate this information to the key therapist skills outlined in later chapters.

To support my statements about the effectiveness of emotion-oriented therapy, I summarize the results of two large meta-analytic studies on humanistic–experiential therapies (HEP) and, more specifically, emotion-focused therapy (EFT). These meta-analyses covered studies completed before 2009 and those from 2009 to 2018 (Elliott et al., 2013, in press). The studies included data from almost 200 studies before 2009, and 91 studies after 2009, on HEP therapies on a variety of populations. Both studies showed large

https://doi.org/10.1037/0000248-003

effect pre–post client gains and controlled effects for the whole group of HEP treatments. Clients in the studies of EFT specifically had the largest pre–post effects of the different HEP therapies. In comparative studies, HEP therapies were statistically and clinically equivalent in effectiveness to other non-HEP treatments (Goldman et al., 2006; Watson et al., 2003). And, in a comparison of EFT alone with other non-HEP therapies, these meta-analyses found a small effect favoring EFT. More specifically, no difference in effect was found between EFT and cognitive behavior therapy (CBT).

Importantly, the general pattern of effects was found to hold across different populations studied, including depression, anxiety, interpersonal problems, substance abuse, eating disorders, and chronic medical conditions. However, a limitation of all comparative results and the ensuing meta-analyses is that researcher allegiance bias has a significant effect on results in comparative trials in psychotherapy (Munder et al., 2013), and most of the comparative studies reviewed were conducted by advocates of one of the approaches under study. All in all, though, the evidence supports the effectiveness of HEP approaches that work phenomenologically with a focus on emotion.

EMOTION ACTIVATION AND EXPRESSION

Empirical research on the role of emotion in therapeutic change has consistently demonstrated a relationship between in-session emotion activation and outcome. And this relationship has also been shown in a variety of different forms of treatment. For example, Jones and Pulos (1993) in the National Institute of Mental Health collaborative study of depression found that the strategies of evocation of affect and the bringing of troublesome feelings into awareness were correlated positively with outcome in both dynamic and cognitive behavior therapies. In another study by this group, an examination of the therapist's stance in interpersonal therapy and CBT of depression, showed that it was important for therapists to focus on emotion regardless of orientation. In that study, Coombs et al. (2002) found that collaborative emotional exploration, which occurred significantly more frequently in interpersonal therapy, was found to relate positively to outcome in both forms of therapy, whereas educative/directive process—more frequent in CBT—had no relationship to outcome. Helping people overcome their avoidance of emotion, focusing collaboratively on emotions, and exploring them in therapy thus appear to be important in therapeutic change regardless of therapeutic orientation.

Research, however, has also shown that venting emotions by expressing them with high arousal by crying, yelling, or pounding to get emotional release was unsuccessful in alleviating disorder. Expressing anger, for example, which was seen as alleviating internal psychic pressure that, if not released, could lead to explosions, dissociations, or disintegration, did not, by itself, necessarily result in good outcomes in therapy (Bohart & Greenberg, 2002; Bushman, 2002; Daldrup et al., 1988; Nichols & Efran, 1985; Nichols & Zax, 1977).

A meta-analytic review found that exposure therapy is a highly effective treatment for posttraumatic stress disorder (PTSD) and that its effectiveness is based on emotional processing (Foa et al., 2003). In a series of studies on behavioral exposure (Foa et al., 1995; Foa & Jaycox, 1999; Foa & Kozak, 1998; Jaycox et al., 1998), positive outcome for PTSD from rape was predicted by the arousal of fear and its expression while retelling trauma memories during the first exposure session and by the attenuation of distress during exposures over the course of therapy. Evidence also suggests that patients with anxiety disorders who are best able to experience anxiety during the therapy session are most likely to benefit from therapy (Borkovec & Sides, 1979). Studies of recovery patterns in sexual and non-sexual assault victims found that, in general, long-term recovery is impeded if the indispensable emotional engagement with traumatic material in therapy is delayed (Gilboa-Schechtman & Foa, 2001). Findings like this indicate that emotional arousal during imaginal exposure is at least a partial mechanism of change across different disorders.

Piliero (2004) investigated clients' experience of the process of affect-focused psychotherapies on outpatient therapies of mixed populations and diagnostic groups. The clients had participated in one of three EFTs: accelerated experiential dynamic therapy (Fosha, 2000), intensive short-term dynamic therapy (Abbass, 2002), and EFT (Greenberg, 2002). Clients' self-reports of their experiences in their treatments were assessed retrospectively. Their reports of having experienced deep affect in therapy were clearly related to both being satisfied with therapy and feeling that change had occurred. A significant relationship existed between clients' recognition of their therapist's affect-eliciting techniques and feelings of satisfaction and change. Piliero (2004) concluded that emotional experiencing may be the final common pathway to therapeutic change.

Recent meta-analytic findings attest to the negative effect of suppressing emotions on therapeutic outcomes (Scherer et al., 2017). They show a significant medium-to-large effect size between the client's emotional expression and outcomes ($d = 0.85$). Third-party rating of emotional expression as opposed to self-report emerged as a significant moderator of outcomes. Pretreatment suppression was found to be the best predictor of nonresponders to treatment rather than reappraisal or diagnosis of a personality disorder. This finding suggests that diagnosis is not a good predictor of outcome and, more specifically, that it is suppression—not reappraisal—that is operative in disorder and needs to be the target of change.

This finding is, to some degree, in line with other studies that have found larger relationships between suppression and psychopathology than between reappraisal and psychopathology (Aldao et al., 2010; Barnow, 2012). It might also be the case that patients with more suppression at the onset of therapy are less able to form a therapeutic alliance with their therapist (Ogrodniczuk et al., 2008). This suggests that training therapists to recognize and facilitate client emotional expression is needed Although many diagnoses have strong affective components (e.g., depression, anxiety, PTSD), researchers and therapists, over the past few decades, have typically privileged changes in behavior as the markers of success. More research is needed to systematically investigate how emotional expression and experiencing relate to therapeutic progress on the way to lasting change (Luedke et al., 2017; Peluso et al., 2012).

PROCESS-OUTCOME STUDIES

Experiencing and expressing emotion appear to be helpful, but not by a procedure of cathartic venting. What, then, is helpful about emotion work? Reviews of process-outcome studies show a strong relationship between in-session emotional experiencing as measured by the depth of experiencing (EXP) Scale (Klein et al., 1969) and therapeutic gain in dynamic, cognitive, and experiential therapies (Castonguay et al., 1996; Goldman et al., 2005; Orlinsky & Howard, 1986; Silberschatz et al., 1986). These findings suggest that it is the processing of one's bodily felt experience in therapy by symbolizing it in awareness that may be a core ingredient of change in psychotherapy regardless of approach. "Symbolizing," here, means making the implicit explicit predominantly by putting inchoate experience into words, although these feelings could, at times, be symbolized in music, movement, or art. Symbolizing is making the implicit available to conscious awareness.

But what is "emotional processing"? Greenberg et al. (2007) defined and developed a measure of productive emotional processing: *client emotional productivity,* which is a person's being mindfully or contactfully aware of a presently activated primary emotion. Emotional productivity was operationalized in terms of the following seven features: attending, symbolization, congruence, acceptance, agency, regulation, and differentiation. This measure discriminated between productive and unproductive arousal in an intensive examination of four poor and four good outcome cases (Greenberg et al., 2007). No significant relationship was found between high expressed emotional arousal, measured over the whole course of treatment, and outcome. Rather, it was the productive processing of the highly aroused emotion that was an excellent predictor of outcome. In a larger study (Greenberg & Watson, 1998) on a sample of 74 clients from the randomized clinical trial of the effects of EFT on depression at York University, Auszra et al. (2013) found that emotional productivity increased from the beginning to the working and the termination phases of treatment. In addition, working phase emotional productivity predicted about 56% of treatment outcome—over and above variance accounted for by beginning phase emotional productivity, working alliance, and high expressed emotional arousal in the working phase of treatment. These results indicated that it is the productive processing of aroused emotion that is important for therapeutic change.

Productive Emotional Processing

An important feature of working with emotion, as noted in Chapter 1, is the distinction between primary and secondary emotion on the one hand, and adaptive and maladaptive emotion on the other. Therapists also need to assess whether a client's emotion is being processed productively. To be productive, primary emotions require a particular manner of processing: being contactfully or mindfully aware of the emotion. A system for measuring this productive emotional processing was developed by Auszra et al. (2013) and found to strongly predict therapeutic outcome.

Referring now to the seven elements of productive emotional processing, at the most basic level, for emotion to be processed productively, the client has to <u>attend</u> to an activated primary emotion to be aware of it. Once a physical or emotional reaction is attended to, it has to be <u>symbolized</u> (generally in words but perhaps in some other form, e.g., painting, movement) to be able to fully comprehend its meaning. For example, consider the following statements from a client attending to his feeling:

CLIENT: I don't know what I feel. It just feels bad.

THERAPIST: Something like, "I feel it was sort of a loss, maybe sad or disappointed." [empathic exploratory response]

CLIENT: Yeah, really disappointed. In some way, it's dashed some of my hopes. [symbolizing]

Next, for a feeling to be <u>congruent</u>, what the client says needs to match how the client feels. Feeling sad is matched with a sad face and voice, not a smile; feeling anger is expressed with some energy in the voice and an assertive posture rather than no vocal energy and a downcast look. Another important aspect of a productive emotional processing is <u>acceptance</u> of emotional experience. In particular, it is acceptance of unpleasant and painful emotional experience that is important.

Emotional experiences also have to be sufficiently <u>regulated</u> for the processing to be productive. The therapist needs to help clients develop and maintain a working distance from the emotion (Gendlin, 1996) so that the emotion is not overwhelming. This distancing enables clients to cognitively orient toward emotion as information, thus allowing for an integration of cognition and affect. Productive emotional processing also involves clients' experiencing themselves as "active agents," rather than as passive victims, of the emotion. This involves a client's taking responsibility for their emotional experience and acknowledges it as a personal experience rather than as something caused by some external agency. With agency, clients feel that they are having the emotion ("I feel sad") rather than the emotion having them ("It takes me over").

To be productive and for emotion utilization and transformation to occur, a client's primary emotional expression has to be <u>differentiating</u> over time. Fundamentally, the client must not be stuck in the emotion but, rather, explores and differentiates new aspects of experience. Their emotional process is highly fluid.

Emotional Expression: Experiencing and Therapeutic Progress

As important and necessary as arousal, acceptance, and tolerance of emotional experience are, they are insufficient for change. Optimum emotional processing also involves the integration of cognition and affect (Greenberg, 2002; Greenberg & Pascual-Leone, 1995). Once clients have achieved contact with emotional experience, they also must cognitively orient to that experience as information and explore, reflect on, and make sense of it. In addition, they must access other internal emotional resources to help transform the maladaptive state.

A recent meta-analysis found an association between clients' emotional expression and treatment outcome (Peluso & Freund, 2018). A significant medium effect size was found between the therapist's emotional expression and outcomes ($d = 0.56$) and a significant medium-to-large effect size between the client's emotional expression and outcomes ($d = 0.85$). Thus, the client's expressions of affect probably prove more important than the therapist's in relation to treatment outcomes.

Although many diagnoses have strong affective components (e.g., depression, anxiety, PTSD), researchers and therapists over the past few decades have typically privileged changes in behavior as the markers of success. Only recently have contemporary researchers begun to systematically investigate how emotional expression and experiencing in therapy can be considered reliable indicators of therapeutic progress on the way to lasting change (Luedke et al., 2017; Peluso et al., 2012).

Further supporting the hypothesis that paying attention to and making sense of emotion are important, process-outcome research on the emotion-focused treatment of depression in EFT has shown that both higher emotional arousal at midtreatment coupled with reflection on the aroused emotion (Warwar & Greenberg, 1999) and deeper emotional processing late in therapy (Pos et al., 2003, 2009), predicted good treatment outcomes. High emotional arousal plus high reflection on aroused emotion distinguished good and poor outcome cases, therefore indicating the importance of combining arousal and meaning construction (Missirlian et al., 2005; Warwar, 2005). Watson and Bedard (2006) also found that higher levels of emotional processing during sessions predicted better outcome. Emotion-oriented therapy appears to work by enhancing the type of emotional processing that involves helping people experience and accept their emotions, and make sense of them.

Core theme-related EXP in the last half of therapy was found to be a significant predictor of a reduction in symptom distress and increases in self-esteem (Goldman et al., 2005). EXP on core themes also accounted for outcome variance over and above that accounted for by early EXP and the alliance. EXP, therefore, mediated between any client individual capacity for early experiencing and positive outcome. In another study, Pos et al. (2003) found that emotional processing—defined here as EXP on emotion episodes—was found to mediate any client individual capacity for early experiencing and positive outcome. The EXP variable was contextualized by being rated only on those in-session episodes that were explicitly on emotionally laden experience.

Early capacity for emotional processing did not guarantee good outcome, nor did entering therapy without this capacity guarantee poor outcome. Therefore, although likely an advantage, early emotional processing skill appeared not as critical as the ability to acquire or increase depth of emotional processing throughout therapy, or both. Late emotional processing was found to independently add 21% to the outcome variance over and above early alliance and early emotional processing.

Warwar (2005) examined midtherapy emotional arousal as well as experiencing in the early, middle, and late phases of therapy. Emotional arousal was measured using the Client Emotional Arousal Scale-III-R (Warwar & Greenberg, 1999). In the study, clients who had higher emotional arousal midtherapy were found to have more change at the end of treatment. And not only did midtherapy arousal predict outcome, but it also predicted a client's ability to use internal experience to make meaning and solve problems, as measured by EXP, particularly in the late phase of treatment. Midtherapy arousal also added to the outcome variance over and above middle phase emotional arousal. The study thus showed that a combination of emotional arousal and experiencing was a better predictor of outcome than either index alone.

The Warwar (2005) study measured "expressed" as opposed to "experienced" emotion. In a study examining in-session client reports of experienced emotional intensity, Warwar et al. (2003) found that client reports of in-session experienced emotion were not related to positive therapeutic change. A discrepancy was observed between client reports of in-session experienced emotions and the emotions that were actually expressed based on arousal ratings of videotaped therapy segments. For example, one client reported that she had experienced intense, painful emotions in a session. Her level of expressed emotional arousal, however, was judged to be low based on observer ratings of emotional arousal from videotaped therapy segments.

Carryer and Greenberg (2010) found that it was a moderate rather than high or low frequency of heightened emotional arousal that added significantly to the outcome variance predicted by the working alliance. That study, however, showed that a frequency of 25% of highly aroused emotional expression was found to best predict outcome. Deviation toward lower frequencies, which indicated lack of emotional involvement, represented the generally accepted relationship between low levels of expressed emotional arousal and poor outcome. Deviation toward higher frequencies, though, showed that excessive amounts of highly aroused emotion are negatively related to good therapeutic outcome. These findings suggest that having the client achieve an intense and full level of emotional expression is predictive of good outcome as long as the client does not maintain this level of emotional expression for too long or too often. In addition, the frequency of reaching only a marginal level of arousal was found to predict poor outcome. Thus, expression that is on the way to the goal of heightened expression of emotional arousal but does not attain it, or that reflects an inability to express full arousal and possibly indicates interruption of possible arousal, appears undesirable.

Development of a Model of Changing Emotion With Emotion

A model of the in-session process of changing emotion with emotion has been proposed and tested (Greenberg, 2002; Greenberg & Paivio, 1997; Herrmann et al., 2016; A. Pascual-Leone & Greenberg, 2007). Clients who resolve their global distress in sessions move from secondary emotions (e.g., "I feel bad") through primary maladaptive emotions based on fear, sadness, or shame (e.g., "I'm worthless," "I can't survive on my own") to primary adaptive emotions (e.g., "I feel resolved," acceptance; Herrmann et al., 2016; A. Pascual-Leone & Greenberg, 2007). Transformation of distressed feelings is thus viewed as occurring by first attending to the aroused presenting symptomatic feelings followed by exploring the cognitive–affective sequences that generate the bad feelings (e.g., "I feel hopeless," "What's the use of trying?"). Exploration of these secondary feelings leads to the activation of some core maladaptive emotion schematic self-organizations.

A. Pascual-Leone and Greenberg (2007) found that clients in states of global distress resolve their distress by moving in one of two directions: into a core maladaptive self-organization based on maladaptive emotion schemes of fear and shame or into the sadness of lonely abandonment. They also may move into some form of secondary expression, one often of hopelessness or a type of rejecting anger. The path to resolution invariably leads to the expression of adaptive grief or hurt and to empowering anger or self-soothing; these expressions facilitate a sense of self-acceptance and agency. More resourceful clients often move directly from secondary emotions directly to assertive anger or healthy sadness, but many of the more wounded clients need to work through their core maladaptive attachment-related fear and sadness or identity-related shame (Greenberg, 2015; Greenberg & Paivio, 1997; Greenberg & Watson, 2006).

A. Pascual-Leone and Greenberg (2007) also found that transformation occurs when core maladaptive states are differentiated into adaptive needs, which act to refute the core negative evaluations about the self that is embedded in their core maladaptive schemes. The essence of this process is that, when mobilized and validated, core adaptive attachment and identity needs (i.e., to be connected and to be validated) embedded in maladaptive feelings of fear, shame, and sadness act to access more adaptive emotions and to refute negative self-messages of being unworthy of love, respect, and connection. The inherent opposition of these two experiences (i.e., "I am not worthy or lovable" and "I deserve to be loved or respected") supported by adaptive anger or sadness in response to the same evoking situation overcomes the maladaptive state. This is done by accessing new self-experience and creating new meaning, which leads to the emergence of a new, more positive evaluation of the self.

Within the context of a validating therapeutic relationship, the client then moves on to grieve, acknowledging the loss or injury suffered (recognizing "I don't have what I need, and I miss what I deserved"), and to assert empowering anger or self-soothing. Depending on whether the newly owned need involves boundary-setting or comfort, clients direct their adaptive emotional expression outward to protect boundaries (i.e., in anger) or inward toward the self (as compassion or caring). This expression often transforms into grieving for what was lost. This grief state is characterized by either sadness over a loss or recognition of one's hurt or woundedness (or both) but without blame, self-pity, or resignation, which characterize the initial states of global distress. Resolution involves integrating the sense of loss with the sense of possibility in the newfound ability to assert and self-soothe. Throughout the process of transformation, moderate-to-high emotional arousal is necessary but at a level that remains facilitative of the healing process. Therapists must facilitate optimal emotional arousal that is sufficient enough so that it is felt and can be oriented to as information but not so much that it is dysregulating or disorienting. The movement depicted in this process—from secondary emotions through primary maladaptive emotion to primary adaptive emotion—represents the core change process by which emotion changes emotion. The measure Classification of Affective-Meaning States was developed and shown to predict good outcome (A. Pascual-Leone & Greenberg, 2007).

A. Pascual-Leone (2018) went on to perform an extensive literature review of studies that examined the preceding model. He identified 24 studies that explored the relationship of the processes in the model and therapy outcome. The studies used a variety of methods and included macro- and micro-observation on 310 clinical cases and more than a 100 subclinical cases. The clinical samples represented seven different treatment approaches, including experiential, psychodynamic, and dialectical behavior therapy, and were on a variety of populations ranging from affective disorders through trauma to personality disorders, thus attesting to the transdiagnostic, transtheoretical nature of the evidence of changing emotion sequences according to the model. The evidence supported that experiencing key emotions in therapy predicts good outcome and that these emotions unfold in a particular sequence. From this review, A. Pascual-Leone found empirical support for the hypothesis that an increase in adaptive emotion predicts good outcome regardless of treatment and that the sequence of moving from global distress through primary maladaptive emotions like shame, fear and sadness, followed by adaptive emotions like assertive anger and grief as well as compassion, were associated with good outcome (Kramer et al., 2015).

Herrmann et al. (2016) examined the relationship between in-session types of emotional experience using a different type of study to test the validity of the emotion changing emotion hypothesis. They defined and operationalized the different types of emotion in the Emotion Category Coding System, which categorized activated in-session emotions as secondary/instrumental, primary maladaptive, primary adaptive, or mixed/uncodable. The different emotion categories were related to reduction in depressive symptoms in a sample of 30 clients who received EFT for depression. Both fewer secondary and more primary adaptive emotions in the working phases of therapy were found to significantly predict outcome. Moderate levels of primary maladaptive emotion in the middle working session were associated with outcome, and the frequency with which clients moved from primary maladaptive to primary adaptive emotions in this session predicted outcome. Results of the study supported the transformational model of changing emotion with emotion in which moving from secondary emotion to primary maladaptive emotion to adaptive emotion is seen to be a key change process.

In this transformation process, the decrease of secondary emotional experience and the accessing and deepening of primary maladaptive emotions to moderate levels of emotional experience played an important role. However, it was the activation of primary adaptive emotions appearing at the end that was especially important in transformation. Therapists thus need to help clients gain access to new primary adaptive emotional resources.

Levels in the different emotion categories in early sessions were not significantly related to therapy outcome and did not show significant interactions with levels later in therapy. Moreover, working phase levels in secondary and primary adaptive emotions were found to significantly predict outcome when controlling for early levels. Emotion categories thus seem to measure ongoing process rather than merely reflect individual dispositions or traits. A higher percentage of secondary symptomatic emotions in the working phase significantly predicted poorer outcomes. What is interesting is that Herrmann et al. (2016) found that the frequency with which clients moved from primary maladaptive emotions to primary adaptive emotions predicted outcome over and above the effect of mere emotional activation on outcome.

It also predicted outcome independently of the effect of secondary emotions. Moreover, the authors found the relationship between secondary emotions in the working phase and treatment outcome to be fully mediated by the proportion of primary adaptive emotions in that phase.

Importance of Accessing Primary Adaptive Emotions

The Herrmann et al. (2016) study validated that reducing secondary emotions, such as hopelessness, in emotion-focused treatment is important but only to the extent that the client succeeds in accessing primary adaptive emotions, such as empowered anger. But primary maladaptive emotions appear to play a central role in the process of therapy because moderate levels of primary maladaptive emotions, such as shame or fear in the middle working session, were associated with outcome. Clients who experienced and worked through primary maladaptive emotions of, say, shame and then accessed primary adaptive emotions, say, empowered anger or sadness, in the middle working session more frequently tended to have better treatment outcomes than those who did not. "Feeling bad" then neither means that this is therapeutically bad or good. What seems to matter is for clients to experience their core painful primary maladaptive emotions at moderate levels, to work through them, and to access adaptive emotional resources. The more frequently this is done, the better.

It seems that a mere focus on reducing symptomatic emotional experience in therapy, such as global depressive hopelessness, symptomatic fear, or secondary defensive anger, is not enough. Focusing on arriving at core primary maladaptive experiences that frequently have become part of the client's identity—such as shame of not being good enough or fear of being too weak to survive alone, or the sadness of lonely abandonment—and then accessing primary adaptive emotional experiences—such as anger against a degrading inner voice, sadness of having lost a happy childhood, pride or self-confidence, or self-compassion—seem of central importance (Kramer & Pascual-Leone, 2016; Kramer et al., 2016).

Of all the variables considered in the Herrmann et al. (2016) study, the proportion of primary adaptive emotions in the working phase was found to be the best predictor of outcome. Clients with good treatment outcome succeeded in accessing more adaptive emotional resources, potentially counteracting and undoing the effect of automatic primary maladaptive and secondary emotional responses, and thus leading to better outcome. Results of the study support the principle of changing emotion with emotion and that primary adaptive emotions play a role in transforming primary maladaptive and secondary emotions.

Timing of Emotional Arousal and Processing in Therapy

Good client process early in EFT trauma therapy has been found to be particularly important because it sets the course for therapy and allows maximum time to explore and process emotion related to traumatic memories (Paivio et al., 2001). Emotional arousal during imaginal exposure is at least a partial mechanism of change (Paivio et al., 2001). One practical implication of this research is the importance—early in therapy—of facilitating clients' emotional engagement with painful memories. Overall, the findings suggest a chain of influence on the degree to which a client processes emotion in trauma. First, the severity of trauma symptoms sets a limiting factor in the facilitation of emotional arousal and processing; next, there is early engagement in imaginal exposure tasks; then, the repetition of exposure tasks over the course of therapy have a successively cumulative impact on functioning at outcome (Paivio et al., 2001; Paivio & Nieuwenhuis, 2001).

Emotional processes also have been studied in three controlled studies (Greenberg et al., 2008; Greenberg & Malcolm, 2002; Paivio & Greenberg, 1995) on resolving emotional injuries and interpersonal difficulties. Emotional arousal during imagined contact with a significant other was a process factor that distinguished EFT from a psychoeducational treatment and was related to outcome (Greenberg et al., 2008; Greenberg & Malcolm, 2002; Paivio & Greenberg, 1995). Research on couple therapy also supports the role of emotional awareness and expression in a satisfying relationship and change in therapy. Couples who showed higher levels of emotional experiencing in therapy accompanying the softening in the blaming partner's stance were found to interact more affiliatively, and ended therapy more satisfied, than couples who showed lower experiencing (Greenberg, Ford, et al., 1993; Johnson & Greenberg, 1988; Makinen & Johnson, 2006). A similar effect of the expression of underlying emotion was found in resolving family conflict (Diamond & Liddle, 1996). Revealing of underlying vulnerable emotion also has been related to session and final outcome in the context of EFT for couples.

In another study, couples rated sessions that contained the revealing of underlying vulnerable emotion significantly more positively than control sessions on a global measure of session outcome (McKinnon & Greenberg, 2013). In addition, following sessions in which underlying vulnerable emotion was revealed, those who witnessed their partners reveal underlying vulnerable emotion scored significantly higher on a measure of problem resolution and a measure of understanding. The revealing of underlying vulnerable emotion was associated with significantly greater improvement in relationship satisfaction at termination.

Emotion Work With Anxiety

Studies on the treatment of generalized anxiety disorder (GAD) found that interventions that focus on clients' affective and bodily experience were more effective in treating individuals with GAD than treatment as usual (Levy Berg et al., 2009). Clients themselves noted that supportive, reflective interventions as well as those that facilitated their emotional expression were helpful. EFT treatment of GAD has been shown to be effective in two sets of repeated case studies (Timulak & McElvaney, 2016; Watson et al., 2017, 2019). The key change process in working with GAD clients in these studies involved accessing core painful feelings, often of attachment insecurity, and transforming them with more adaptive emotions. The overall therapeutic process involved, first, the formation of an empathic relationship. Once a therapeutic relationship was developed, therapists shifted the focus to how anxiety was generated by using two-chair dialogues between a worrier, the anxiety creator, and the experiencing self who feels the impact of the anxiety and worry. In this process, clients see that they are the agents rather than the victims of anxiety. This serves to empower them and give them a sense that they can change (Watson & Greenberg, 2017).

The overall effectiveness of working with emotion in the treatment of anxiety is also supported by studies that looked at social anxiety (Elliott, 2013; Elliott & Shahar, 2017; Shahar, 2014; Shahar et al., 2015). In addition to systematic case studies (MacLeod et al., 2012; Shahar, 2014), two outcome studies of emotion work with social anxiety showed good effects (Elliott, 2013; Elliott et al., 2014; Shahar et al., 2017). The effect sizes obtained for EFT were quite large and superior to effects found in comparable studies of CBT and medication. These two studies provided evidence supporting that emotion-focused work is promising for social anxiety and offers large benefits for clients. The key change process in EFT for social anxiety involved accessing and activating shame so that it could be restructured within a secure, accepting, validating therapy relationship. Clients were helped to access their sense that they are defective, worthless, or inferior and then to deepen it to their core pain (e.g., deep brokenness, isolation) so that it could be transformed by experiencing and expressing adaptive emotions, such as self-soothing/compassion, assertive/protective anger, and connecting sadness (Greenberg, 2011). These adaptive emotions strengthen socially anxious individuals and help them to connect with important needs that have been missing in their lives, thus encouraging them to reestablish relationships and fulfill authentic life goals and values.

Conclusions of Process-Outcome Research

The evidence from psychotherapy research indicates that certain types of therapeutically facilitated emotional awareness and arousal, when expressed in supportive relational contexts and in conjunction with access to new adaptive emotions and some conscious cognitive processing of the emotional experience, are important for therapeutic change despite, in general, the type of client or disorder. It appears that the process of change is similar regardless of diagnostic grouping. It thus seems that (a) arriving at emotion by attending, accepting, and symbolizing, and (b) leaving emotion by changing emotion with emotion, are transdiagnostic processes. Emotions, at times, need to be accessed and used as guides; at other times, they need to be regulated and modified; and yet, at other times, emotions need to be transformed by other emotions. Cognitive processing of aroused emotion in therapy has been found to be helpful to make sense of emotions and to create new narratives.

Arousing emotion or regulating it depends first on factors, such as whether the client's emotion is over- or underregulated and whether the emotion is a sign of distress or of working through the distress (Greenberg, 2002; Kennedy-Moore & Watson, 1999). The role of arousal and the degree to which it could be useful in therapy also depend on what emotion is expressed, by whom, about what issue, how it is expressed, to whom, when and under what conditions, and in what way the emotional expression is followed by other experiences of emotion and meaning-making (Greenberg, 2002; Whelton, 2004). Nonetheless, for effective emotional processing to occur, the distressing affective experience must be activated and viscerally experienced by the client, and new emotions are needed to change old emotions.

RESEARCH ON THERAPIST PROCESS

There has been limited research on specific therapist interventions that facilitate emotional processing. In general, empathic attunement to affect is the key skill and is discussed throughout this book. Since Rogers (1957) identified empathy as an important variable in therapy, it has been found to be a consistent predictor of client change (Bohart et al., 2002; Bohart & Greenberg, 1997; Elliott et al., 2011). For example, Watson et al. (2014) found a significant direct relationship between therapists' empathy and therapy outcome. This finding suggests that clients' perception of their therapists as empathic is an important mechanism of change in psychotherapy.

In addition, Adams (2010) tracked moment-by-moment client–therapist interactions and found that therapist statements that were high in experiencing influenced client experiencing and that depth of therapist experiential focus predicted outcome. More specifically, if the client was externally focused and the therapist made an intervention that was targeted toward internal experience, the client was more likely to move to a deeper level of experiencing. Adams's study highlights the importance of the therapist's role in deepening emotional processes. Given that client experiencing predicts outcome and that therapist depth of experiential focus influences client experiencing and predicted outcome, a path to outcome is established, suggesting that therapists' depth of experiential focus influences clients' EXP, and this relates to outcome.

Another important development in the articulation of therapist process has been in the area of therapeutic presence. Specifically, developments have been made in the conceptualization and provision of therapeutic presence in EFT. This is seen as a continuation of a tradition that began in client-centered (Rogers, 1980) and Gestalt therapy (Perls, 1973) and was further developed within the emotion-focused relationship by Geller and Greenberg (2012). Geller and Greenberg (2002) developed a measure of therapist presence and established it as an important condition related to outcome. Watson and McMullen (2005) studied key aspects of the EFT therapy process and also compared them with CBT. Watson and McMullen found that CBT therapists taught more and asked more directive questions, whereas EFT therapists offered more support. In their examination of the complex relationship among empathy, affect regulation, and outcome reporting, Watson and Prosser (2002) found that the effect of therapist empathy on outcome was mediated by changes in clients' affect regulation.

CHANGING EMOTION WITH EMOTION

Empirical evidence has mounted to support the importance of a process of changing emotion with emotion. Parrott and Sabini (1990) early on found that mood repair occurs by people recalling events that counteract both sad and happy moods, and this recollection is done without awareness. In a further interesting line of investigation, positive emotions have been found to "undo" lingering negative emotions (Fredrickson, 1998; Fredrickson &

Levenson, 1998). Studies have clearly shown that positive emotions (e.g., joy, love) can be used to undo the effects of so-called negative emotions like anger and sadness (Fredrickson, 2009). For example, Fredrickson (2001) showed that a positive emotion may loosen the hold that a negative emotion has on a person's mind by broadening a person's momentary thought action repertoire. The experience of joy and contentment were found to produce faster cardiovascular recovery from negative emotions than a neutral experience.

Fredrickson et al. (2000) found that resilient individuals cope by recruiting positive emotions to undo negative emotional experiences. The basic observation is that key components of positive emotions are incompatible with negative emotions. In a further study, Tugade and Fredrickson (2004) found that resilient individuals cope by recruiting positive emotions to regulate negative emotional experiences. These individuals manifested a physiological bounce back that helped them to return to cardiovascular baseline more quickly. Bad feelings appear to be able to be transformed by happy feelings—not in a deliberate manner by trying to look on the bright side or by replacement, but by the evocation of meaningfully embodied alternate experience that undoes the physiology and experience of negative feeling. In a therapy analogue study dealing with self-criticism, Whelton and Greenberg (2000) found that in two-chair dialogues, people who were more vulnerable to depression showed less resilience in response to self-contempt than people who were less vulnerable to depression. The less vulnerable people were able to recruit positive emotional resources like pride and anger to combat the depressogenic contempt and negative cognitions. These studies together indicate that emotion changes emotion.

In a line of research on the effect of motor expressions on experience, Berkowitz (2000) reported a study on the effect of muscular action on mood. Subjects who had talked about an angering incident while making a tightly clenched fist reported having stronger angry feelings, whereas fist-clenching led to a reduction in sadness when talking about a saddening incident. This finding indicates both the effects of motor expression on intensifying congruent emotions and on dampening other emotions. Thus, it appears that the muscular expressions of one emotion can change another emotion. In addition and in line with the James–Lange theory of emotions, Flack et al. (1999) demonstrated that adopting the facial, postural, and vocal expression of an emotion increases the experience of the emotion whether the subject is aware of what emotion they are expressing. The experience of an emotion, to some degree, can be induced or intensified by putting one's body into its expression. Interestingly, there are individual differences in this capacity; those who are more body sensitive show this tendency to a greater degree.

A more general line of research in social psychology on the effects of role playing on attitude change also supports the idea that performing actions in a role brings people's experience and attitudes in line with the role (Zimbardo et al., 1977). Role playing can transform what is, at first, not real into something real, just as saying something can lead to believing it (Myers, 1996). Thus, a possible way to evoke another emotion is to have people role-play its expression. As they express an emotion, it will change their experience toward the expression.

In psychotherapy research, it has been found that music is helpful in evoking alternate emotions and even more helpful than imagery for changing emotion (Kerr et al., 2001). Right frontal electroencephalogram (EEG) activation typically associated with sad affect was shifted toward symmetry by both massage and music (Field, 1998). Shifts to more positive mood or at least to symmetry between sad and happy affect were accompanied by shifts from right to left frontal EEG activation in both mothers and children (Field, 1998).

Results of a number of single-case investigations of therapies of depression (Watson et al., 2007) combined with larger group studies that compared therapies of depression (A. Pascual-Leone & Greenberg, 2007), along with others more generally relating emotional arousal to outcome (Greenberg, 2015; Herrmann et al., 2016), supported the principle that emotional arousal and the attendant transformation of emotion with emotion occurred significantly more in cases with recovery of their depression than in poor outcome cases with no recovery of their depression. In a number of intensive analyses of good outcomes, Watson et al. (2007) found reductions in shame and fear and increases in anger, sadness, contentment, and joy. The patterns of emotional transformation, however, were idiosyncratic. Which emotions replaced which were idiosyncratic to each case.

CONCLUSION

In addition to the studies reviewed in this chapter, it is heartening to note an emerging theoretical approach to a unified treatment: Barlow et al. (2004) postulated the existence of a *negative affect syndrome*, which manifests differentially as depression, anxiety disorders, or even as eating disorders in different patients. They identified three basic principles that may cause distress to patients regardless of disorder and that should therefore be targets of a transdiagnostic approach to therapeutic change: altering antecedent reappraisals, modifying emotion-related action tendencies, and overcoming emotional avoidance. In the concluding chapter, "Looking Ahead: A Unified Approach to Psychotherapy," I discuss more emerging directions and offer a fuller vision of what lies ahead for emotion work in psychotherapy. For now, I summarize by stating that the relationship between therapeutic benefit and emotional experience, expression, or specific therapy processes is not a simple one. However, many indicators do suggest the benefits of a trans-theoretical clinical approach with emotion at its center.

3

CHANGING EMOTION WITH EMOTION

In this chapter, I discuss *changing emotion with emotion*—that is, the process of transformation by the synthesis of opposing emotions. I also look at the *theory of memory reconsolidation*, which shows how introducing new present emotional experience can change old memories through the process of memory reconstruction. It is new emotional experience that allows automatic connections (unconscious) at a neuronal level (schematic) to sculpt new ways of feeling and being.

It is important to understand that in discussing changing emotion with emotion, we clinicians are talking about changing underlying emotions from the past that influence the present to improve real-world coping. So, for example, we work to change the painful emotion schemes that have been developed from past experience that produce emotions, such as fear of abandonment, shame of unworthiness, or sadness of empty aloneness. These are the feelings that form the basis of presenting problems, including low self-worth, interpersonal problems, or global distress. Changing emotion with emotion is done by accessing underlying maladaptive emotions and transforming them with new adaptive emotions.

https://doi.org/10.1037/0000248-004
Changing Emotion With Emotion: A Practitioner's Guide, by L. S. Greenberg

We are not talking about direct modification of presenting symptomatic behavior—for example, overcoming the anxiety that prevents one from going to the mall or reducing angry outbursts. We also are not working to reduce symptomatic emotions by habituation or exposure to reduce arousal. Rather, the work is to transform underlying painful emotions—often not initially in awareness or expressed—that are the underlying determinants of the presenting problematic arousal or symptoms. The necessary first step in changing emotion with emotion is to *increase* the dreaded painful underlying emotion rather than *reduce* the presenting symptomatic emotion. The aim is not the extinction of the activated underlying emotion but, rather, its transformation with new experience.

MODELS OF CHANGE

Learning theory models of change view change as occurring by *extinction*, which involves modifying automatic processing by some form of new conditioning. Change is seen as occurring by inhibition of associations (Craske et al., 2014). New learning takes place that suppresses the original learning rather than transforming it, leaving the old learning intact. Cognitive therapy still embracing learning theory has added the view that people are not only reactive processors governed by prior conditioning but also are influenced by goals and expectations. Stimuli are seen not only as leading to behavioral responses but as activating beliefs, which then influence emotions and behaviors.

Foa and Kozak (1986) developed an emotional processing model that proposed that the mismatch between what was expected based on prior knowledge and current learning was one of the necessary conditions for new learning to occur. This perspective led to exposure as a main form of treatment; however, it did not take memory change into account. Thus, left open is the question of whether exposure simply strengthens inhibition of old memories or leads to change in memories. Are old memories inhibited or transformed so as to erase the old memory? The fact that people often relapse after exposure treatments suggest that the memory has not changed, but is only being inhibited and is ready to be reactivated—if the conditions are right.

In contrast to learning theory, Greenberg and Safran (1987), adopting a neo-Piagetian developmental point of view, proposed that change occurs by a dialectical synthesis of opposing emotion schematic memories of past painful experience. This view has been supported by the subsequent development of reconsolidation theory (Lane et al., 2015; Nader et al., 2000), which I elaborate later. This theory proposes a different process in which the memory is actually transformed by new experience. Memory change and extinction, then, are two different, mutually exclusive, processes. Here, I present the theory of changing emotion with emotion as a transformational process in which emotional memories are changed—not inhibited—by the experience of new emotional responses. Memory reconsolidation involves both activation of the emotion memory and generation of a new emotional response to change the old emotional response.

In addition to the debate about transformation versus suppression of memories and their emotions, a belief commonly held in modern acceptance-based and other third-wave cognitive behavior therapy approaches (Hayes et al., 2008) is that change occurs by experiencing and accepting emotion or by accessing and expressing. The acceptance of the disowned was a view originally proposed by humanistic–experiential approaches (Perls, 1973; Rogers, 1959), but, in my view, it is a simplification that can be detrimental to therapeutic change. This view is based on a notion that mere acceptance of emotion helps clients to overcome what, in cognitive behavior therapy language, has come to be called "experiential avoidance" or what humanistic therapy had originally referred to as "disowned feelings" (Perls, 1969; Rogers, 1957). In the acceptance or reowning view, problems are seen essentially as being caused by avoidance or denial of emotion.

In an insight-oriented view of change, emotions or impulses are seen as being kept out of awareness by habitual defenses, and therapeutic change is seen as being effected by overcoming defenses and acknowledging feelings. In their affect phobia approach, McCullough et al. (2003) blended psychoanalytic and behavioral views, essentially seeing psychological problems as arising from fear of emotion. Based on this viewpoint, they proposed a type of exposure and response prevention theory to emotional change. It is this: Exposure to the client's fear of and anxiety about their feelings as well as response prevention (i.e., not avoiding or giving up defenses) help clients overcome avoidance, put aside defenses, and experience deep emotion long enough that the anxiety subsides.

Some psychodynamic views also propose that clients also develop enough of a self-observing capacity and self- understanding that they are able to see their defenses coming up and, in the course of ordinary life, are able to make different choices. In these views, therapists thus need to help the client access unprocessed feelings, experience them deeply enough to break the conditioned anxiety, and then, through understanding, consciously choose to overcome the avoidance or defense (see, e.g., Hayes et al., 2008) and see choice as an important factor in change.

As important as acceptance of previously disclaimed emotions and action tendencies are, the view that I propose here differs. I see clients as changing by having new emotional experience that is discrepant from old experience. Changing emotion with emotion is not exposure, is not associationism or conceptual learning, and is not understanding or insight. Rather, changing emotion with emotion is new procedural learning by having new emotional experience in the session that transforms old emotional memories and responses. This involves implicit psychological processes of change by the automatic synthesis of old elements of experience (which have been stored as emotion schematic memories) with new experience in the session. It works by the brain's making new implicit linkages as opposed to accepting or making conscious, previously denied feelings or by counterlearnings as proposed by learning theorists.

EXPANSION OF THE EMOTIONAL RESPONSE REPERTOIRE

As noted in the Introduction to this volume, Alexander and French (1946) and Goldfried (1980) proposed that providing clients with new, corrective experiences is a common therapeutic strategy and a core change principle regardless of approach. What I am proposing, although in the same spirit, differs from these proposals by specifying a unique process: that of changing emotion with emotion as at the core of corrective emotional experience. This, I am suggesting, is a transtheoretical process that is applicable across orientations. It necessitates working at an experiential level with visceral bodily experienced feelings. These feelings change only after a bodily felt shift occurs that then is symbolized in language and formed into narrative meaning to consolidate the experiential change. I suggest that the change takes place neuronally as the brain lays down new pathways to form new emotion schemes that represent the new lived experience. Furthermore, regardless of approach—be it experiential, cognitive behavioral, or psychodynamic—when change takes place, it is because of new emotional experience changing old emotional experience. In addition, this change process is applicable transdiagnostically regardless of disorder because most disorders are disorders of emotion and emotional processing.

Useful change comes not from what we tell ourselves, what our minds invent to soothe our anxieties, or even what we are told by others but by close contact with new experience. This is why this type of process is called *experiential*: It involves learning from experience, not from a therapist, not from reasoning, and not from new understanding. The therapeutic task becomes to facilitate new experience but not by psychoeducation, skill training, or interpretation. Working in this way to help clients have new emotional experiences to change the old emotional experiences involves the ability of the therapist to handle (i.e., contain) the client's fear of their dreaded experience as well as the therapist's own fear of the client's emotions.

New experience is what is change producing. In this process, conscious change in beliefs, narratives, and decisions comes relatively late in the sequence of change and only after an emotional shift has occurred. The emphasis is not on just experiencing previously disallowed emotions; rather, the broad goal of change is arriving at previously disclaimed, dreaded emotion to make them accessible to transformation by new emotions. People have to feel emotions to change emotions. They need to feel fear to change fear, feel shame to change shame. To achieve change, therapists need to promote experience of new emotions to change old emotions. This goes beyond the more restricted goal of only making contact with and accepting emotions. The simple experience and expression of emotions, although important, are not enough.

As described briefly in Chapter 1, in this book, I focus on two basic aspects of working with emotion: "arriving at" emotion and "leaving" emotion. To heal, people have to allow themselves to fully experience what it is that they are feeling; but, if that's all they do, then they just end up feeling their maladaptive fear, shame, or sadness. What is now needed is to leave these emotions. Transformation of these reowned maladaptive emotional responses happens when people are able to access new primary adaptive emotional responses to change the old, now obsolete, responses. So, we have a two-step process: arriving and leaving. In the first stage, the therapist helps the client to reown the disowned feelings, reclaim the disclaimed action tendencies, and articulate and explore their emotional significance.

In the second stage, having arrived at a core maladaptive feeling and having articulated its personal meaning, the goal is to help the client access a more adaptive emotional resource as an antidote to the maladaptive feeling. One of the most effective interventions to help access a more adaptive emotional response is asking clients what their feelings need to feel better. The therapist might ask, "What does this deep feeling of hurt and distrust need?" The client might respond, "I just need to be held and to be comforted. I do so want some of the warmth." Accessing a feeling of deserving to have a previously unmet adaptive need met is a central part of the change process of accessing new feelings to undo old feelings (Greenberg, 2002, 2011). Once new adaptive feelings are accessed, therapists focus on facilitating the construction of new narratives.

Therapists, for example, can help depressed clients reown their maladaptive feelings of shame of rejection by guiding them to an episodic memory in which this emotion had been strongly evoked. Clients may, for instance, be asked to imagine themselves as a frightened child who has been left alone, and once the emotion is felt, to focus on what is needed. They need to arrive at the feeling of lonely abandonment before they can leave this feeling. Transformation occurs when people are able to access new emotional responses to the old situations. A client first has to reexperience, for example, their shame and fear as they remembers their abusive father and scenes related to the abuse. That client then needs to generate new emotional responses, such as anger at violation, sadness of grief, and compassion for the pain their younger self suffered. Transformation results in an expansion of a person's emotional response repertoire (Greenberg, 2011) that enables the expression of more adaptive action tendencies and new story outcome. Although a feeling has to be felt to be changed, change involves more than just feeling an emotion; it also requires experiencing a new more adaptive feeling and developing a new narrative.

Emotion work of this type involves a combination of following and leading. Following to arrive at the emotion is seen as taking precedence over leading, which is especially the case with clients having greater internal locus of control, or those with more oppositional styles who are more reactive to control, or more fragile clients who need more safety. More distressed and more avoidant clients, however, often benefit initially from more leading. Leading takes the form of process guidance and emotion coaching in which the therapist consistently guides toward emotion. It includes a form of emotional "re-parenting" in which therapists offer validation, soothing, and compassion in response to clients' emotions. Often the clients who need this type of response had never received it before. Therapists need to fit the degree of leading and following to each client.

Although there may be something to be said for the more traditional ways of thinking about changing emotion, such as acceptance, expression and completion, habituation, extinction or, reflective understanding, I have found, based on my research of studying actual change events in therapy (Greenberg, 1984, 2007), that changing emotion with emotion is a more accurate description of how emotional change actually takes place. Reason is seldom sufficient to change automatic emergency amygdala-based emotional responses. Darwin (1897), on having automatically jumped back from the strike of a glassed-in snake, noted that having approached it with the determination to not move back, his will and reason were nevertheless powerless against the imagination of a danger that he had never even experienced.

Maladaptive emotions are impenetrable to reason and are best transformed by other emotions. An analogy in nature is fighting fire with fire. In *King John*, Shakespeare wrote, "Be fire with fire; threaten the threatener and outface the brow of bragging horror" (V, i, 48–50; Staunton, 1898). In other words, respond by using a similar method, match kind with kind; so, here: change emotion with emotion.

Neuronal Change in the Synthesis of New Experience

The repeated or sustained coactivation of a more adaptive emotion along with a maladaptive emotion to the same stimulus helps to synthesize a new experience, thereby transforming the maladaptive emotion. There appear to be a number of aspects of the process of transformation through the coactivation of different emotional states to synthesize new emotional responses. At the most fundamental level, the action tendencies in the new emotion oppose the action tendencies in the old one, leading to a novel response. A person cannot withdraw in fear if anger with a tendency to thrust forward is coactivated. This is not a process of one emotion *replacing* another emotion; rather, it is that one emotion *undoes* or *transforms* another emotion by a process of a dialectical synthesis to produce a new form of experience. Just as yellow combines with blue to make green, so do approach tendencies combine with withdrawal tendencies to make a new response tendency— possibly of boundary setting or calm.

At the schematic level of processing, different schemes synthesize to form higher level schemes. As Hebb (1949) stated, the first law of neuroscience is that neurons that fire together wire together and continue to fire together. So, new emotion schemes are formed by the synthesis of two or more schemes coactivated by the same stimulus. With new action tendency, and new scheme formation, there is new bodily felt experience and changed orientation to the world. This new feeling is now consolidated by the construction of a new narrative, which leads to new meanings and new articulated views of self, world, and other.

In therapy, maladaptive fear, once aroused, can be transformed into security by the more boundary-establishing emotions of adaptive anger or disgust or by evoking the softer feelings of the sadness of loss, compassion, or forgiveness. Similarly, maladaptive anger can be undone by adaptive sadness and result in letting go and accepting. Maladaptive shame can be transformed into self-acceptance by accessing anger at violation, pride, and self-worth or by self-comforting compassion, or all of these. In this manner, emotions that lead to withdrawal are transformed by approach emotions from another part of the brain. Once emotion changes, cognition and narratives also change. Now, people, neglected as children, who no longer feel unworthy change their narratives: Where once they were unlovable, now the narrative specifies that others were incapable of love. Where once people who were abused blamed themselves and felt ashamed or guilty about the abuse, now they see themselves as not responsible.

The Undoing, Not Replacement, of Emotion

It is intuitively clear to most people that feeling good can change feeling bad, but we are not talking primarily about replacing so-called negative emotions with positive ones. Rather, in therapy, we are talking about *undoing* the maladaptive emotion with another emotion that has an opposing action tendency. For example, anger is frequently used to battle against fear and helps people overcome fear by changing the experience of situations. In life, anger changes behavior and enables one to take a greater risk, whereas fear hinders risky action. In therapy, one way to transform fear from prior abuse is to experience one's previously inaccessible anger at violation, which leads to more assertive experience. If, for example, a client imagines an abusive father, and doing so evokes his fear from memories of prior abuse, then if he comes to experience his adaptive anger at violation and expresses it to the imagined father, he has a corrective emotional experience in which he now feels stronger and more able to assert himself. Anger influences cognition; it triggers a more optimistic view of oneself than sadness and biases a person toward feeling and seeing the self as powerful and capable. By way of contrast, fear is adept at reducing anger. The action tendency to withdraw will dampen the forward-thrusting action. In life, angry decision makers typically process information in ways that fail to consider alternative options before acting. Introducing the emotion of fear makes them overestimate danger and holds them back from action. In other words, fear modulates anger. Clearly, emotions change emotion and change cognition, too.

Probably the most important way of dealing with maladaptive emotion in therapy involves not only its acceptance, understanding, or regulation but also its transformation by other emotions. I have found that the primary maladaptive emotions most in need of change that arise in most therapies are fear of danger, fear of separation, shame of unworthiness, and the sadness of lonely abandonment. And the adaptive emotions that help in the transformation process are empowered anger, the sadness of grief, and compassion (Greenberg, 2015). An important goal in working with emotions, then, is first to arrive at the maladaptive emotion—not to accept it for its good information and motivation—as if it were an adaptive emotion (because it does not provide such emotions) but to make it accessible to transformation. In time, the coactivation of the more adaptive emotion along with or in response to the maladaptive emotion helps transform the maladaptive emotion. The paradox of this path to emotional change, however, is that it does not start with trying to change emotion. Rather, it's the opposite: to fully accept the painful emotion. Emotions must be fully felt and their message heard before they are open to change by new emotions. Emotion acceptance always precedes emotion transformation: You have to feel an emotion to heal an emotion.

The process of changing emotion with emotion differs from such notions as catharsis, exposure, extinction, or habituation in that maladaptive feelings are not purged, nor are they attenuated by people feeling them. Rather, another feeling is used to transform or undo the old feeling. Although dysregulated secondary emotions, such as the anxiety in phobias, obsessive–compulsiveness, and panic, and the fear-laden intrusive images from trauma may be overcome by exposure, in many situations, primary maladaptive emotions (e.g., the shame of feeling worthless, the anxiety of basic insecurity, and the sadness of abandonment) are what underlie symptoms and are best transformed by accessing emotions with opposing action tendencies.

People who suffer from social anxiety, for example, may have core underlying primary maladaptive emotions of shame of inadequacy or fear of abandonment from their developmental history, and it is these that lead to withdrawal. Change is produced not by exposure to social situations but by first accessing the underlying painful emotion and then by coactivating an incompatible, more adaptive approach experience, such as empowering anger or pride, or compassion for the self. The new emotion undoes the old response (Fredrickson, 2001) rather than attenuate or replace it. This involves more than simply facing feelings or accepting feelings of anxiety to diminish them. Rather than involving efforts to modify the anxiety by, say, exposure, in-therapy emotion work involves accessing and staying in contact with the withdrawal tendencies of the underlying primary maladaptive fear or shame and coactivating the approach tendencies in anger or in comfort-seeking sadness.

Which Emotions, When, and How?

An important issue in any treatment is what emotion should be activated to transform the maladaptive emotion. Here, there is no formula. It depends on the idiosyncratic experience of the client and on what adaptive emotions are available and can be evoked. This accessing of adaptive emotions involves the therapist's empathic attunement to what emotions seem to emerge in the process. This is an exploratory, not a prescriptive, process. Other important questions are, "When should painful emotions be activated and when should they be regulated? And exactly which emotions are to be regulated— and how?"

Underregulated emotions generally are either secondary emotions, such as despair and hopelessness, or primary maladaptive emotions, such as the shame of being worthless, the anxiety of basic insecurity, and panic that are currently not able to be connected to adaptive cognition because they are so overwhelming. When emotional arousal is too high and outside the client's zone of tolerance, emotion no longer informs adaptive thought and action, so it then needs to be regulated (Greenberg, 2002). In such situations, clients benefit from interventions that help create a working distance from the intense emotions to prevent being overwhelmed by them.

In some cases, avoiding or suppressing aroused feelings can produce a rebound effect or a bottle-up–blow-up syndrome. Disengagement in many situations is not helpful. In other cases, however, people can effectively disengage from emotion, and this disengagement can facilitate learning and memory. Too much emotion at too high an intensity can be countertherapeutic (Carryer & Greenberg, 2010). A crucial clinical judgment is when to distract and down-regulate, and when to facilitate emotion approach and intensification. I deal with this topic in greater depth in Chapter 11.

PATHS TO EMOTIONAL CHANGE AND THERAPY SEQUENCES

In illuminating the process of arriving and leaving, it is helpful to understand that there are two different paths to emotional change. Those paths depend on whether the previously disclaimed emotion the client is helped to arrive at in therapy is (a) an adaptive emotion like unacknowledged grief or assertive anger; or is (b) a maladaptive experience of feeling, say, fear-based anxious insecurity, the sadness of lonely abandonment, or shame-based worthlessness. The first path—denying an adaptive emotion, which provides adaptive information and action tendencies that can be used as a guide to change one's behavior—is simpler to work with therapeutically. This work involves a two-step process of moving from secondary reactive to primary adaptive emotions—like from secondary anxiety to underlying adaptive anger. The client is helped to reown the adaptive emotion, accept it, and experience it in the therapy—not just talk about it or have insight but have the bodily-felt experience of feeling empowered and asserting the right to not be violated. Informed and transformed by this emotion, the client symbolizes it in words, reflects on the emotion to create new narrative meaning, and decides how to act.

A number of important recognizable two-step sequences occur. The first is one in which secondary anger often is a reaction to, or sometimes a defense against, an original or more primary feeling of sadness, hurt, or vulnerability. Another major two-step sequence flows in the opposite direction to the preceding sequence. This is where secondary sadness masks the more primary anger. In the first case, when clients have learned that it is unsafe to experience or share—or both—their sadness–hurt–vulnerability and cover it with anger, therapists first need to validate the client's secondary anger and then focus on the experience of sadness beneath the anger. After the client has acknowledged the anger, they need to acknowledge and process the original hurt.

One way to reach the original hurt is to invite clients to pay attention to what they feel immediately after they have expressed their anger because a window to the original primary feeling of hurt or sadness often opens following expression of the secondary feeling. Other ways to approach the primary feeling are to either empathically inquire into or to conjecture about the original feeling that might have led to the client's anger. For example, the therapist might say, "Something must have hurt very deeply to leave you feeling so angry. How did you feel when that happened?" or "Angry but also maybe hurt by what she said?"

When, however, newly accessed primary painful emotions are not a source of good information or do not provide adaptive orientation to the current situation, they are maladaptive and need to be changed. When working on this second, more complex, path, therapists first need to help their clients arrive at the previously disclaimed painful, maladaptive emotion. This involves a three-step sequence. This sequence begins with the client in a symptomatic state and involves moving from secondary reactive to primary maladaptive emotions to adaptive emotion—for example, from secondary social anxiety to underlying maladaptive shame and then to a transformative primary adaptive emotion, say, assertive anger (Greenberg & Paivio, 1997). When clients are already in their primary maladaptive emotions, there also is a two-step sequence from primary maladaptive to adaptive—say, from shame to adaptive anger.

The major three-step sequence involves first acknowledging secondary distress, hopelessness, or anger. The second step is accessing the primary maladaptive feelings of shame, fear, or sadness beneath the first state.

Once the primary painful emotion has been accepted and symbolized in awareness, the third step involves accessing more adaptive emotions, usually healthy anger or sadness that were overregulated or were not readily accessible. This frequently is followed by a sense of compassion for the suffering of the self. States, such as a shame-filled sense of worthlessness, an anxious sense of basic insecurity, or a paralyzing state of traumatic fear, often are found beneath more surface despair, hopelessness, or rage. These avoided states need to be approached and faced. This two-step sequence from secondary to primary maladaptive emotion, however, is not yet fully therapeutic. The third step of accessing another set of healthy emotions and motivations is needed to move beyond the maladaptive states. These three steps embody the basic change process involved in changing emotion with emotion and have been shown to predict outcome (Herrmann et al., 2016; A. Pascual-Leone & Greenberg, 2007).

It is important to recognize unproductive sequences, however. A frequent, unproductive, three-step sequence often occurs when there is a conflict around feeling a newly accessed primary adaptive emotion. Thus, clients may present with a sadness or hopelessness, and through exploration, they may access healthy anger at violation but then feel guilt or anxious about their anger. Here, the third emotion interrupts and prevents the second emotion that is the healthy adaptive response.

Maladaptive emotions, such as the anxiety of basic insecurity or the fear of abandonment, or of annihilation from past childhood maltreatment, are transformed into security, calm, or even love or happiness by the activation of more empowering, boundary-establishing emotions of adaptive anger or grief at what was missed and compassion toward the self. Similarly, maladaptive fear can be undone by adaptive sadness. Maladaptive shame, which was internalized from the contempt of others, can be transformed by accessing anger at violation at the abuse one suffered, which enhances self-assertion and pride and self-worth, and by accessing self-compassion for the pain suffered. Anger at being unfairly treated or thwarted helps overcome hopelessness and helplessness (Sicoli, 2005). The thrusting-forward tendency in presently accessed anger at violation or the reaching out for contact and comfort in sadness transforms the tendency to shrink into the ground in shame or collapse in helplessness. After the new emotion is accessed, it undoes the original state, and a new state is forged. Introducing new present experience into currently activated memories of past events leads to transformation through the assimilation of new emotional material into past emotion memories during memory reconsolidation (discussed later in the chapter).

NEW EMOTIONS, NEW SELF-ORGANIZATION

How does the therapist help the client access new emotions to change old emotions? A number of ways have been outlined (Greenberg, 2002). Therapists can help the client access new emotions in the present by a variety of means, including shifting attention to *subdominant emotions* that are currently being expressed but are only on the periphery of a client's awareness. The subdominant emotion is often present in the room nonverbally in tone of voice or manner of expression.

I have found that focusing on what is needed is a key means of activating a new emotion (Greenberg, 2002, 2015). Asking clients what they need to resolve their pain when they are in the pain of their maladaptive state is the most powerful way of activating a new emotion. Raising a need or a goal to a dynamic self-organizing system opens a problem space for implicit processing to search for a solution. At the affective level, it conjures up a feeling of what it is like to reach the goal and opens up neural pathways both to the new feeling and the attainment of the goal. Organisms are motivated to survive and thrive, and by paying attention to and experiencing their pain. In so doing, they mobilize to eliminate the pain.

The essence of this process is that when clients' core maladaptive emotions of fear, shame, or sadness are accessed, core needs for connection and validation are mobilized. Emotion is generated by appraising the situation in relation to a need. When the need is raised in salience, the brain, which automatically evaluates that the need was not met generally, generates anger or sadness. Once the need is articulated, clients can be helped to feel deserving of the previously unmet need by the therapist's validating the need— for example: "Yes, as a child, you deserved protection, love, and safety." Once clients feel that they deserved to have the need met, a more adaptive emotion related to their needs not being met is generated automatically. When clients feel that their need to be loved or protected was valid and that they deserved to be loved or protected, the emotion system automatically appraises that needs were not met and generates either anger at having been unfairly treated or sadness at having missed the opportunity of having one's needs met. These new adaptive feelings become a new emotional response to the old situation, and they act to transform the more maladaptive feelings.

The result is an implicit refutation of the sense that the person does not deserve love, respect, and connection. The opposition of the two experiences "I am not worthy or lovable" and "I deserve to be loved or respected," supported by adaptive anger or sadness in response to the same evoking situation, produces a reorganization that undoes the maladaptive state and leads to a new self-organization. These new feelings were either felt in the original situation but not expressed, or are felt now as an adaptive response to the old situation. For example, accessing implicit adaptive anger at violation by a perpetrator can help change maladaptive fear in a trauma survivor. When the tendency to run away in fear is transformed by both anger's tendency to thrust forward and by sadness's tendency to reach out for comfort and care, the abuser is able to be held accountable for wrongs done. Thereafter, there is a grieving for the loss of what was missed, and self or other comfort is more likely to be experienced. Accessing one's adaptive needs acts automatically as disconfirmation of maladaptive feelings and beliefs. In this way, new experience changes old experience. The newly accessed, alternate feelings are resources in the personality that help change the maladaptive state.

Often a period of validating and making sense of the painful emotion is needed before the activation of an opposing transforming emotion. It is essential to symbolize, explore, and differentiate the primary maladaptive emotion, especially in the case of fear, and to regulate it by breathing and calming before accessing the new, more adaptive emotion—often, anger.

Expressive Enactments

Other methods of accessing new emotion involve using enactment and imagery to evoke new emotions, remembering a time an emotion was felt, changing how the client views things, or even the therapist's expressing an emotion for the client (Greenberg, 2002). *Expressive enactment* entails asking people to adopt certain emotional stances and helping them deliberately assume the expressive posture of that feeling, and then intensifying it to help evoke the experience of the emotion. Therapists might use psychodramatic enactments and instruct clients, for example, "Try telling him I'm angry. Say it again. Yes, louder. Can you put your feet on the floor and sit up straight?" The therapist coaches the client to express until the client experiences the emotion.

A number of experimental social psychology studies lend support to the notion that expression activates emotion. Berkowitz (2000) found that people who made a tightly clenched fist while talking about an angering incident reported stronger feelings of anger. However, clenching a fist while talking about a sad incident led to a reduction in sadness. These findings showed that motor expression intensified congruent emotions and dampened other emotions. The bodily expressions of one emotion can change another emotion.

Similarly, Flack et al. (1999), in line with the James–Lange theory of emotions (i.e., that action leads to emotion), showed that adopting the facial, postural, and vocal expression of an emotion increases the experience of the emotion being expressed regardless of the person's awareness of the emotion they are expressing. Thus, the experience of an emotion can, to some degree, be activated or intensified by body expression. Interestingly, people who were more body sensitive showed this tendency to a greater degree. Research on the effects of role playing on attitude change also supports the idea that performing actions brings people's experience in line with the role (Zimbardo et al., 1977). Playing a role can evoke emotion.

New Emotions Provided by the Therapist and Therapy Relationship

Remembering a situation in which an emotion occurred can bring the memory alive in the present. The therapist can ask the client, "Remember a time when you felt happy or sad? What was it like?" Cognitively creating a new meaning by changing how one views a situation or talking about the meaning of an emotional episode often helps people experience new feelings. Therapists also can express the new emotion for the client, such as outrage, pain, or sadness that the client is unable to express, and this helps the client experience their own emotion.

The therapy relationship can generate new emotion. A new emotion can be evoked in response to new interactions with the therapist that disconfirm pathogenic expectations. The client can undergo a corrective emotional experience with the therapist that repairs the traumatic influence of previous relational experiences. Corrective emotional experiences with the therapist are happening constantly whenever clients experience their therapists as attuning to and validating their internal experience. Therapy repeatedly offers opportunities for the regulation of distressing emotion via the soothing effect of an empathic therapist who helps break the client's feeling of isolation because the client is in contact with the therapist and is mirrored. Overall, the genuine relationship between the patient and the therapist, and its constancy, is a corrective emotional experience. In addition, therapy provides new self-experience through more intrapsychic experiences in which new, alternate adaptive emotion schemes that can potentiate new emergent self-organizations are activated.

Specific new emotional experiences with the therapist that supply an undoing of specific patterns of interpersonal experience provide the other form of corrective experience. People's core emotion schemes change by positive interpersonal experience, disconfirming pathogenic ways of being like not trusting or feeling controlled or diminished. Clients often disconfirm pathogenic ways of being by testing them directly in the therapeutic relationship (Weiss et al., 1986). Thus, clients who fear abandonment may test to see if the therapist will not abandon them; clients who fear being controlled test limits. If the therapist provides, in the first case, a new experience by caring and, in the second case, by giving freedom, these become corrective emotional experiences that help alter past experience.

Mastery Over Emotions

The goal is for clients, with the help of safety in therapy, to experience mastery in reexperiencing emotions they could not handle in the past. Clients in therapy thus can reexperience events differently than they did originally. Now, the client can express vulnerability or anger with the therapist without being punished, and can assert without being put down. This new experience allows clients to feel that they are no longer powerless children facing powerful adults.

Furthermore, the therapist can be seen as a transitional conductor promoting an experience of transitioning from one emotional state to another just as a caretaker does with an infant in distress. With a distressed infant, the caretaker first soothes the feeling, thus validating the presence of the feeling. Then, when the infant has calmed down, the caretaker introduces some novel stimulus like a rattle or teddy bear to evoke a new emotion. The infant learns implicitly two things: that emotional distress can be soothed and, maybe even more importantly, that it is possible to transition from a negative to a more positive state. A great number of fragile clients have never experienced this type of soothing and transitioning. Their experience has taught them that if you enter a negative state, it is a vortex that sucks you in. When the therapist validates the painful feeling and responds empathically, the client has a new experience and begins to internalize not only the soothing but also the possibility of transitioning. Therapy thus provides two new experiences: It is possible for emotional pain to be soothed, and it is possible to transition to more salutary states and escape the painful emotion.

MEMORY RECONSOLIDATION

Memory and the impact of the past on our current lives play a central role in working with emotion. Previous theories of memory stability, grouped under the traditional name "memory consolidation," argued that once short-term memory was consolidated into long-term memory, it would become stable.

In the past 20 years, a new memory process referred to as "memory reconsolidation" has been proposed and studied. Introducing new present experience into currently activated memories of past events has been shown to lead to the assimilation of new material in the present into memories of the past (Nadel & Bohbot, 2001; Nadel et al., 2012; Nader & Hardt, 2009).

The standard view of memory suggested that immediately after learning, there was a window of time during which the memory was labile, and, after sufficient time had passed, the memory became more or less permanent. During what was called the "consolidation period," it was possible to influence memory formation; once this time window had passed, however, the memory could not be changed or eliminated. Developments in memory research, however, have shown that every time a memory is activated, the underlying memory seems to be labile once again and requires another consolidation period (Nadel & Moscovitch, 1997). This reconsolidation period allows for another opportunity to disrupt the memory. Nader et al. (2000) demonstrated that conditioned fear can be eliminated in rats by blocking reconsolidation, but it also appears that the new experience needs to occur not immediately but only about 10 minutes after the activation of the memory. Also, it has been shown (Hupbach et al., 2008) that when memories in humans are reactivated through reminders, they are open to modification through the presentation of similar material that then becomes incorporated into the original event memory.

Because memory reconsolidation only occurs once a memory is activated, it follows that emotional memories have to be activated in therapy to be able to change them. Thus, emotional memories can be changed by activating the experience of the memory in a session, and, if, after about 10 minutes of working on the painful experience related to this memory, a new emotion is experienced, it will in some way be incorporated into the memory and can change the experience of the original memory (Greenberg, 2019). By being activated in the present, the old memories are updated by the new current experience.

The new experience comes both from the safety of the therapy relationship and through the activation of more adaptive emotional responses in an in-session enactment of reacting to the old situation in a new way using new adult resources. Incorporating these new elements, the memories are reconsolidated. This process of memory reconsolidation offers a possible view of a general therapeutic change process for transforming experience of past emotional injuries. Introducing new present experience into currently activated memories of past events can lead to transformation via the assimilation of new material into past memories during memory reconsolidation (Lane et al., 2015).

It is important to distinguish "memory reconsolidation" from "behavioral extinction," though. *Reconsolidation* is assumed to change components of the reactivated memory, whereas *extinction* is assumed to merely create a new memory that overrides the previously trained response. Thus, an "extinguished" response is not really gone because it can spontaneously recover over time or be reinstated if the organism is exposed to a relevant cue in a new context. Recent work has shown that cellular and molecular differences exist between the two processes. Whether reconsolidation or extinction occurs depends on the temporal dynamics of the test procedure and how recently the memory in question was formed, reactivated, or both (de la Fuente et al., 2011; Inda et al., 2011; Maren, 2011). At this time, it is clear that reconsolidation and extinction represent distinct reactions to reactivating a memory (Lane et al., 2015).

To exemplify the change process in a nutshell, consider the following synopsis of a course of therapy. Doug, a 52-year-old man suffering from panic, reported a life marked by abusive relationships with his father. With support from the therapist, Doug revisited difficult moments in his childhood. When he did so, memories were activated, and he made contact with his core fear and with his unmet needs for support and protection. After a number of sessions, Doug also accessed empowering anger toward his father in conjunction with his fear. Assertive anger, with its function of protecting an individual's boundaries and its behavioral tendency toward facing and fighting, allowed him to experience himself as an agent able to survive— something he had never felt before. Instead of fleeing or freezing with fear, he synthesized new emotions into his memory, adding anger to the previous fear, strengthening the self, and feeling more confident. He also experienced compassion toward himself and his remembered self, a frightened child. This important emotion was reconsolidated in Doug's memory. Coupled with the experience of empathy and compassion from the therapist, Doug built new emotional memories.

SESSION TRANSCRIPT

This section includes a session transcript that demonstrates changing emotion with emotion with a client suffering from anxiety. Underlying this 60-year-old woman's anxiety (she was diagnosed with generalized anxiety disorder), with which she had grappled all her life, was her fear-based basic insecurity and the painful sadness of lonely abandonment from having a mother who had died of cancer. Her mother had languished slowly over many years of the client's childhood. In therapy, these painful maladaptive feelings were transformed by accessing a different type of sadness: the sadness of grief and accompanying feelings of assertive anger. The anger came from a sense of having deserved to not have the burden of an incapable mother and to have deserved a more normal childhood.

Near the end of the transcript, note that the client finally feels compassion for herself. Her feelings of being alone and afraid at the base of her weak self-organization are thereby transformed to a more secure sense of self. New feelings strengthen her sense of self, and new emotions undo her insecure sense of self. Her compassion toward her wounded-child sense of self undoes her anxiety, leaving her feeling calmer and more comforted and safe. By the end of treatment, she grieves for what she missed and assimilates her loss into a new narrative. In addition, as her self-organization changes, new and more positive memories become accessible; these new memories counterbalance her old, negative ones.

The transcript that follows is from Session 16. Early sessions focused on her symptomatic anxiety, provided empathic attunement to her feelings of vulnerability, and helped her to unfold her narrative, which fairly quickly zeroed in on her childhood growing up with a mother who was bedridden and dying of cancer. To help the client regulate her anxiety, the therapist had her focus on her breathing when she was anxious. From Session 3 onward, the therapist began a process of guiding the client to pay attention to her feelings and connect them to her anxiety. A good alliance was developed, and the client commented that she felt safe and liked coming to the sessions, but it was difficult helping the client face her underlying feelings.

The segment that follows starts close to the beginning of Session 16; it is provided so the reader can see how the session theme was established. The segment then skips to minute 17, when the therapist guides the client to talk about her relationship with her mother.

Arriving at the Ache

CLIENT: I get tired. Well, that always happens. Remember: (*Therapist: Yeah.*) I told you the (*Therapist: Yeah.*)—when the sun comes down (*Therapist: Mm-hmm.*) and it starts getting darker, I always feel this, ah, you know the feeling of (*Therapist: Mm-hmm.*) emptiness (*Therapist: Yes.*), and—and, like, it—it's not really a pain but like an emptiness in my stomach.

THERAPIST: Yeah, an empty, ah, an ache. That happens inside.

CLIENT: Yeah, some kind of an ache. Yeah (*Therapist: Yeah.*) and, um, and—and it seems like, ah, in my mind, um, things come—come in like, I worry (*Therapist: Mm-hmm.*) about my son, my daughter, my husband, all the problems, you know?

In the next 12 minutes or so, the client talks about feeling down and depressed as well as not really appreciated by her children. When she returns to talking about her feelings of lonely abandonment, the therapist guides her toward the therapeutic focus based on the coconstructed case formulation: that her anxiety is based on underlying feelings of isolation and abandonment by her mother. Up until now, in previous sessions, they worked on her paying more attention to her bodily felt feelings in general and more specifically when her anxiety is triggered. In addition, they have, to some degree, talked about her feelings toward her mother, but the client has never experienced those feelings in the session. The first part of the session involves arriving at the emotion.

THERAPIST: Yeah (*Client: Yeah.*), in terms of, ah, last week, something that, um, we were talking about that seems like—I mean, let me tell you what I'm thinking about in terms of where (*Client: Yeah, yeah, yeah.*) I think we need to go in the next few sessions and see what you think. So, there's this feeling that you keep trying to get rid of, right? And this really seems like the—the place that, ah, a lot of—of the sadness comes from, right, and the anxiety? And this—this place is kind of—if there is—if there would be something that would be good for us to work on, it might be kind of around that (*Client: That feeling.*)—that ache you know (*Client: Yes, yeah.*), and that ache, as we have said, certainly goes back to the childhood (*Client: Yeah, yeah, yeah.*) time. And I wonder about your mother in terms of revisiting your mother. Like I understand it's hard, but I kind of get the sense that it's hard to say anything bad about your mother. It's like you feel, "I don't blame her for being sick," and you know. [guiding to a focus]

CLIENT: How can I say it (*Therapist: Yeah.*), sure it was not her fault (*Therapist: Yeah.*), what happened to her. [cancer]

THERAPIST: But what I wonder at the same time: It's not whether it's someone's fault or not. I wonder at the same time if it's that those needs you had still weren't met.

CLIENT: Mm-hmm. I—I never—never—never thought (*Therapist: Mm-hmm.*) this was her fault. Never. (*Therapist: Mm-hmm.*) I might have been sometimes upset because, you know (*Therapist: Mm-hmm.*), I didn't—I didn't have her the way I wanted, but, ah (*Therapist: Mm-hmm.*), you know, I just had to deal with it.

THERAPIST: What about what it was like for you. I mean, I think this might be . . .

CLIENT: I never talked to her or anybody about these things (*Therapist: Yeah, yeah.*). No, no.

THERAPIST: And I don't mean in a blaming way, but I mean, would it feel okay to try that—to talk to her about what it was like for you?

CLIENT: You mean, now, ah (*Therapist: Yeah.*), how?

THERAPIST: Imagining her. (*Client: Yeah, yeah.*) Like it—it—would that feel okay? Or . . .

CLIENT: Yeah, I mean it (*Therapist: Yeah.*) should. Yeah, okay.

THERAPIST: We'll try it and see. So, just close your eyes if you like and imagine your mom (*Client: And . . .*), if you could just—just take a minute and just (*Client: Yeah.*) slow it down, and just take a minute and take in some breaths. And just sit with it for a second, and just try to get a picture of her. (*Client: Yeah, yeah.*) And just—just see what—what comes up when you f—when you start feeling something and try to put words to it.

CLIENT: Ah, yeah, I'm trying to remember when I was young and, ah . . .

THERAPIST: Mm-hmm. Try to picture her. How old were you?

CLIENT: 6 to 8 to 9, yeah, yeah.

THERAPIST: So, you can kind of—so, you can kind of picture—how about picturing the mother that she was?

CLIENT: Yeah, but, yeah, I can see when I was 6 years old (*Therapist: Yeah.*), and she was a lot younger, and, ah (*Therapist: Mm-hmm.*), and, um, and I couldn't—she couldn't take—make to the movies. I had to go with somebody else if (*Therapist: Okay.*) I could.

THERAPIST: So, what does (Client: *You know [sighs].*) it feel like inside? When you see this. [focusing internally]

CLIENT: It felt like, ah, I was alone.

THERAPIST: What's it feel like (*Client: Ah.*) when you say this?

CLIENT: Ah, I feel that, um—um something is missing.

THERAPIST: Something is missing.

CLIENT: I want her to be there, you know.

THERAPIST: What do you miss?

CLIENT: I miss like that she was there with me. (*Therapist: Mm-hmm.*) You know, taking care of me, and (*Therapist: Yeah.*), ah, and I didn't have her next to me (*Therapist: Mm-hmm.*) when I was going to the movies with my friends and her mother. (*Therapist: Mm-hmm.*) And I felt like I was, yeah, I was a tagalong with other people.

CLIENT: The—the, I don't know, I felt like I went along with them like but didn't belong.

THERAPIST: A third wheel.

CLIENT: Third wheel. Yeah, exactly.

THERAPIST: Tell her, "I'm 6 years old, and I (*Client: Ah.*)—I tag along."

CLIENT: Yeah, yeah, I had to tag along with other people (*Therapist: Yeah.*), yeah, yeah, and, um (*Therapist: Yeah.*), and, of course, my father couldn't do much. (*Therapist: Yeah.*) He did a few, you know, things for me, but, ah (*Therapist: Mm-hmm.*), he had other things to do (*Therapist: Mm-hmm.*) because he had to be father and mother. [accessing emotion schematic memories of loneliness]

THERAPIST: Mm-hmm. (*Client: Right.*) Try to stay with this feeling of being alone. [focusing internally]

CLIENT: With her.

THERAPIST: Yeah (*Client: Um.*), try to stay with this feeling. So, what did it feel like to be—to miss not having her there? I mean, in physical being she was there, but to really not have her, (*Client: Yeah, yeah.*) she was really not really there. (*Client: Yeah.*) What did that feel like? [focusing internally]

CLIENT: Well, it was—it was—it was lone—it was lonely! (*Therapist: Mm-hmm.*) It was the—the sadness.

THERAPIST: If you could tell your mom, "I feel lonely because (*Client: Yeah.*), as your 6-year-old . . ."

CLIENT: I felt so—I feel so lonely because you're not there for me. (*Therapist: Yeah.*), ah, and sometimes I wish you were because

I (*Therapist: Yeah.*)—some people say things that I didn't like, or (*Therapist: Yeah.*)—and maybe you would have been there just to defend me but, ah (*Therapist: Mm-hmm.*), you couldn't because you couldn't (cries), and I felt so alone. I felt afraid, unsafe. [accessing emotions, schematic feelings of sadness and fear; arriving]

THERAPIST: "And it left me feeling so scared and alone."

CLIENT: I felt like I didn't know what to do. Maybe I wouldn't have these inadequacies now if those—if those things never happened. Maybe if I, ah—ah—ah—I would have felt loved, felt a lot, ah, more secure (*Therapist: More secure, yeah.*), more self-assured, ah (*Therapist: Yeah.*), but, um, I don't blame her. I don't blame her because she's sick. It's not her doing. I mean, she's sick (*Therapist: Mm-hmm.*) like that, and I can't help her.

THERAPIST: Yeah, so I don't blame her, and at the same time, it doesn't take away that I missed something. (*Client: Yeah.*) Is that it? Yeah. (*Client: Yes, yeah.*) What would you want to say to her?

CLIENT: You know, I—I don't blame you because you're like that— you're (*Therapist: Mm-hmm.*)—you have a physical problem, um (*Therapist: But . . .*), a mental (*Therapist: There's still a but, yeah.*) problem. I don't want to say that, but (*Therapist: Right.*) it's that what it was, and I never want to tell her that, but I would say, "You have a mental problem."

THERAPIST: So, you weren't there. I don't blame (*Client sighs.*) you because you didn't have control over it but, I needed you and you weren't there emotionally, mentally. (*Client: Yeah.*) That's what it comes down to.

CLIENT: Ah, I need, yeah, I needed you, and you weren't there. (*Therapist: Yeah.*) And many times, I felt alone (*Therapist: Yeah.*) and, um, and—and—and alone and—and insecure and afraid. (*Therapist: Yeah, afraid.*) Afraid—yes. [need]

THERAPIST: Can you tell her about that fear? (*Client: Yes, yes.*) Tell her about that fear. [focusing on core maladaptive fear]

CLIENT: Ah, I felt afraid, like in my stomach, a kind of queasy feeling because, ah, I was always surrounded by people that weren't, ah, my family (*Therapist: Mm-hmm.*), and I needed you to be with me! (*Therapist: Mm-hmm.*) I—in—in—in school, you know, when they had, ah, you know, the plays or whatever (*Therapist: Mm-hmm.*). You know, they—I needed you (*Therapist: Yeah.*), and—and, ah, you didn't help me because sometimes you didn't sew my—my—my dresses for me and for—for (*Therapist: Mm-hmm.*) me and for the stage and everything, but, ah (*Therapist: Yeah.*), you should have been there. So, the—the teachers—the teachers had to do, yeah, the teachers had to fix it for me. Um . . . [arriving at fear plus need]

THERAPIST: Get a sense of her and tell her again, "I needed you to be there for me."

CLIENT: Yeah, I needed you to be there for me.

THERAPIST: How does that feel when you say that to her.

CLIENT: Yeah, I feel guilty. (*Therapist: Yeah.*) [secondary emotion]

THERAPIST: So, it feels bad to say this to her because . . .

CLIENT: Yeah, it's still that's—that's what happened for me, that's what happened. (*Therapist: Yeah, yes.*) And, um, ah, whenever I pray, I was always praying that, ah, please, you know, bring her back to me (*Therapist: Mm-hmm.*) the way she was. I never knew how she was before (*Therapist: Mm-hmm.*), but, ah, bring her to me normal.

THERAPIST: Yeah, like I wanted you to be something different. (*Client: That's right.*) I needed you to be something different.

CLIENT: Something like a friend, you know, who, like, you could talk to and . . . [need]

THERAPIST: Yeah, tell her what you needed from her. What did you need from her? [focusing on need]

CLIENT: And, ah—eh—eh—you know, I need you to—to take walks with me, take me for ice cream (*Therapist: Yeah.*) like, you know, um (*Therapist: Mm-hmm.*), and maybe we could just fix the garden together. (*Therapist: Mm-hmm.*) Ah, you know those things that the mothers and daughters do (*Therapist: Mm-hmm.*), but, ah (*Therapist: Mm-hmm.*), we never did even though you were home. (*Therapist: Yeah.*) And, yeah, you did show me how to sew, but . . . [need]

THERAPIST: That's the most painful part (*Client: Yeah.*), right? The most painful part is that, as you said last week, "You know I had a mother, but I really didn't."

CLIENT: No, no, I really didn't. (*Therapist: Yeah.*) No, no. (*Therapist: Yeah, and she . . .*) She was there, she helped me for, ah—eh— you know, she helped me, she showed me, she sometimes tried to teach me.

THERAPIST: Yeah, so I (*Client: Um.*) appreciate that you did (*Client: Yeah.*), um—um, yeah, it's not that it wasn't all bad, but when it came down to the important things . . .

CLIENT: Yeah, when it came to the important things, you weren't there (*Therapist: Mm-hmm.*), like, ah, more like personal (*Therapist: Mm-hmm.*) things (cries). [arriving]

THERAPIST: Yeah, tell her (*Client: This.*) more about that. What other things you would have liked to have had from her? What else would have been nice?

CLIENT: You stopped cooking, um (*Therapist: Mm-hmm.*), so my dad had to cook. (*Therapist: Mm-hmm.*) So, he cooked whatever he could, mostly—ha ha—barbecues because he (*Therapist: Mm-hmm.*), you know, he—he wasn't, ah, really a cook. (*Therapist: Mm-hmm.*) But, ah, when you—when you—I remember when you used to cook, and I used to love the things that you used to make. (*Therapist: Mm.*) Ah, you used to make a preserves and things that (*Therapist: Mm-hmm.*) I loved, you know. (*Therapist: Mm.*) Ah, but then (*Therapist: This child missing these things.*)—yeah, yeah, I—I remember that, but (*Therapist: Yeah.*) you stopped doing them.

THERAPIST: That important part of my childhood, it was gone, so try to get a sense for here, I know, it's kind of hard, so try to picture her there and tell her what it was like when she stopped doing things.

CLIENT: Yeah, ah—ah, I don't remember exactly (*Therapist: Mm-hmm.*) when you stopped. . . . Maybe I was 7 or 8. I was, busier. I had to do a lot more homework (*Therapist: Mm-hmm.*), and I didn't have time, and . . .

THERAPIST: But I knew there was something missing. You were gone. (*Client: Yeah.*) You vanished. (*Client: Yeah.*) Is that what I'm feeling? (*Client: Yeah, yeah.*) Tell her what that felt like.

CLIENT: Yeah, it felt like, ah, you abandoned me, you know. You know, you just want to choose to be in bed, that's all. (*Therapist: Yeah.*), and I felt so abandoned.

THERAPIST: And still sits inside (*Client: Yes.*). I feel it now when I (*Client: Yes.*)—when the sun goes down (*Client: Yeah [weeps].*), and I have to come in from playing. (Client sighs deeply.) I feel that in—it's the—it's here (points to stomach).

CLIENT: Yeah, it's in my stomach, yeah (*Therapist: Yeah.*), yeah. [arriving]

THERAPIST: And can you (*Client: This.*) speak from that like that's almost where the abandonment sits? Can you speak from that place and tell her?

Naming the Need, Leaving, and Changing the Narrative

With the emergence of the need, the session now enters the leaving phase.

CLIENT: I needed you to come to me? Mm (*Therapist: Yeah.*), why don't you come and talk to me and (*Therapist: Yeah.*) be a mother. (*Therapist: Mm-hmm.*) Ah, be my friend. (*Therapist: Mm-hmm.*) Um, when I had problems with my other girlfriends that they— they used to fight and I'd come home, and I would never have anybody to talk to, or (*Therapist: Mm-hmm.*) nobody would just give me any sympathy because nobody was there to do that. (*Therapist: Yeah.*) My dad didn't want to hear about all these things (*Therapist: Mm-hmm.*), but, ah, you—you know, you won't—you won't hear it. Yeah, you won't hear it. Ah.

THERAPIST: So, what do you feel as you say this?

CLIENT: I feel angry. [new transforming emotion; leaving]

THERAPIST: Tell her what you resent.

CLIENT: I resented you chose your bed over me. I needed you. I resented you preferred your bed to me, you never spoke to me, let me come into your room. It was like I didn't exist. I resented you didn't care. I felt like you didn't care.

THERAPIST: I felt so uncared for. You were the one who I needed to be, yeah, yeah, and I felt abandoned. I (*Client: Yeah.*)—and it was almost—you vanished, and because of that, I felt?

CLIENT: I feel alone—alone—very, very, very lonely. I was scared and alone.

THERAPIST: Very alone (*Client: Mm-hmm.*). I felt alone and—and, scared I wouldn't have felt that way if you had been there.

CLIENT: If you were, yeah, if you had been there, yeah (*Therapist: Yeah.*), I would have been, ah, you know, with my mother. (*Therapist: Mm-hmm. Mm-hmm.*) And that's, ah, that's an important— I missed so much. (*Eyes fill with tears. Gets a tissue.*) I needed a mom.

THERAPIST: What do you feel as you say this?

CLIENT: So sad, and it was so unfair to be robbed of my mother. I feel mad I resented not having a mom when all the others had moms who picked them up after school, took them to movies. I was robbed of a normal childhood. [leaving, transforming anger; leaving]

THERAPIST: So, sort of angry at how unfair it was. Yeah, life dealt you a hard blow, losing your mom emotionally like that.

CLIENT: Yeah, I feel sad that I missed out on having a mother to take care of me. I needed her to be there for me, too (*eyes fill with tears*), and I deserved to have a mom, and I missed having a childhood free of those fears. [emerging sadness of grief; leaving]

A few minutes later in the session, the dialogue shifts to what the mother would have said to the 6-year-old. The therapist says to the client, who is now in the mother's role:

THERAPIST: Okay, so let's put—let's try to put this into words when you see that 6-year-old, what do you want to say to that lonely girl?

CLIENT: Well, you know, yes, I'm sorry—I'm . . .

THERAPIST: I'm sorry, yeah, yeah.

CLIENT: But I'm here anyways, and, ah, if you and I do my best . . .

THERAPIST: So, it's like doing the best I can. (*Client: Yeah.*) Is that what she's saying?

CLIENT: Oh, I feel very, very sorry.

THERAPIST: Your mother (*Client sniffles*) feels very, very–feels very sorry.

CLIENT: I feel myself very, ah, looking at (*Therapist: Mm-hmm.*) myself, I'm now 60 years old. You know, I feel (*Therapist: Yeah.*) that I missed that a lot. [sadness of grief]

CLIENT: (*Speaks as mother*) I'm sorry that you had to miss so much because, um, ah, I wasn't there for you. (*Therapist: Uh-huh.*) I wish—I was okay, ah (*Therapist: Yeah.*), I wish I could, you know, be more with you, and I could have been more, you know (*Therapist: Mm-hmm.*), of a mother, but, unfortunately I (*Therapist: Mm-hmm.*)—it was something that I couldn't do.

THERAPIST: So I wish I could have been there. What do you—what—what do you wish you could have done?

CLIENT: Mm, well, be more of a mother. Be more (*Therapist: Mm-hmm.*), yeah, take you for ice cream in the summertime when you were on holidays and, ah (*Therapist: Mm-hmm.*), play more with you. You know (*Therapist: Yeah.*), I remember you used to bring a couple of friends that they were really nice, and (*Therapist: Mm-hmm.*) they didn't mind me, and, um (*Therapist: Yeah.*), and you used to play with the hose and, you know (*Therapist: Mm-hmm.*), and . . . [compassion for self]

THERAPIST: I remember those moments. (*Client: Yeah, yeah.*) I remember when we were (*Client: I remember, yeah, yeah.*) together. And it (*Client: Yeah.*) felt good. (*Client: Yeah.*) Is that what she's saying to her?

CLIENT: Those—those—those—those moments were good, yeah.

THERAPIST: So, I missed (*Client: Yeah.*) those moments, too.

CLIENT: And she even baked—she even baked a couple of times (*Therapist: Yeah.*). You know, I remember, a couple of times she baked cookies (*Therapist: Mm-hmm.*), and she baked a couple cakes, whatever. (*Therapist: Mm-hmm.*) And, um, and we had a good time, yeah. [accessing positive memories]

THERAPIST: What about this when you were 6, though. I mean, when you were 6, that's when it really . . .

CLIENT: Well, she did buy me things to (*Therapist: Yeah.*)—and I was, you know, some days, she was okay, yes, but some days, she would (*Therapist: Mm-hmm.*), just like I said, talk to herself and, ah (*Therapist: Mm-hmm.*), the poor woman, she never talked to anybody, so she had to talk to herself. (*Therapist: Mm-hmm. Yeah.*)

THERAPIST: So, you really feel for her. Yeah.

CLIENT: And she would just stay in bed as much as she could (*Therapist: Yeah, yeah.*) because she probably . . .

THERAPIST: How does the 6-year-old feel when she hears that?

CLIENT: Yeah, I would feel that, um, yeah, it's true. She should have done more me. (*Therapist: Mm-hmm.*) Uh, you—you did do that (*Therapist: Mm-hmm.*). I mean, she could have done it. (*Therapist: Mm-hmm.*) But in some ways, you—you—you—you were in a cocoon, I don't know (*Therapist: Mm-hmm.*), for some reason.

THERAPIST: Untouchable to me. I see . . .

CLIENT: Yeah, she was hidden somewhere. She just (*Therapist: Mm.*)—she hid herself from everybody. (*Therapist: Mm-hmm.*) Ah, it seems like, well, yeah, it must have been, ah—ah—a problem that she had. (*Therapist: Mm-hmm.*) You know, like a condition, but, um, maybe if she tried a little harder, she would, you know, I know . . .

THERAPIST: Mm-hmm. (*Client: Um.*) But you could have tried.

CLIENT: (*Speaks to remembered mother*) You could have tried.

THERAPIST: You could have done something different, maybe. Yeah.

THERAPIST: Tell her what—that you would have liked.

CLIENT: It would have been great. (*Therapist: Yeah.*) I would have more memories of my childhood. (*Therapist: Yeah. Mm-hmm.*) Better memories. [deserving]

THERAPIST: Better memories.

CLIENT: Yeah, because I really, I think I erased a lot of memories, you know, because (*Therapist: Mm-hmm.*) they weren't nice, so (*Therapist: Mm-hmm.*), um.

THERAPIST: So, I remember the bad. I mean there's bleeding (*Client: Yeah.*), but I really remember the alone abandoned, lying in bed.

CLIENT: I remember that, but, ah, I don't dwell on that. I've always tried to remember the—the good things, you know. (*Therapist: Mm-hmm.*) But, ah, those things, of course, come up to (*Therapist: Mm-hmm.*), but, um, I think I was always an . . .

THERAPIST: Can you tell her about this place?

CLIENT: I—I have this feeling because—because of you, actually. (*Therapist: Yeah.*) Yeah, yeah, because . . .

THERAPIST: I have this feeling. Tell her (*Client: Yeah.*) again. Can you say that again?

CLIENT: Yeah, you, because of the way she was (*Therapist: Yeah.*) and because the things that—that I were missing in my life. (*Therapist: Mm-hmm.*) I had always this feeling of emptiness (*Therapist: Mm-hmm.*) and, eh, that aches inside me. (*Therapist: Mm-hmm.*) And that, eh, always applies to everything in my life. (*Therapist: Mm-hmm.*) It applies to my—my husband, my family, my way of life. (*Therapist: Yeah.*) My everything.

THERAPIST: Everything. It touch—it taints it, colors it everything.

CLIENT: It's—it's exactly. So, it seems like I'm never going to be able to be happy. (*Therapist: Yeah.*), and I was never really happy. I deserved to have a mom who took care of me, not one I had to care of.

THERAPIST: Yes. It wasn't my responsibility. I was just a kid.

CLIENT: Yeah, I was just a child. [changing the narrative]

THERAPIST: Let's try something. Come over here. Remember—remember about a bunch of sessions ago, I don't remember the number, you were imagining as if you could be an older sister (*Client: Mm-hmm.*), and you could see that 6-year-old, and you could almost, like I remember you—you (*Client: Yeah, I remember.*) just wanted to hold her. (*Client: Yeah.*) Can you, I mean, if you picture that 6-year-old girl who is just sitting there with that ache, what comes up for you? I mean, is this—this, I mean, if you could be that big sister, then . . . [self-soothing]

CLIENT: No, well, I would just grab her and, you know, and hug her and just kiss her and say, you know, don't worry about anything. (*Therapist: Mm-hmm.*) Everything is going to be all right. (*Therapist: Mm-hmm.*) Ah, you're always going to be looked after. You're always going to have (*Therapist: Mm-hmm.*), you know, whatever you need. Um . . . [self soothing]

THERAPIST: You say that ache is here (*points to stomach*). That's where— that's where it sits. A lot of people are walking around (*Client: Yeah.*) with big holes in their stomachs. You can't see them.

CLIENT: Is that right? (*Therapist: Oh, yeah.*) I'm not the only one. And that—and that is where—and that's where—where it stings. That's why I feel that thing.

THERAPIST: Right in the gut.

CLIENT: A sickness or something. Like a physical problem that I—like when I had ulcers, and I said, Well maybe when my ulcers go away (*Therapist: Yeah.*), this will go away as well, but no, ha ha.

THERAPIST: Yeah. (*Client sniffles.*) Like people describe it in different ways: It's like a hole. It's like a wound. (*Client: Yeah, yeah.*) That yours is an ache (*Client: Yeah.*), a painful ache sometimes.

CLIENT: Yeah, yeah, and a hole to, like, you know, like an emptiness there (*Therapist: Yeah, yeah.*) that aches. Yeah. You know what I realize too? (*Therapist: Mm-hmm.*) That this gave me a great— great inferiority complex. (*Therapist: Yeah.*) I feel—you know (*Therapist: Yeah [sniffles].*), yeah, so part of you was, like, I feel so—I just—like I'm not good enough and—no—yes—and, on the other hand, it's like I'm angry.

THERAPIST: Right, okay. So, there's this inadequacy (*Client: Yeah, yeah.*) like here, and then if you went underneath, that inadequacy, it's like the pain and hurt (*Client: Yes.*) because if she had been there, would this even exist? You know, would you even have the ache? [narrative reconstruction]

The session ends with self-soothing in the form of an imagined older sister and restorying her experience and realizing how the ache affected her sense of self. Crucial was accessing her core maladaptive feelings of fear associated with being abandoned and the attendant sadness of loneliness (emotion schematic processing), and through accessing her need, she begins to feel sad about what she missed and anger at not having a mother. Her sadness is a central aspect of grieving her loss and is a healthy adaptive emotion that helps her assimilate the loss. It differs from the sadness of lonely abandonment, which is a more passive, helpless state. Her anger strengthens her sense of self and helps her to feel deserving of what she missed that she had not felt before.

The new experiences of grieving what she missed and feeling more deserving undo her "weak me" feelings of fear and loneliness. She cannot believe she is unlovable or inadequate while she feels deserving of love. She ends up validating her needs and feels compassionate to herself. A process of change has begun. After having arrived at her core lonely abandonment and fear, she is able to change these emotions with the adaptive sadness of grief, with assertive anger, and with self-compassion. The different emotion schemes synthesize at an implicit level to help her leave these painful states by producing a new state: one of confidence and calm, a truly novel experience for her from all her years of anxiety.

CONCLUSION

I hope to have shown how changing emotion with emotion is a key change process. It helps people who present with symptoms based on underlying maladaptive emotions, first arrive at their core painful feelings, accept them, tolerate them, and symbolize them in awareness. Then, it helps them access new adaptive emotions to transform the old maladaptive feelings they arrived at. It is not just accepting emotion or overcoming avoidance of emotion that is change producing. Rather, it is experiencing new emotion to oppose old emotion that is central in changing maladaptive emotion. This change, achieved by a synthesis of the old and the new, is consolidated into a new narrative and gives a people a more salutary view of self, world, and other. This process of new emotional experience changing old experience is a transtheoretical process in line with Goldfried's (1980, 2012) proposal that providing corrective experiences is a midlevel strategy of change shared by all approaches.

In addition, changing emotion with emotion is best viewed not only as a transtheoretical process but also as a transdiagnostic process applicable regardless of the disorder. Whether one arrives at core shame in depression or social anxiety, or attachment-related anxiety in generalized anxiety disorder, or destructive anger in addictions, it is the access to adaptive feelings that help bring about a transformation to a new emotional state regardless of diagnostic category. All disorders are based on emotional disorder, and all require emotional change by the process of changing emotion with emotion.

4

ESSENTIAL THERAPIST SKILLS FOR PRACTICING EMOTION-BASED APPROACHES

Before unpacking the clinical processes of helping clients arrive at and leave painful emotions, regulate emotions, and construct new narratives, I want to first describe the mind-set, background knowledge, and basic skills I have found to be most facilitative in practicing emotion-based approaches. I have most often had success when adopting a mindset that is open to the opportunities and limitations that my own in-session emotional disclosures present to therapy. When working with emotion, therapists frequently must discern whether, when, and how it may be appropriate to disclose their own emotions with clients in a session. Part of this discernment process involves thinking through how the content and manner of the disclosure might be received, which depends, among other factors, on the therapist's and client's intersecting cultural identities (e.g., nationality, ethnicity, race, religion, gender identity, sexual orientation). I expand on this theme in the first part of this chapter.

Regarding background knowledge for working with emotion, I have found it helpful to focus on information that helps increase my comfort in "sitting with" an ever-increasing variety of emotions. Not only do therapists need to sit nonjudgmentally with their own and their clients' emotions, they

https://doi.org/10.1037/0000248-005

also need to apply a transcultural frame to evaluate which emotions are most distressing to the client or in what terms the client will feel most comfortable expressing emotion. I go into more depth on these topics in the second part of this chapter.

Despite my view that, at core, people are all pretty much alike emotionally, therapists cannot simply assume the universal applicability of our models unless the issues of culture, race, and gender that permeate every aspect of life are embedded in our treatment framework. We thus need to always consider who we are working with, where we are conducting our therapy, and to whom our research applies. Accordingly, the last section of the chapter focuses on recognizing how institutionalized racism is baked into so many of our social structures, including scientific research, and indeed into the very psychotherapy models we practice. I conclude by advocating that therapists confront systemic racism by adopting the role of social change agent in their work.

Having worked now in many world cultures, I am convinced that although cultural upbringings and the rules of emotional expression vary, what people feel inside and the prototypic, existential situations are all experienced in similar ways across cultures (Capps et al., 2015). All people, regardless of culture, react internally, emotionally, and in a similar fashion to death, loss, loneliness, meaninglessness, and to issues of freedom as well as issues of abuse, intimacy, attachment, and dominance and submission. What leads to these difficulties and how people express their emotions may be different because of culture, but what is felt is similar. In addition, I have found that emotional problems, such as unfinished business, destructive self-criticism, and interruption of emotion, manifest and can be framed and resolved in therapy in similar fashion regardless of culture.

Around 2007, when I began doing training in China, I subscribed to the stereotype that Chinese people were inscrutable and would not express much emotion. I was wrong! Working among groups of trainees on personal issues in the emotion-friendly environment of experiential training, where permission was given for emotional expression, it was more a case of how to dampen down expression rather than how to activate it. When I first went to Norway to train, some of the Norwegians said that "this soft empathy stuff won't wash with Norwegians because they are tough and won't respond to this caring stuff." How wrong that was, too. In Turkey, people had difficulty opening up in the self-experience component of the training until we talked about it. They said that, in Turkey, they were used to getting criticism and advice, so they had learned to close up as a means of self-protection. Once my team and I set the ground rules of listening and empathy rather than advice and criticism, our Turkish trainees and clients, delighted with the opportunity to speak their truths, went to great emotional depths. All people respond to being listened to and understood, and when they feel safe enough, all people regardless of culture have painful feelings that benefit from airing and attention.

KNOWING WHETHER TO DISCLOSE EMOTIONS DURING SESSIONS

As noted in Chapter 2, the past several years have seen a growing interest in the study of therapist emotions. In part, this interest stems from a broader attention to studying therapists' effects on outcome in general. In a recent meta-analysis of the effect of therapists' emotional expression on outcome (Scherer et al., 2017), a significant medium effect size was found between the therapist's emotional expression and outcomes ($d = 0.56$). This finding validates that therapists' emotional expression in therapy has value and needs further understanding, and that training therapists on emotional expression is warranted.

Nearly every therapist has probably experienced an intense emotion during a client's session and possibly even cried (Blume-Marcovici et al., 2013). Perhaps it was grief as a client described the death of her 5-year-old son. Maybe it was anger triggered by the client who consistently showed up late or sadness at the termination of a therapy. Imagine the following scenarios: Your panic client takes her first ride in an elevator. *How do you feel?* A patient tells you that his therapy with you is going nowhere, and he wants a referral. *How do you feel?* You have a new client who reminds you strongly of your estranged, hostile mother. *How do you feel?* Your client makes a fortune on his annual bonus while you are struggling economically. *How do you feel?*

How should therapists best deal with such emotions and with the myriad of other emotions they experience in sessions? Should they or shouldn't they express them? Deciding whether to disclose emotions, such as anger or sadness, with clients depends on many factors, including the client's emotional state, the amount of time left in the session, and the therapist's clinical assessment as to how the patient will handle the emotion.

Ensure Disclosed Feelings Are Relevant to What's Happening in the Session

I disclose quite a bit of my personal feelings about things that pertain to me— if they come up in the session and seem relevant. I, for example, expressed anger toward an insurance company's handling of a flood in my office when a client asked me how the flood had been managed. And when a client arrived and saw me standing in the street watching an ambulance take away a neighbor, I expressed how my own anxiety about having a heart attack was activated as I observed what was happening. This type of expression usually would take place at the beginning of a session as part of the meet-and-greet phase of a session or maybe at the end if it was about something that came up in the session. The client and I might get into a brief discussion about some of what was happening in the world, like the effects of the COVID-19 pandemic, but soon I would redirect the conversation back to the client's experience. I believe that it helps clients feel more trusting and safer talking to me when they see me reacting to things in a human way.

If a client asks me how I felt or would feel in certain situations that they encountered, I may share more personal feelings or thoughts; however, I am careful to say it in a way so that I do not imply that this is what the client did, or should, feel. Usually, my expression involves a type of validation of the universality of what most people may feel in that type of situation. I also might show my feelings in response to a highly emotional or self-relevant topic the client is talking about. For example, a new client came for therapy because her 12-year-old son had recently been killed when, as a pedestrian, he was hit by a car. This woman's grief was so raw—she talked to me for an hour about the last time she saw her son, from getting the call from the coroner's office, going to identify his body, and describing how he looked when she saw him at the morgue. It was absolutely heart wrenching to listen to her story and to witness her grief. I had lost my wife a number of years earlier in a similar fashion, and I found myself close to tears several times until, at some point, she said something that was particularly impactful, and I showed some tear drops. To not respond with sadness, to not share that I had suffered a similar, although different, tragedy would have been inhuman. We have to allow ourselves to be human, but we also have to stay focused on our clients' emotions.

Consider Whether the Feelings Might Build or Disrupt the Therapy Relationship

Therapists have all kinds of feelings. So-called negative feelings, such as anger or fear, may signal an alliance rupture, which therapists then need to identify, explore, and work through (Safran & Muran, 2000). Feelings like shame or guilt also may occur when the therapist makes a mistake or is criticized. If therapists avoid contact with such feelings or discard them, they unwittingly ignore clues that may indicate that something important is going wrong in the relationship. Therapists' emotional reactions to clients' behaviors also often are a consequence of client behavior. Asking oneself questions like, "How does what I feel now relate to what the client is doing with me?" will help the therapist understand aspects of the interaction that they have not yet identified. Therapists who know more about their feelings and are good at exploring the origins of those feelings as well as their effects on the relationship will be able to use the information in treatment. Thus, the therapist's emotional reactions can provide valuable clues for identifying clinically relevant client behavior.

The therapist's own emotional history could also be the source of their reactions; they need to take into account the possibility of so-called counter-transference reactions (i.e., emotional reactions to one's client). Attraction to, admiration for, or boredom and irritation with a client may be related to the therapist's personal experiences, sensitivities, or preferences that are not relevant to the client's problems. Or a therapist may feel that ethical or religious commitments are threatened by the direction therapy is taking. It is important that therapists be alert to such confounding factors because they affect their ability to help the client.

Therapists are often trained to limit self-disclosure about their personal thoughts and feelings as well as to manage their countertransference. At the same time, they are trained to be authentic, genuine, warm, and trustworthy. To hold these opposing views in mind can be tricky, and different therapists choose to practice in different ways. The best approach, in my view, is to be genuinely present and focused on the client in an empathic way. Showing feelings about what the client is saying can be a sincere and helpful response. Simultaneously, therapists must learn how to avoid expressing their reactive secondary emotions—for instance, getting angry at someone who has led one to feel diminished.

Some clinicians believe that a therapist should never express anger or grief in front of a client. But therapists who express emotion with a client model integrity, and doing so encourages more open communication and often reinforces a client's instincts. Therapists need to show emotions that they believe will be most helpful for progressing in therapy. That would mean, then, that the therapist would be genuinely excited if a client made progress with things that were worked on in therapy, but the therapist would not necessarily share the frustration they were feeling if the client had not followed through on an action they had committed to in a previous session. Feelings disclosed by the therapist should be, at any given moment, the best response for the client in the situation so that, from that experience, the client learns that sharing one's inner feelings and thoughts can be worthwhile.

Practice Self-Awareness of Emotion

To facilitate the emotional work of clients, therapists have to be engaged in their own emotion awareness and development process. Probably the best training in this process of being aware of one's emotions is to be in emotion-oriented personal therapy or some form of self-experience process that focuses on emotion. It is only through working with one's own emotions that one can help others to do that work. It is only by allowing and accepting our own emotions that we can see that emotions do inform and organize us. It is only by learning to discriminate between our own adaptive and mal-adaptive emotions, as well as by learning to tolerate our own unpleasant emotions, that we can experience that they do come and go. It is only by suffering our own pain and finding that we survive and are resurrected that we truly know that this is possible for our clients. Thus, we might rephrase the saying "Physician, heal thyself" as "Therapist, deal with thine own emotions." Therapists have to train themselves, or receive training, in identifying and staying with their own emotions. They have to learn by experiencing their own emotions, symbolizing their own feelings in words, and identifying their own painful maladaptive emotions. And they need to experience accessing adaptive emotional resources to transform and soothe their mal-adaptive emotions.

Psychotherapists should undergo psychotherapy themselves and reclaim their own unresolved feelings and psychological needs. This work will help them better understand their clients' emotional dynamics and ensure that their own psychological dynamics do not interfere with accessing clients' emotions or impede their ability to be truly helpful to their clients. Therapists who find themselves becoming overly personally upset, defen-sively insecure, embarrassed, or fatigued by their work with clients should explore how the contact with their clients may be triggering these emotions. They need to examine doubts about their own sense of identity, negative self-evaluations, unpleasant memories, painful feelings, and other uncomfort-able experiential states that may not necessarily be pertinent to understand-ing and healing the client's own psychological issues.

When therapists openly explore and resolve their own psychological issues, they can then view clients in a more compassionate, empathically under-standing manner and thereby respond to clients in a more appropriate, truly therapeutic way. Although reactivity by the therapist can be an impediment to effective psychotherapy, taking a cold, detached, uncaring, "professional" stance toward clients also can detract from the effectiveness of psychotherapy work. Clients who pick up that kind of coldly detached attitude may likely feel uncomfortable baring their intense feelings, needs, and experiential dynamics. A lack of caring, empathic communion between client and therapist also can prevent awareness of blocked feelings that the client does not feel comfortable sharing with a therapist perceived as coldly detached and uncaring. However, when the client experiences genuine warmhearted, caring, compassion, empathic understanding, and deeply invested "good listening" from the therapist, that warm caring can function like a melting process. It helps the client become unfrozen and blocked emotions to become more fluidly available and to flow more freely so that the client can move toward core painful feelings.

Use Facilitative, Congruent Responses

Emotional awareness and emotional authenticity in therapists promote the same in their clients. Therapists need to be aware of their own internal experience, and they need to be transparent and able to communicate to their clients what is going on within when it is therapeutic to do so (Rogers, 1957). If, however, therapists find themselves often feeling anger toward particular clients, it is important for them to explore if their reactions toward their client are coming from their own unresolved issues or concerns and to seek supervision or therapy. Congruence involves being aware of what one is feeling and disclosing it in an effective manner.

There are two central components of congruence (Greenberg & Geller, 2001). The internal-awareness component is the easiest aspect of the concept to endorse as universally therapeutic. If therapists are not aware of their own feelings in their interaction with their clients, that is likely to impede therapeutic progress because they will be ignoring important information generated by their emotion system about what was happening between them and their clients. It would be akin to a surgeon's operating in the dark.

The second aspect of transparency, the communication of what one is feeling, is much more complicated than the self-awareness component. Being able to be facilitatively transparent involves a variety of interpersonal skills, such as the ability to express not only what one is truly feeling but also to express it in a nonthreatening way. Genuineness is a higher order concept for a complex set of interpersonal skills embedded within a set of therapeutic attitudes. This ability to be genuine in a facilitative way seems to depend on three factors: (a) the therapist's attitudes, (b) certain processes, and (c) the therapist's interpersonal stance (Greenberg & Geller, 2001). To be facilitative, congruent responses need to be communicated nonjudgmentally. It helpful to use the word "facilitative" to qualify the word "congruent." The therapist's expression of themselves needs to be done for the client's benefit, not for the therapist's.

Therapists need to communicate their primary feelings genuinely and in a disciplined manner rather than impulsively blurting out whatever they feel in the moment. First, they need to be aware of their primary experience, which may take exploration and reflection as well as time. They also need to be very clear on their intention for communicating what they are feeling: that this sharing is not for themselves but to help clients or to improve the relationship. In addition, therapists need to be sensitive to the timing of the disclosure and not disclose if they sense the client is closed or too vulnerable to receive it. Disciplined genuineness thus involves the therapist's not simply saying whatever they are feeling in the moment and communicating core primary feelings rather than secondary ones.

Another important aspect of congruence that makes it helpful is *comprehensiveness*, which means "saying all of it." The therapist needs to express the central or focal aspect that is being experienced. But, they also must express the experience of what they are feeling about what the client may be experiencing in response to what the therapist said as well as what they, the therapist, is feeling about what they said. Thus, saying that one feels irritated or bored—even if done to take full responsibility for it as their own feeling, as in "I find myself reacting with some irritation" or "I'm finding it hard to stay connected and involved"—does not compose comprehensive communication. Therapists also need to communicate their concern about such revelations being potentially hurtful. For example, one may say, "I am anxious that this not be hurtful [or "I am concerned about this being hurtful"], but I want you to know I'm saying this to help me deal with this feeling, so we cannot let it get in the way of our relationship." Therapists communicate that they are revealing their emotions out of a desire to improve their connection, not damage it. This is the meaning of "saying all of it." Being therapeutically congruent, in addition to the skill of being aware of one's feelings, involves the interpersonal skills of knowing one's primary feelings, being nonjudgmental, disclosing for the good of the client, and being disciplined and comprehensive in one's communication.

The therapist's interpersonal stance is important in helping understand how to be facilitatively transparent. The key aspect that makes transparency facilitative is that the communication comes from an affirming and disclosing position. Responses in supportive therapies are generally affirming, but a transparently genuine response of what one is feeling, to be facilitative, needs to be expressed as a disclosure. It is not the content of the disclosure that makes a response facilitative; rather, it is the interpersonal stance of disclosure that is important.

Disclosure implicitly or explicitly communicates a willingness to, or an interest in, exploring with the other person what one is disclosing. For example, attacking when one is angry is different to disclosing that one is feeling angry. Therapists take responsibility for their feelings by using "I" language that helps disclose what they are feeling, not "you" language, which is blaming. The key aspect of openly disclosing vulnerable feelings, be they fear, or hurt, or even anger, is that the communication does not involve going into a one-up, power position. When a therapist is experiencing nonaffiliative, difficult feelings, such as anger or a loss of interest, it is being able to disclose those feelings in a stance that is affiliative—and that is helped by communicating that the therapist does not wish to feel this way. Therapists thus might reveal these feelings as problematic feelings that are getting in the way of their being able to be as present as they would like. They also might explain that they are attempting to repair the distance so they will be able to feel more understanding and feel closer to the client. The key to communicating what could be perceived as negative feelings in a congruently facilitative way is generally occupying an interactional position that involves disclosing in an affiliative and nondominant manner.

SITTING WITH ALL TYPES OF EMOTION

Therapists conducting emotion-focused therapy need to be able to sit within their clients' feelings, be able to dwell in them, and accept them whatever they are. For many helping professionals, especially younger ones in Western "fix-it" cultures, this can be difficult. In current psychotherapy, doing something to modify the problem quickly is favored over acceptance, which is a longer process. Evidence of this quick modification, at least in the United States, can be seen in the confusing array of insurance policies that cover only "medically necessary" behavioral or mental health care and often only a few sessions at that. Although many mental health practitioners do not work with insurance companies, it would be hard to deny that public policy has some influence on training programs and individual therapists' service offerings.

In addition to policies that are inhospitable to emotions, the human impulse to self-preserve—even when it plays out as a well-meaning desire to help—can impede emotional work. After all, it is difficult to sit in the poignant moment when the client is experiencing painful feelings, such as the shame of being a "failure," or is feeling powerless or hopeless. The ability to be with painful emotion is a skill that therapists must learn to be most helpful and to deepen the therapeutic process. Having helped the client arrive at the painful place, therapists can then help them not by giving advice or correcting errors but by helping them explore, pay attention to internal alternatives that arise on the edge of their awareness, and create new meaning from their new experience. As Chapter 5 reveals, therapists can be most helpful by being sensitively attuned to clients' feelings and assisting them to stay focused on their internal tracks so they can face what causes them pain. This work cannot be done if therapists fear emotion— an attitude that, in my opinion, has become too prevalent with the advent of providing coping skills. Helping clients simply regulate emotion or remove symptoms works against deepening emotion to get to core painful feelings so they can be made amenable to new input.

Learn to Be Vulnerable

In general, society has seen emotion as being weak and has not seen vulnerability as a healthy possibility. Vulnerability essentially is about showing up and being seen. It is tough to do that when people are terrified about what others might see or think of them. Learning to be vulnerable in one's own life is important if one is going to carry this message to clients.

This denial of vulnerability is undergoing a change with the growth of emotion-oriented treatments, especially in couple therapy in which disclosing vulnerability is seen as a key change process (Greenberg & Goldman, 2008; Wile, 1992). The work of Brené Brown (2012), who is a proponent of the benefit of vulnerability, has popularized the idea that the courage to be vulnerable will transform the way we live. Men now cry publicly, and needing support and getting it from others are viewed as important.

I, however, still supervise therapists who are trying with the best of intentions to help people by using self-soothing or emphasizing the positive when clients clearly are in pain. For example, when clients are feeling worthless and like failure, the therapist might try to help the client stand up to their negative voice by saying, "The reason you are still trying and haven't given up totally means you are standing up for yourself." Although the therapist thinks this is therapeutic, their positive framing goes counter to the aim of deepening into the core feeling of shame to access it so that it can be made amenable to new input. Essentially, therapists are often afraid to go into the hopelessness to get to the shame; instead, they try to save clients from the pain produced by their punitive voices. But, in working with emotion in most cases, the only way out is through. Therapists have to help clients face, rather than run away from, their dragons.

Learn How Culturally Informed Views of Self Influence Emotion

A frequent limitation noted in research publications on therapy is the homogeneity of the population examined: predominantly White, educated, and middle class and above. Clinicians need to recognize that people of different cultures may differ in their emotional responses. White therapists, in particular, cannot necessarily accurately read the emotions of a client of color if trying to understand from the White experience. Likewise, the emotions of gender nonbinary people cannot necessarily be fully understood from the heteronormative experience.

The predominant model of the self in the Western world, which is implicit in most if not all psychotherapy, is one of an independent self (Markus & Kitayama, 1991). From this perspective, personhood involves being separate and distinct from others, and behaving as such, and groups are viewed as existing to promote an individual's well-being. Western culture is, therefore, viewed as an individualist culture in which each person's uniqueness is important. People are encouraged to express their feelings, wishes, and thoughts, and effectiveness is seen as being able to influence others. All affect how therapy is conducted to promote assertiveness and self-esteem.

In East Asian contexts, the main model of the self, however, is one based on interdependence. From this perspective, being connected to others is fundamental to what it means to be a person as well as be responsive to situational demands. The central unit of society is the group, and for social harmony to be maintained, individuals must adjust themselves to the group. Thus, Eastern culture is viewed as a *collectivist culture* in which individuals attempt to modify themselves to fit into the group rather than try to influence others. Western psychotherapy has more recently been strongly influenced by Eastern traditions and now promotes acceptance and awareness (mindfulness).

There appears to be a real difference in the way people view themselves and their place in society as a function of cultural upbringing. In a classic study comparing American and Japanese students (Cousins, 1989), U.S. subjects were significantly more likely than Japanese subjects to describe themselves by means of individualistic psychological attributes (e.g., friendly, cheerful). Japanese participants were more likely to describe themselves with references to social roles and responsibilities (e.g., a daughter, a student). Cultures that ascribe to an independent model of self encourage people to express themselves and influence others by, for example, trying to change their environments to attain their own goals and to fit their own beliefs and desires. In contrast, people brought up in a culture that has an interdependent model of self are taught to suppress their own, goals, beliefs, and desires, and to adjust to others.

Markus and Kitayama (1991) argued that these different cultural models of self influence how people in Western and East Asian contexts feel. For example, Western culture has been found to value high arousal emotions, which are ideal and effective for influencing others and, therefore, are valued, promoted, and experienced more often in the West. Eastern cultures, on the other hand, value low arousal emotions and consider adjusting and conforming to other people as desirable. To meet this goal, low arousal emotions work better than high arousal emotions and are, therefore, valued, experienced, and preferred more than high arousal emotions. These differences influence how readily people of different cultures will be to experience and express high and low arousal emotional states.

Other studies have revealed some of the cultural aspects of emotion experience and expression. In a study of somatization comparing Korean and American subjects, Choi et al. (2016) found that Koreans somatize emotions more than Westerners do, and, more importantly, somatizing emotions compared with verbally naming emotions elicits more empathy from the other. Similarly, the Ghanian language has a preponderance of somatic references in the communication of emotion, which suggests that embodiment features prominently in Ghanaian cultural scripts of emotions (Dzokoto et al., 2013). Thus, cultural differences in use of somatization may reflect differences in ways of communicating and responding to distress in different cultures (see Ye, 2002).

Culture also regulates emotion at the individual level by making emotional responses that are in line with cultural models of emotion more readily accessible (Mesquita & Albert, 2007). In this way, culture increases the likelihood of an emotional response when it is consistent with the model and decreases its likelihood when it is inconsistent with the model. There are also culture-specific emotion syndromes. In Korea, Hwa-Byung, with the literal meaning of "anger disease" or "fire disease," is a culture-related syndrome related to suppressed anger that is characterized by unique symptoms of a fire in the chest or heart (Lin, 1983; Min et al., 2009). Another example of cultural differences includes higher levels of alexithymia among Chinese Canadian versus Euro Canadian outpatients. This finding has been explained by group differences in one component of alexithymia—externally oriented thinking (EOT)—possibly because Chinese cultural contexts may encourage EOT given a greater emphasis on social relationships and interpersonal harmony rather than on inner emotional experience. In a study of alexithymia, Chinese Canadians showed higher levels of EOT than did Euro Canadians. Those results suggest that cultural differences in alexithymia may be explained by culturally based variations in the importance placed on emotions rather than on deficits in emotional processing (Dere et al., 2012).

Given that emotion is not only biologically determined but also is influenced by the environment, cultural differences do need to be understood. Culture clearly does constrain how emotions are expressed. It influences how people should feel in different situations and the ways people should express their emotions. And because emotion is not only biologically determined, culture, to some degree, influences emotional experience and even more strongly influences emotional expression. Therapists, therefore, need to be culturally sensitive.

Being a culturally sensitive therapist involves first recognizing and understanding that their own culture influences them, and then, that it influences their relationships with clients. Subsequently, they need to understand and respond respectfully to the culture that is different from their own. Given that a main principle of an emotion-oriented therapy is to understand and be empathically attuned to the client's feelings, this baseline stance provides a general safeguard against imposing one's culturally biased views on others. Still, it is important to be on guard against enacting our cultural biases because they often may be more implicit than explicit.

Learn How Culture Influences Which Emotions Are Appropriate

One major issue in which different cultural assumptions can cause confusion in therapy is the role of assertion and boundary setting. Because preserving social harmony is a major concern in Asian culture, interpersonal conflict, for example, in marital relationships, is not a common presenting problem. It has been found that American partners are more apt to express anger and argue than Japanese partners (Kitayama et al., 2000). For example, in Japan, an individual does not say "no" in direct response to the other's opinion or suggestions. To do so would be viewed as hostile. Instead, to avoid conflict, a response is phrased as a positive sentence or a polite "yes," or by silence. The listener is then expected to determine if the answer is a definite agreement or simply a polite no. In East Asia, indirect communication that is possibly ambiguous is, therefore, deemed more appropriate and seen as maintaining group cohesiveness and harmony.

As a result of an interdependent perspective on self, the expression of emotions is significantly shaped and influenced by a consideration for how it will affect others (Hwang, 2006; Markus & Kitayama, 1991). For example, expressing anger to defend the self, which is independent of the other, is not uncommon in Western cultures. This emotion is less prevalent for those with interdependent selves for which there is not much of a sense of being separate from the other. In this cultural context, self-serving motives are usually replaced by what appears as other-serving motives (Markus & Kitayama, 2001). In addition, because Japanese people place high value on emotions that are low on the arousal spectrum, calmness, serenity, and tranquility are encouraged (Ruby et al., 2012), and similarly "powerful" emotions, such as anger, contempt, and disgust, are discouraged (Safdar et al., 2009). Japanese individuals thus may often minimize negative self-expressions in an effort to preserve social harmony. This presents a challenge for therapists working within a Western individualist model that views authentic self-expression (i.e., want and needs) as an essential step toward change in therapy and toward creating a strong connection between people.

UNDERSTANDING THE RULES OF EMOTIONAL EXPRESSION

My experience in conducting individual therapy in a variety of cultures is that although different cultures have different rules of expression, when therapists get to core issues, the emotions and the processes of change are the same. I mention "individual therapy" because modality does affect how much attention needs to be given to culturally informed rules of emotional expression. Doing individual therapy, therapists predominantly are not dealing with communication between partners and resolving current relational conflict for which rules of expression would be more important. Rather, we are dealing with the effect of clients' own painful emotion histories on their lives. Couple therapy needs to deal much more with rules of expression and the meaning of communication, which are more culturally laden than dealing, in individual therapy, with people's experience of their own emotions.

Emotions are a given of human existence and are experienced by all people regardless of culture. However, the expression of emotion as opposed to the experience of emotion is highly influenced by culture, including influencing whether an emotion is perceived as healthy or problematic. Western approaches to psychology need to be careful to not pathologize the way different cultures experience and express emotion. Different ways of perceiving, experiencing, and expressing emotion can be healthy within one cultural context but often be oppressive and problematic in another. Cultural knowledge, therefore, can be instructive in helping therapists develop the necessary skills to work with client emotions in a culturally sensitive manner. For example, consider my observation about emotional arousal: When Turkish clients in Germany present their problem, they show more intense emotion than German clients in similar situations. Both Turks and Germans feel anger and sadness, yet it appears that in the Turkish context, one needs to show a lot of emotion to indicate the seriousness of the problem. If a person does not weep or express their anger, they might not be taken seriously. So, cultural rules of expression influence what people do.

Be Open to Positive and Negative Interpretations of Anger and Shame

Anger is probably the emotion with the strongest differences in cultural prohibitions. How therapists talk to clients about anger may need to be adjusted in more collectivist cultures by saying, for instance, "I don't like" or "I feel it's not fair" rather than directly encouraging clients to say, "I'm angry." It is almost forbidden to express anger at one's parents in collectivist cultures, and this prohibition is even stronger in cultures like Thailand and Vietnam, where there is ancestor worship.

People in different cultures do acquire different views of emotions and do carry those views into therapy with them, so it is useful for therapists to be aware of them. In Eastern cultures, shame is generally considered a good emotion; it can be seen as modesty or embarrassment, and it shows propriety, humility, and that one knows one's place in the world. Experiencing and showing shame when one has violated cultural norms are seen as ways of repairing norm violation. In Western cultures, shame, however, is often more associated with failure and frequently results in behaviors that are destructive for self and relationships. Westerners withdraw in shame and do not want to be seen. It is not just that the same emotion is valued differently; the view of emotion is different. How one experiences shame, whether one reaches out or withdraws, and how shame impacts one's reputation and relationships are all culturally specific.

I had the experience of lecturing on self-criticism in Japan, and it was from a question in the audience that I realized when I said "self-criticism," it implied something good to many audience members, when, in my Western context, it automatically meant something bad. I had to qualify and talk about destructive versus constructive self-criticism. In the same way, therapists can broaden their view to see that there can be both adaptive and maladaptive shame. Although the feeling of shame is universal, therapists need to be sensitive to what it means in the client's cultural context.

Shame is so unbearable in individualist cultures that it is often turned into anger. When people who want to be seen as independent feel ashamed, they feel bad about themselves. And they do not think to question, "How important is it that I feel good about myself?" If people took some distance from the culturally set goal of feeling high self-esteem and independence, then they could live with shame. Understanding how one's emotions are culturally influenced does provide the possibility of options to feel different.

Help Clients Find Their Own Solutions

While working in Hong Kong, which has mixed Asian and British influences, I encountered the influence of culture in interesting ways in dealing with the perennial problem of the "mother-in-law." In an Asian context, I observed, the mother-in-law may come into the married couple's kitchen and cook. The daughter in-law may feel this as an intrusion or may accept it as normative. How should she handle this? The harmonious Asian way is to value harmony above assertion, which will lead to acceptance with goodwill. The Western way would be to prioritize assertion and boundary setting and would involve directness and possible conflict.

When working on their own intrapersonal conflict about how to manage these situations, those daughters-in-law who held harmony as an integrated, intrinsic, cherished value resolved the conflict in favor of harmony. Those who were more Westernized and valued individual rights favored assertive solutions. The problems arose for those who had adopted harmony as a "should" rather than as an intrinsic value. They became depressed and unhappy. In helping clients work on their internal conflict between harmony and assertion, it was important for the therapists to not be biased in one direction or another but, rather, to help the client find her own solution. It would have been countertherapeutic to assert a more individualistic, Western view that one should stand up to one's mother-in-law with a client who had harmony as a core value.

Develop Safety and Trust

The way in which cultural difference can affect relationship formation in therapy is meaningful because alliance formation and how to create trust do differ across cultures. In therapy in an Asian context like Japan, where saving face is important and concern about not shaming the other is a priority, it is crucial in creating an alliance to work on emotion and to be direct about the importance of self-disclosure (Greenberg & Iwakabe, 2013). At the start of therapy, the therapist can lay out that in the therapy session, it is counterproductive to save face, so the client needs to disclose their underlying feelings whenever possible. Also, it can be helpful to note that the purpose of therapy is not for the therapist to give advice (which often is the client's expectation) but, rather, to help the client with their emotions—and that therapy is a place to experience and resolve painful emotions. Some psychoeducation on emotion often is needed to encourage clients to express emotion. Given the difference in view on arousal and given the importance of saving face, in general, as well as harmony and filial loyalty in Asia, it frequently takes longer to develop safety, trust, and an alliance to work on these emotions.

As another example of how emotions involved in forming the therapy relationship need cultural sensitivity, I learned from my work with Indigenous cultures in North America that empathy and questions can be experienced as intrusive and lead to withdrawal. To survive, small, close-knit communities needed to avoid conflict. Because they lived in close proximity while maintaining privacy, it was important not to interfere with one another. Asking questions, giving advice, or being too familiar could be experienced as interfering. Thus, an aboriginal client could experience empathy as unwanted; the more therapists would try to engage clients in this way, the more the clients would close up.

Working with any person from any culture to develop an alliance to work on emotion involves dealing with the same universal fear of emotion: It is dangerous because it is not fully in one's control, and it comes unbidden and can take control of behavior, and be seen by others. Different cultures teach different ways of dealing with the uncontrollability and exposure to others of emotion: the West, with rational control; the East, with observational distancing. But one thing is clear: All cultures have the same feelings that humans have been grappling with for thousands of years.

Recognize How Societal Oppression Influences Emotional Expression

Gender, race, culture, and class all combine to encourage and suppress the expression of certain emotions as do societal oppression and institutional power structures. The socialization process of emotion and its expression are also known to be different for both men and women, and for people of different races and ethnicities. It is important to recognize how these intersections affect working with emotion in therapy.

It is known that women express emotion more freely than men, both more positive feelings and more internalized negative feelings, and they cry in front of others more than do men (Gard & Kring, 2007). Men, on the other hand, express more anger and aggression than do women. However, when their physiology, such as blood pressure and cortisol level, is measured, it is higher than women's, which suggests that men feel but do not express; they tend to keep their emotions bottled up inside (Gard & Kring, 2007). Although, undoubtedly, people regardless of gender feel all emotions, the degree of emotional expression and which emotions are expressed in therapy will be somewhat different according to gender (Brody & Hall, 2008; Fischer & Manstead, 2000).

Race also exerts a strong influence on emotional expression, especially in the context of racism. Members of marginalized racial or ethnic groups have reported fears that expressing emotion is dangerous and evokes negative stereotyping (Richman & Leary, 2009; Wingfield, 2010). Because of these fears, African American children, for example, are socialized to not express anger so they will not be judged as violent. It is generally more dangerous, especially for African American men, to be assertive in public, and it is potentially lethal to be so with police. The terrible paradox is that anger, which is a healthy response to injustice and violation, is denied to African Americans, and, yet, they have the most cause to feel angry about social injustice. Therapists, in working with anger with African American clients, need to understand that it is dangerous for them to express anger because of racial stereotyping. People of color are in much greater danger of the use of force against them if they express anger, whereas White people have the privilege of being able to express anger without prejudice or fear of being penalized for being angry.

We therapists who have been trained to work with emotion have had to learn to get comfortable with difficult feelings. It is imperative, then, that we deal with our own difficult feelings related to racism so we can serve and improve our clients' lives—and not perpetuate their problems. It has become clear that, in the dominant, White culture, people in general and specifically therapists find talking about race uncomfortable. This discomfort is a fear-based feeling that needs to be faced. As therapists who promote digging into uncomfortable feelings for transformation, we need to engage in the antiracist work of self-transformation.

Dominant culture therapists need to recognize that racism has been—and is—a major problem and be able to sit with their own discomfort as well as explore questions about racism that make them uncomfortable, questions such as their own privilege. They need to address their own guilt and complicity in perpetuating systems that have worked to their advantage but have oppressed others and have made people of color feel negatively about themselves and their place in the world (Kendi, 2019; see also Morin, 2020).

TAKING THE ROLE OF SOCIAL CHANGE AGENT

White, heterosexual, educated, and middle-class therapists need to be better at acknowledging the impact of their own and others' silence when it comes to the experiences of people of color. Therapists need to understand their own privilege in ignoring racism and their own unearned power by virtue of being White. In sessions with their clients, they also need to speak out against racism. Healing from internalized whiteness is needed. To do this, therapists need to be aware of the prevalence of systemic racism and listen to clients of different races, cultures, and genders to understand their experience of disempowerment. However, these are only the first steps.

The next step for therapists is to adopt the position of educators, raising the awareness of both their White and African American clients of how they have been affected by systemic racism if they are not already aware of it. It is important for therapists to be able to discuss the effect of race when their clients are ready and open to it but also not to impose this conversation on clients who do not wish for it.

At this time in history, with the visibility of recent horrifying examples of systemic racism in police murders of people of color and accompanying protests, the world is being called again to confront this injustice, which has existed for centuries in most European countries. This form of prejudice and institutionalized racism were made explicit for many years in the modern era by the South Africa apartheid system but was kept more hidden in European countries. Now, systemic racism is being named and needs to be included in therapeutic dialogues, including unequivocally stating how racism has damaged one's clients. Racism in its systemic structural, institutional, and interpersonal forms is a threat to mental and public health.

Therapy needs to address the emotional issues of racism that people of color have had to suffer. Therapists need to do more than be supportive; they need to take the role of a social change agent by teaching and raising awareness of the effects of systemic racism. This means engaging in a more directive stance around these issues—a stance that is somewhat different to following responsively and being empathic. Every good therapist, in some ways, needs to be a revolutionary, questioning the lies widely accepted within any cultural context and helping people extricate themselves from social constraints and oppression.

This more proactive stance involves helping people face issues created by society. What needs to be discussed are problems that people of color may have experienced that relate to the pressure they experienced to identify and conform to White culture rather than learn about and identify with their own racial heritage. Their experience of questioning White culture and showing an interest in their own racial group needs to be encouraged as does their experience of possibly wanting to withdraw from White culture to delve into their own racial history in the effort to define a new identity. Therapists also may help clients who wish to integrate with the dominant culture without compromising aspects of their own racial or ethnic identity work on balancing all aspects of their heritage.

Clarify Who the Self-Critic Is

Clients who are members of racial and ethnic minority groups possess a unique set of lived experiences that may drastically differ from that of the dominant culture. Failure to recognize these differences can cause ruptures to the therapeutic alliance and hinder the effectiveness of therapists' interventions. An example of one major issue that needs attention in an awareness-raising context is the chronic stress related to stigmatization from negative societal attitudes toward minority individuals in a racist/White/heterosexist privileged society. Many feel shame induced by the internalization of hostile criticism, discrimination, and violence to which others have subjected them. This influences their sense of self.

For a person of color growing up in a dominant, White culture, there is not only an internalized personal self-critic but also an internalized external societal oppressor. Here, the behavior of others has diminished, disempowered, or destroyed the person's self-confidence and invalidated the person's identity by communicating messages of core unworthiness (Wong et al., 2014). It is essential in therapeutic work that individual self-criticism and social oppression not be confused with each other. The internalization of a critical voice of a parent, for example, that produces shame differs from the internalization of systemic racial oppression and marginalization of the self by the society one lives in. The latter aspect develops through living with one or more marginalized identities in the dominant culture.

Therapists thus need to work with clients to clarify who the self-critic appears to represent. Is it a personal, psychological, criticism, or is it the internalization of societal invalidation? If it is an internalized personal self-critic, work needs to proceed to resolve the self-criticism and shame induced by it and work toward self-compassion and negotiation or integration between different internal voices. If, however, it is the introjection of external, dominant culture or criticism, assertion of self through adaptive anger needs to be supported and encouraged followed, possibly, by self-soothing to strengthen the self.

Attend to Chronic Stress and Trauma

Another important topic for therapist to attend to is unresolved racial trauma or race-based stress. Many people of color experience danger from real or perceived experience of racial discrimination, such as threats of harm, humiliation, and the witnessing of harm to other people of color from racist attacks. Although similar to posttraumatic stress disorder, racial trauma is unique in that it involves ongoing individual and collective injuries resulting from exposure and repeated exposure to race-based stress (Comas-Díaz et al., 2019). *Historical trauma*, the cumulative psychological wounds that result from historical traumatic experiences, such as colonization, genocide, slavery, dislocation, and other related trauma, has intergenerational effects such that racial trauma may accompany people of color throughout their whole life.

Although African Americans are more exposed to racial discrimination than are other ethnoracial groups (Chou et al., 2012), many Indigenous people, Latinx, and Asian Americans also suffer from race-based stress. Therapy needs to help clients work through the emotional wounds caused by racial trauma to find relief, gain awareness, and cope with systemic oppression while encouraging resistance and protection from the external forces that cause ethnoracial trauma.

CONCLUSION

Does emotional experience and expression come first because of in-wired programs, or is emotion determined by culture? In the dialectical constructivist view of emotion that I have sketched out in this and previous chapters, the answer is that both views are valid. Although there are basic emotional expressions before culture, there are not many adult expressed emotions that are separate from a person's culture and learning. Emotional experience is a synthesis of inborn, basic, psychoaffective motor emotion programs in interaction with previous lived experiences, learned expectations, and social knowledge plus what is happening in the moment.

When, for example, shame is discussed, many elements are similar regardless of culture. For instance, shame includes a wanting to disappear and an idea that "I am not good enough." Clearly, elements in the experience of emotions are universal and recognized across cultures—both types of situations and types of meanings that are similar in different cultural contexts. But emotions also are not totally independent of social context or culture, and feelings do not always feel exactly the same across different situations or different cultures. Therapists need to be empathically attuned to what this person in this culture is saying about their feelings. They also need to ensure that any self-disclosure of their own emotion respects these differences and does not invalidate the client's concerns or reinforce oppressive power structures.

There are different differences between different cultures. Latinx cultures are more expressive than more Anglo Saxon, British, and Swedish cultures, which are more restrained (Hareli et al., 2015). Also, certain cultures have more masculine-derived philosophies of being strong, with notions of "don't whine or be a baby." These cultures, or possibly subcultures in many cultures, put down vulnerability in favor of being tough or value the virtues of a stiff upper lip. But all these differences are more at the level of rules of expression and not at the level of more basic emotional experience. I have not found a lot of difficulty in applying my work with emotion across different cultures provided I am aware of what my own Western biases are and know a bit about the culture I am working in.

In North America, when a White therapist meets with an African American client, race is in the room and needs to be dealt with. White people typically avoid Black spaces, but Black people are required to enter White spaces. Both the therapy room and training room are White spaces where Black people are constantly required to navigate as a condition of their existence (Anderson, 2015). The experience of otherness by virtue of being a member of a non-White group living in a predominantly White society is impossible for people of color to avoid. Thus, therapists need to negotiate the rapids of how to acknowledge their clients' collective experience of unfairness and oppression while not denying the person's individuality and personal experience. Therapists need to bear witness to the person's experience of injustice without thereby exacerbating feelings of otherness. In developing this skill, therapists seek not only to be better helping professionals but also to become agents of social change.

PART **II** ARRIVING AT
EMOTION

5 EMPATHIC ATTUNEMENT TO AFFECT

As we introduced in Part I, therapy to change emotion follows a two-stage approach of arriving at and then leaving emotional experience (Greenberg, 2002). In the first stage, the therapist listens to the client's narrative and lets the story and its emotional significance emerge. In this first stage, the therapist works to activate core emotion schemes to access painful maladaptive feelings. They do so in various steps, the first of which—empathic attunement to affect—is the subject of this chapter.

Empathic attunement to affect involves a kinesthetic and emotional sensing of another's inner world, knowing their rhythm, feeling, and experiencing by metaphorically being in their skin. Empathically following affect is more a right brain process than a left brain, analytic one. It functions at levels beneath conscious awareness and involves being with the client rather than doing to the client. It is helpful to distinguish between "empathic understanding" and "empathic attunement to affect." Both are therapeutically important, but empathic attunement to affect goes beyond empathic understanding to create a two-person experience of reciprocal *affective resonance*, a responsiveness that creates a feeling of unbroken connectedness in which the focus is clearly on affect, not meaning. This type of connection allows for the coregulation of affect.

https://doi.org/10.1037/0000248-006
Changing Emotion With Emotion: A Practitioner's Guide, by L. S. Greenberg

Rogers (1957) famously introduced the idea of empathy as reflection of feeling, but what he called "reflections" were more predominantly reflections of meaning. Before his death, he said he wished he had used the term "checking his understanding" instead. Empathic understanding involves imaginative entry into the world of the other plus the ability to turn this understanding of the other's inner world into words. It is a crucial therapeutic skill (Watson, 2016). Empathic attunement to affect, however, goes beyond empathic understanding because the focus is not only on conveying understanding but also on focusing on and mirroring affect. "Feeling felt" by another creates a resonance of minds that is essential to survival, is pleasurable, and helps in regulating one's affect.

Another way of describing the process of empathic attunement to affect is by an analogy with the experience of musical attunement in which a singer matches their pitch with that of another singer or musical instrument. Using this metaphor, listening to the client in an affectively attuned manner would mean to attune with the client's affective experiences in the here and now or, extending the metaphor a little, attune with the melody (or tune) of the client's internal affective experience. That is, through empathic attunement to affect, the therapist vibrates to or resonates with the client's melody that is emanating from their being in the immediacy of the therapeutic encounter. The pitch and rise, energy, rhythm, and tone of the therapist's voice, and the expression of the face and eyes, and their contours over time, all mirror the client's affective experience of tiredness, excitement, anger, or sadness. This does not occur by deliberate means but automatically out of being fully present, interested, and attuned. Unpacking the meaning of the word "interest" is helpful because its use in the previous sentence conveys the special sense of the kind of presence needed. The word, broken into its components in Latin is: est, "to be" and inter, "among." Thus, one is "among" the other. One needs to be fully absorbed and curious.

The addition of the words "attunement to affect" to "empathic" emphasizes being spontaneously tuned into, interested in, and harmonizing, with the rhythm and contour of the client's emotional experience (Stern, 1985). Given that the goal of working with emotion in therapy is to facilitate people's ability to deal with their emotional pain, it is important that therapists focus on their clients' moment-by-moment emotional states. The ability to be attuned really comes down to how present therapists are to their clients' affective states in the moment and how successfully they mirror those states so that a connection that goes beyond words is felt. The client will then feel felt.

As well as conveying understanding of clients' meanings and feelings, therapists also need to mirror their clients' bodily based physiological experience.

Therapists need to respond to their clients' facial expressions, the way they sit and hold their bodies, their micromovements, their breathing, and their vocal tone. Therapists can achieve synchrony with their clients by being attuned to their clients' physiological processes. The therapist's pacing and the tempo of the interaction needs to match the client's state; their biorhythms become coordinated. This is expressed in a matching of language use, vocal tone, skin conductance, pauses, and other nonverbal behaviors (Watson, 2019). And all of this is occurring automatically.

Affect attunement is an embodied phenomenon. Neuroscience research demonstrates that this type of attunement is a whole-body experience (Gallese, 2009). The discovery of mirror neurons suggests that human and primates' brains run a type of embodied simulation that allows people to understand the experience of others' feelings, sensations, emotions, and intentions without words and at a sensory-motoric level (Watson, 2019). This simulation is not a deliberate or conscious process; rather, it is nonconscious and prereflective. It is through the simulation of others' intentions, which are conveyed mainly by bodily actions and facial expressions, but also by understanding the context that the emotions of others are sensed and recognized. In other words, the brain runs a type of simulation of what it's like to do what the other is doing in the situation described.

In therapy, the more vivid the description the other provides, the more the therapist can imagine the experience and the more their brains will be able, automatically, to run a simulation, thus giving the therapist a sense of what it was like for the client. Therapists need to actively imagine clients' stories and actively imagine what clients experience. Therapists' empathy is enhanced when they can deliberately imagine and sense clients' experience (Greenberg & Ruchanski-Rosenberg, 2002; Watson & Greenberg, 2017).

It is important that in both empathic attunement and empathic understanding, therapists do not feel what the other feels. Rather, we experience, bodily, a type of metaexperience, feeling what it feels like to feel a feeling but not actually feel the feeling. Thus, if my client feels shame, I do not feel a taste of shame with its action tendency to withdraw. Rather, I feel what it feels like to feel this, always keeping distinct that this is what it feels like for the other rather than feeling it myself. What I might feel as my own emotional reaction might be something quite different. For example, when my client feels shame, I do not feel shame. Rather, I may feel compassion or even a sense of anger or sadness at what the client has suffered. A study of what therapists felt when they were being highly found that only 11% of the time did therapists report feeling the same feeling as the clients empathic (Greenberg & Ruchanski-Rosenberg, 2002). The majority response about

40% of the time was that therapists had a vivid image of what the client was saying, and they read the feeling of what was depicted in the image.

Affect attunement is a profound process. The question becomes: How do we learn it, how do we do it in therapy, and how do we train people to improve their capacity to be empathically attuned to affect? We probably learn empathic attunement to affect by a combining some innate ability to recognize emotion with having had our own affective experience empathically mirrored and, over time, internalizing this capacity at a procedural level.

One could say that a caregiver's attunement to their infant's affect provides the building blocks to how children learn to be connected to others, build relationships, and be attuned to affect. A caregiver's ability to be attuned is important to children's ability to learn to regulate their nervous systems and deal with distress. The consistent failure of caregivers to be attuned to infants' ever-changing affective states results in poor affect regulation and poor abilities to deal with affect in others. In addition, then, to our personal experience of attunement throughout our life that has given us some capacity for attunement now as helping professionals, training in being present is a way to enhance attunement.

THERAPEUTIC PRESENCE

Therapeutic presence involves the ability to be fully in the moment with the client in the fullness of their experience (Geller & Greenberg, 2012). Therapeutic presence is not a technique; rather, it is a way of being with the client. It involves therapists' being open and sensitive to their own, and to their clients', moment-by-moment changing, awareness, and experience, and responding from this state of inner receptivity. *What* the therapist does is almost not as important as *when* the therapist does it; being present to the moment enhances attuned responsiveness. Therapeutic presence entails being fully immersed in the moment with the intention of being in service of the client's healing process while maintaining a sense of groundedness in one's own personal existence and a connection with the other. This state is enhanced when therapists suspend or defocus from their own needs, hopes, concerns, beliefs, or assumptions, and instead focus with their full attention on the client's process and what is occurring between them in the moment.

This quality of being in the moment provides a foundation for attunement to affect. All emotion occurs in the present, so therapists need to be in the present to be aware of their client's emotions. Primarily, *presence* is a way of meeting the client that is free of the therapist's preconceptions, judgments, and agendas. I like to describe my experience of presence this way: When I am sitting in front of a client, if a sunbeam is shining through the window, I see the sunbeam, and if a speck of dust drops between us, I see the speck of dust. Likewise, if the client's eyes film over before tears appear, I see the change in the reflected light in the eyes. Therapeutic presence is a way of being fully open to clients in the depth and complexity of their internal emotional, cognitive, and spiritual world.

Geller and I (Geller & Greenberg, 2012) defined *therapeutic presence* as bringing one's whole self into the encounter with a client by being completely in the moment on a multiplicity of levels: physically, emotionally, cognitively, and spiritually. Presence involves (a) being in contact with one's integrated and healthy self while (b) being open and receptive to what is poignant in the moment, and immersed in it, with (c) a larger sense of spaciousness and expansion of awareness and perception, and with (d) the intention of being with and for the client in service of their healing process. The inner receptive state involves a complete openness to the client's multidimensional internal world, including their bodily and verbal expression, and openness to the therapist's own bodily experience of the moment to access the knowledge, professional skill, and wisdom embodied within. Being fully present, then, allows for an attuned responsiveness based on a kinesthetic and emotional sensing of the other's affect and experience as well as one's own intuition and skill, and the relationship between.

Therapists can train to become more present by engaging in different exercises of present-centered awareness. In the 1950s, Gestalt therapy, drawing on Zen Buddhist practice, introduced exercises in present-centered awareness. These exercises essentially involved practicing being in the moment by saying, "Now I am aware of . . ." and shuttling between awareness of outer sensation, involving perceptions beyond the skin, inner sensation and perception within the boundary of the skin, and what was called "middle zone awareness"—thought, expectation, memories, and so forth—that involved conceptual processing. This conceptual processing was meta to or beyond the experience of present sensory-motor awareness. *Mindfulness meditation*—which has gained popularity since the 1990s—is another form of practice in being present to what is occurring; it also trains attention to focus on present internal experience within. These and other forms of Eastern practice, such as tai chi and yoga, aid the development of the capacity to be in the moment without memory, thought, or desire—what Bion (1967) suggested as the ideal state for therapists to be in during therapy.

THE EXPERIENCE OF ATTUNEMENT

Attunement implies a type of communication that occurs between two people who each have a body gifted with a sense of direction. I use my bodily felt sense of direction to guide each of my clients to become what they are but what they may never have been able to become by themselves alone. In this process, I am not reducing the other's experiences to mine, but, rather, I am simultaneously making explicit my experience and also my client's experience as it is conveyed to me. I try to understand the other's experience through my own (see, e.g., Merleau-Ponty, 1945/1962). It is something like the two of us—my client and I—are one—like my body and the other person's body are one whole, two sides of a coin, and my body inhabits both bodies simultaneously. My client's emotions like anger, fear, shame, hate, and love are not hidden at the bottom of their awareness. Rather, they exist as possibilities *in* the specifics, *in* this person's description, *on* this face or *in* these gestures, not hidden behind them. The client's feelings and meanings are embodied, and my empathic attunement to affect is a lived bodily experience in which I develop a "felt sense" of the other's "interior." I sense something by resonating with my client's sense of intention.

This sense is given to me spontaneously in a passive construction of felt meaning. As I listen, my client's private world shows through, permeating the fabric of my own experience, and, for a moment, I sense what it feels like. As Merleau-Ponty (1968) described it in his book *The Visible and the Invisible,* "My private world has ceased to be mine only; it is now the instrument which another plays" (p. 11). It is precisely my body that perceives the body of another and discovers in that other body a miraculous continuity of my own intentions, a familiar way of dealing with the world. I reach into this shared bodily experience and sense what it feels or felt like. Doing this, I pronounce, "You must have felt so lonely, or afraid, or even humiliated," even though the client has not said any of this explicitly.

Transposing myself into the other's experience does not mean actually putting myself in the place of the other person and thereby displacing the other's experience with my own. Rather, it consists of being myself and, only in this way, bringing about the possibility of being able to go along with my client while still remaining other with respect to them (Heidegger, 1953/2000). I go along with the other through imaginative identification, transposing myself into the other's way of being. This going-along-with means directly learning how it is with this experience for my client and discovering what it is like to be this person with whom I am going along in this way.

When I am talking with my client, attunement involves relying on the resonance I find within my own body. I pay attention to what I feel called to do by the other. I try to say what would capture all that the other feels, wants, and intends. Feelings and emotions always refer to something; therefore, to fathom my client's emotional or mental states, I also try to understand their mental representations or the contents of their narrative to capture what their mind is directed at. There is an "aboutness" or "directedness" to emotional mental states, and it is this that I am trying to understand. Attunement to affect is not just naming a feeling but capturing the whole state, its felt meaning, and its sense of direction. It is not just "You are sad" but "You are sad about missing or losing this, and you want or need this." In this way, I try to capture the whole feeling, what it is about, and what it implies as well as its sense of direction. I ultimately try to put into words the need or want that is embedded in the emotion.

THE EFFECTS OF ATTUNEMENT

Attunement to affect in therapy has similar effects as it does in human growth and development. There is a right-brain to right-brain form of communication between people that is constantly helping to regulate affect through both verbal and nonverbal aspects of communication. The client's brain is constantly reading and responding physiologically to patterns and, most importantly, to moment-by-moment changes in patterns of vocal and facial features. The voice is soothing; the face, reassuring; the eyes, concerned. It's not just the look, or the face, or the tone of the voice but the way it is changing moment by moment. The brain reads change over time, not just static features. It is not the smile alone that affects us, it the speed with which it emerges and how rapidly it decays that is being read, and it is this that provides information as to its authenticity.

Porges (2007) demonstrated that affect is regulated interpersonally by a direct face-to-heart connection. The brain is constantly processing inter-actions to determine safety, and the reading of the facial and vocal patterns of the person with whom we are interacting bypasses the cerebral cortex and goes directly to regulate our sympathetic and parasympathetic nervous systems. People relax automatically in the presence of the right nonverbal patterns of the other.

In his book *The Polyvagal Theory*, Porges (2011) showed how the vagus nerve, which connects the heart and brain, serves as a type of brake that can be switched on or off to either calm or activate a person's protective action.

As people's brains neuroperceive safety and danger, their body reacts. *Neuroception* describes how neural circuits discern safety and danger based on information outside awareness. When there is a *neuroperception* of safety, individuals feel calm and soothed, and protective action is inhibited. This state of safety and calm is communicated by means of posture, gaze, attention, vocal quality, care, warmth, and attunement to the client's experience. As a result, the client's heart rate may slow down. To add to Porges's (2011) findings, from a philosophical perspective, Levinas (1969, 2000), the French post-Martin Buber philosopher, emphasized how compelling the face is in human relationships. He insisted that the face of the other demands a response from us and pulls for a reaction automatically at the nonverbal and neuronal levels. We know that gazing into the eyes of another automatically activates specific areas in the brain.

Therapists, therefore, need to keep their fingers on the client's emotional pulse, moment by moment; respond to the client's momentary shifting states; and recognize when the attunement and the safety it produces are lost. This means that the therapist may sense through a client's body posture, pitch rise in their voice, disconnected eye gaze, or tight facial expression that they are not feeling safe. The sensing helps therapists understand that they may have said something that has led the client to not feel heard, and they adjust accordingly. Therapists, thus, are reading both the client's and their own bodily felt sense and action tendencies moment by moment, and then they are intervening to try to correct any misattunement. They watch to see if their next response causes the client's facial expressions to soften and leads to deeper breathing, and if the client again feels safe in the relationship and that a tear in the alliance has been repaired.

To work with affect, one has to learn that less is more and that attunement to affect is profoundly helpful and central to transformative experience. This lesson can be difficult to accept for beginning therapists, especially in the current era in which fix-it therapies fit into in a fix-it culture. It is easy to feel the pressure to do something to help their clients in distress. And it is reassuring to have techniques to modify and to psychoeducate—all more deliberate efforts to change what a person does to relieve their suffering. However, what therapists most need to learn is the power of communicating to their clients that their experience matters. When clients see that the therapist is attuned to and interested in their affective experience, this helps them deal with their emotional pain. One of the core beliefs that develops for many clients as a result of early childhood betrayal and trauma is that they and their experience do not matter, that others are not interested in their experience, and that having feelings gets in the way of surviving. In the face of that reality, having someone who is affectively attuned, interested, and accepting is the beginning of the development of trust, which may in itself be a profound fundamental change.

THE SKILLS OF EMPATHY AND EMPATHIC ATTUNEMENT TO AFFECT

Therapists can learn a number of skills in addition to practicing being present to help them become more empathic and more attuned to affect. These skills include the creation of an alliance to work on emotion, internal tracking, perceptual skills, fluency in different types of empathic responses, and compassion.

An Alliance to Work on Affect

Working on affect assumes that an alliance has been created to do so. The collaborative aspect of the alliance requires both an agreement on goals and on tasks. The goal is to transform emotion, and the task, in this instance, is to accept empathy and empathic attunement. However, given that emotion work involves approaching painful, dreaded emotions, clients often have adopted a self-protective strategy of not feeling. Thus, forming an alliance to work on emotions can be a major task. Clients might believe that it is better to put their feelings in a box and shut the lid tightly, and also that to talk about feelings just feels bad and is a waste of time. To clients with those beliefs, vulnerability implies weakness, and being strong has been their main mode of survival. This means that, initially, certain clients will not respond well to an empathic style and to a focus on emotion because they see both as counter to their method of coping: to "be strong" and to steer away from emotion. So, how does one kindle an alliance to work on emotion in these circumstances?

First, therapists need to understand and validate clients' concerns about going into their emotions. Clients need to feel neither pushed nor confronted. Rather, the therapist's presence, and the provision of enough safety, leads clients to feel able to access their emotional experience. Providing safety can mean spending time providing a detailed rationale for approaching emotion in therapy. Two of the main objections that clients often raise are: "How can feeling bad lead to feeling good?" and "It's all in the past. You can't change the past, so what's the use of going into it?" Therapists need first to provide a rationale for how "feeling bad can lead to feeling good" and then how "going into the past" can be helpful. These rationales help motivate clients to overcome their avoidance of emotion.

All the material on the theory of how emotion works and on memory reconsolidation forms the basis of these rationales. Therapists can say, "Emotion gives you information about what is good and bad for you, and about what needs are being met or not." Metaphors like the following are often more communicative:

> Emotion is like the warning light on the dashboard of a car. When it goes on, it tells you something is wrong in the engine or another important system like the brakes, and you best pay attention to what it is saying.

Another is to liken emotion to how a GPS helps you navigate on a journey: Emotions are like an emotional positioning system, or EPS: They provide us with information on whether where we are is meeting our needs. Yet another rationale, developed initially in Hawaii, where, of course, surfing is king, is to liken emotion to a wave coming at you. As all experienced surfers know, it is best to dive into and under the wave rather than try to swim away from it. If you try to escape, the wave upends you, but if you go through it, you come out the other side into calm. This image illustrates the idea that the only way out is through.

Regarding past memories, therapists can tell clients that the past influences the present, emotion memories are formed at a young age when they could not be adequately processed, and those past memories pop up to affect the present. Therapists also can say evidence shows that by going into the memory and working on it, how one experiences the past can be changed (memory reconsolidation). Events in the past will not change, but the way we think and feel about them, the way we see ourselves in relation to the events, and the way our bodies react can all change.

This process of developing an alliance to work on emotion is the sine qua non of emotion work. Clients have to be helped to see the relevance of talking about their feelings. This is achieved partly by developing a safe, trusting bond and partly by providing a rationale to those clients who are closed or openly opposed to going into their emotions. Another way to help clients feel safe is to have a mutually agreed on formulation of the underlying painful emotions. That is, therapist and client coconstruct a way to describe the presenting difficulties that puts emotion at the center.

One client, a 30-year-old man in therapy for social anxiety, said he was "allergic to emotion." He declared that his emotions were dangerous and overwhelming, so he did not want to talk about them. Instead, what he wanted to do was stop being so anxious: "So, please don't talk to me about my emotions." Despite any of the rationales given by the therapist, he remained opposed to talking about how he felt. In such situations, therapists have their work cut out for them to help clients see that focusing on emotion can be helpful and the way to heal. Eventually, after about eight sessions, this client came to see the usefulness of emotions.

It happened by a strange route. He first began to understand something about his wife's emotions. He noticed how her feelings led her to behave, and this opened him up to see that his own emotions led him to behave in certain ways. Then, a few sessions later, he came in and reported that, one day, as he was sitting in his car and was feeling anxious, he suddenly remembered having this feeling when he was kid and his parents were fighting. This feeling memory just came to him out of the blue, so to speak. The therapist gently explained that, although the memory had come on suddenly, it actually was the result of the slow increase in the man's attention to emotion that had been taking place over the 12 weeks of therapy up to that point. Now, the therapist and client were able to truly collaborate. They agreed on the goal of therapy as greater facility with emotion, on the task of paying attention to what he felt in the moment, and on evoking his childhood emotion of anxious insecurity that was at the root of his current social anxiety.

Internal Tracking

First and foremost in learning the skills of attunement to affect is to make the distinction between "internal" and "external" tracking. In terms of a psychotherapy process coding system called the *narrative coding system* (Angus et al., 1999), one can categorize client narratives as being in one of three landscapes: (a) the landscape of action "what happened"; (b) the reflexive landscape "what it meant"; or, most important, (c) the "landscape of feeling "what it felt like." Clients, in general, talk initially in the landscape of action of what happened, and therapists often respond by following this external track; conveying their understanding of what happened; or, in some cases, responding in the landscape of meaning by offering a response focused on what this meant. The first important skill in being attuned to affect, however, is to not respond by reflecting an understanding of the content of what occurred or its meaning. Rather, it is to respond to the client's experience—to the internal track in the landscape of feeling.

Say a client says, "My husband's never there for me. He doesn't pay attention to what I say. At dinner, he looks at his phone repeatedly and barely looks at me, and I just handle this now by having another glass of wine." The therapist has options in how to respond. If the therapist were to respond by focusing on what happened rather than what was felt by saying, "So, you husband is just so inattentive, looking at his phone, barely looking at you, and all you can do to manage this is turn to drinking," the client is likely to continue with more of a description of what happens; for example: "Sometimes I ask him to put his phone away, but then he does it reluctantly and just gets morose, and we still don't talk." Although allowing the client to elaborate on a sequence of events is not wrong in and of itself, it belabors the therapeutic process.

To start getting to the work at hand, therapists need to respond to the client's internal track and say, "It must leave you feeling so unimportant, so lonely and terribly hurt, and maybe kind of angry, too." This response focuses the client on her internal track, and she might respond, "Yes, hurt and angry. I'm basically feeling hopeless," and the narrative now unfolds in the landscape of feeling. In a study of therapist responses, my colleagues and I (Adams, 2010; Adams & Greenberg, 1996) showed that clients are 8 times more likely to deepen their experience in their next talk turns when responding to a therapist's statement that focuses on the client's internal track than when responding to a therapist's empathic reflection on the client's external track. The internal track gets to a deeper level of experience; the external track is at a shallow depth of experience (EXP).

The key skill is applying a gentle, persistent focus on the client's internal track—on the client's bodily sense of experience. A helpful technique is for the therapist to adopt the position of seeing the client as providing a movie of what happened: a description of events and behaviors. The therapist runs in parallel a movie of the client's internal track, extracting from what happened, what it must have been like for the client, and what must possibly have been experienced. The therapist does this not by focusing on the actions of the actors but, rather, by listening to the music—the client's voice and nonverbal manner of expression—accompanying the narrative. It is the voice and nonverbal manner of expression that carry the affect accompanying the contents and actions. In a movie, we see the actor peering around the door, but it is the music, slow and scary or light and happy, that conveys the affective tone. It is the music, not the content, that needs to be responded to and put into language. This is following the internal track.

In conjunction with a focus on the client's internal track is the important tenet that clients are experts of their own experience. Their internal stream of experience has a direction. The client knows what hurts the client and is an active agent who tries internally to make sense of their experience. For this reason, the therapist follows their internal track rather than imposes a sense of direction from outside that may distort this process of client-guided internal search. How, then, can therapists be process guiding if following is so crucial? By guiding toward the client's internal experiential track, the therapist helps the client get closer to their own experience. Whatever the therapist does by being attuned and by guiding is based on the understanding that the client has an internal track of experience, and this is the path therapists want to guide them along.

This focus on the client's internal track is achieved by both the therapist and the client's engaging in the detailed unfolding and exploration of sensations and emotions, which emerge in the retelling of an event. Working in the landscape of feeling and focusing on the internal track, there is an elaboration of subjective feelings, reactions, and emotions connected with an event. This addresses the question of "What do I feel?" during the event. In the following example, a client talks about a visit from her mother, and the therapist's focus on the internal track guides the client to pay attention to her bodily felt sense.

THERAPIST: Mm-hmm. So, how does it make you feel when she [the client's mother] acts like this?

CLIENT: I feel like she's intruding. I mean, she's the guest. I don't know, I just want to scream, I get so frustrated. She treats me like a little kid. There is no point telling my husband. He just sides with her. I just get really upset—just feel like one of the kids when she's around. [external track, moderately low EXP; giving limited emotional reactions]

THERAPIST: Leaves you feeling, I guess, kind of criticized but so hopeless and powerless. [focusing on internal track at a deeper level of experience]

CLIENT: Yeah. Like when she cleans or says that I'm not dressing my kids right. It's so aggravating. No matter how hard I try, I can't please her. [semi-internal; still just emotional reactions]

THERAPIST: I just can't please her. A kind of helpless, hopeless feeling. A sinking inside?

CLIENT: More of a jittery, shaky feeling. Like I think I'm starting to experience panic attacks when I know she's coming for a visit. I do feel helpless.

THERAPIST: Jittery. Feeling panicky anticipating not being able to please her. Just so helpless.

CLIENT: Like before she arrived, I had a headache for a week. My stomach was in a knot, and I could hardly eat. I just felt really tense and nervous. I just know that she will find something to criticize me about, and I will feel like I've failed again. Yes, that's what I feel—failed again and can't do anything about it.

Here, we see the therapist running the internal track movie and responding in the landscape of feeling. The client is struggling with making sense of her experience, and the therapist is helping her arrive at this internal sense of feeling helpless and failing again. She has now arrived at what she feels, always a first step in problem solving. Now that the client experiences and knows what she feels, she can begin to work on what she needs and wants to do to move on and solve this problem.

Perceptual Skills

It is the therapist's perceptual skills that are so important in enabling moment-by-moment attunement to affect. First, as a client tells the therapist their story, the therapist must listen both explicitly and implicitly for what is the client's most poignant and painful emotional experience. The therapist focuses on those stories that are emotionally tinged and, in some way, touch or move the therapist; these stories are deepened and further explored to identify core painful emotions. As clients talk, therapists hear from among all the things clients are saying those things that stand out because the way they are expressed has more force or concern behind them. Something captures the therapist's interest and attention, compelling them to focus on that point. What makes it stand out might be a sigh, a look on the face, the voice, a change in breathing, or a stronger emotional intensity in the body— all indications of poignancy. The therapist may feel a twinge in their chest or an anticipatory holding of their breath that indicates internally that something is important or meaningful in what the client is describing. Therapists can recognize when an emotion is adaptive because there tends to be a natural body rhythm, and the person's whole system appears coordinated and congruent. Therapists also need to use their knowledge about universal emotional responses as well as knowledge of their own emotional responses to understand their clients' emotions.

Therapists also need to attend to clients' emotional processing styles. These styles indicate client's emotional accessibility and how currently amenable they are to an emotion-focused treatment, or whether more specific work is needed to increase their emotional accessibility. Various features and dimensions of manner of processing are to be considered in this process. First, when there is an activated client emotional expression, the therapist and the client together need to determine whether the emotional expression is primary, secondary, or instrumental (Greenberg, 2011). For emotional processing to be productive, primary emotions need to be accessed. Thus, the therapist must know how to determine what type of emotion is being expressed in the differences between primary adaptive, maladaptive, secondary, and instrumental emotions (see Chapter 1 for a more detailed discussion of emotion types).

In observing how clients are processing emotion, client vocal quality, degree of emotional arousal, levels of experiencing, and degree of productive processing of emotion are all important. Client vocal quality, a crucial guide to the type of processing the client is engaged in, has been divided into four mutually exclusive categories describing a pattern of vocal features that reflect the momentary deployment of attention and energy of the speaker (Rice & Kerr, 1986; Rice & Wagstaff, 1967). Each of the four categories— focused, external, limited, and emotional—describes a particular type of processing of experience. *Focused* voice indicates that clients are tracking their internal experience, their eyeballs are turned inward, and they are attempting to symbolize their experience in words. *External* voice has a prerehearsed, speechlike quality with a "talking at," lecturing quality; this voice lacks spontaneity. It has an even, rhythmic tone and a quality of energy turned outward. It is unlikely that content is being freshly experienced. *Limited* voice is low energy and often comes out high pitched. Anxiety leads to tightening in the throat, indicating that affect is being strangulated and that it is difficult for these clients to trust. The clinical picture, thus, is one of wariness. *Emotional* voice is indicated by emotion breaking through in the voice as the client talks. Focused and emotional voices have been found to predict good outcome in experiential therapy (Rice & Kerr, 1986; Watson & Greenberg, 1996).

Aspects of speech patterns identified by Rice (Rice & Kerr, 1986; Rice et al., 1979) that characterize the different voices just described are (a) accentuation pattern, (b) regularity of pace, (c) terminal contours, and (d) whether there has been a disruption of speech patterns. *Accentuation pattern* refers to emphasis patterns in sentences. In the English language, accentuation of words tends to occur in particular ways in sentences. This can either give the effect of a regular beat that can be more pronounced than usual for the English language, analogous to a sermon (e.g., "We are gathered here today to . . ."). Conversely, accentuation patterns also can be more irregular than usual. *Regularity of pace* refers to the variation of pace within a particular utterance. For example, a person may begin speaking quickly and continue the last half of their phrase in a slower manner. *Terminal contours* involve aspects of pitchlike evenness: rises or drops in pitch. Contours can be used in an accentuating speechmaking way, or they can give the total intonation pattern a more ragged, unexpected sound. *Disruption of speech pattern* refers to the extent to which the regular speech pattern is disrupted or distorted by emotional overflow.

Moving from vocal features, another important aspect of client process that predicts outcome is expressed emotional arousal. As defined in the Client Emotional Arousal Scale-III-R (Warwar & Greenberg, 1999), emotional arousal depends on the degree of intensity in the voice and body, and the degree of restriction of expression. Research has shown that moderate levels of emotional arousal in combination with deeper experiencing to make sense of the arousal, rather than pure high emotional arousal, predict positive outcome in experiential therapies (Carryer & Greenberg, 2010; Missirlian et al., 2005; Warwar & Greenberg, 1999).

Client EXP (Klein et al., 1969) has been studied extensively (Klein et al., 1986) and has been related to positive outcome in therapy. EXP differs from arousal by describing clients' ways of talking about their inner experience to make sense of it as well as to achieve self-understanding and problem resolution. In this seven-level scale, at early levels (1 and 2), the speaker's content and manner of expression is impersonal, and feelings are avoided. This moves to description of events in external or behavioral terms with emotional reactions. At Level 4, the quality of involvement in speech content clearly shifts the speaker's attention to the subjective felt flow of internal experience rather than to events or abstractions. At the higher level (6), the client synthesizes newly discovered feelings and meanings to resolve emotional problems related to the self.

Findings by Warwar and me (Warwar & Greenberg, 1999) indicated that higher emotional arousal at midtreatment predicted outcome, but, as clinicians, we knew that some emotional arousal was productive and some was not productive, and the correlation between arousal and outcome was around .33. This left a lot of the outcome variance unaccounted for. We knew that the therapists in the study discriminated between good and poor arousal, so unproductive process was curtailed because the therapists worked to facilitate more productive forms of emotion processing. We, therefore, set out to develop a measure to discriminate productive from unproductive emotional processing.

As mentioned earlier, the main elements of productive emotional processing are attending, symbolization, congruence, acceptance, agency, regulation, and differentiation. See the section Productive Emotional Processing in Chapter 2 for a detailed description of these elements.

Fluency in Different Types of Empathic Responses

This approach to working with emotion grew out of Rogers's (1957) non-directive approach combined with Perl's (1973) more active Gestalt approach. I blended the two interactional styles into one in which following and leading are combined synergistically into a sense of flow. Elliott and I (Greenberg & Elliott, 1997) delineated different types of empathic responses, and therapists can use these types to focus predominantly on affect by helping clients focus on their affective experience. These types range from purely empathic understanding responses, to validating and evocative responses, to exploratory ones, and to conjectural and refocusing responses (Greenberg & Elliott, 1997). These types are described in this section. Remember that "affect attunement" means that added to the words is the therapist's bodily felt resonance that is communicated in the rhythm and tone of the response as well as the content.

The empathic responses to be described shortly increase in the proportion of leading over following as one goes down the list. One of the fundamental skills of working with emotion is being able to effectively combine following and leading in a seamless manner. In working with emotion, I recommend that therapists take a not-knowing position. See clients as being experts on their own experience. They know what hurts, and we, as therapists, need to follow their pain because it will point the process in the right direction. Clients, however, also protect themselves from experiencing their dreaded emotions. They can benefit from suggestions by a guide who points them toward that place where they feel their feelings and also helps evoke painful emotions, in the safety of the therapeutic situation, which makes clients amenable to change. Later in therapy, as the bond develops, more process-directive interventions are added using guided imagery and psychodramatic enactments.

Empathic Understanding

This involves a type of interchangeable understanding by reflecting on the main point of the client's message (Elliott et al., 2004). Here, the therapist is most strongly following the client. Empathic reflection seeks to demonstrate understanding to help build and maintain a safe, therapeutic relationship. It provides an underlining of the important meaning of what the client is saying. The empathic understanding response carries the flavor of, "Is this what you mean? Do I understand? Do I get it?" The therapist is trying to understanding the main thing the client is saying.

Empathic Affirmation

Here, the therapist's response goes beyond understanding to validation, support, and confirmation of the client's experience. This is especially helpful when the client is taking about a painful emotion related to self. Buber and Rogers disagreed on this point (Merrill, 2008). Rogers (1957) said he just wanted to convey understanding and the client would then be able to eventually grow. This was a more an intrapsychic, as opposed to an interpersonal, process. Buber, on the hand, emphasized the interpersonal aspect in which it is the therapist's confirmation of the other that helps the other come into being, as captured in the Swahili greeting, "I see you," to which the response is, "I am here." We exist in the eyes of the other, which adds validation to understanding. A good example of this type of response is the no-wonder response. A generic example is: "No wonder you felt this way given what happened." Here, the therapist validates that the client's experience makes sense. This helps the client bear their painful experience because they feel the therapist's support and validation. The end result is feeling stronger. A further example might be: "Yeah, it's really hard to stay with the sadness because it rips you apart inside. How else could it be? It was such a devastating loss."

Empathic Evocation

Evocative empathy involves communicating understanding via metaphors, connotative language, and expressive speech to help activate experience. It brings experience alive emotionally and helps clients reenter past scenes and reexperience what was felt. Evocative reflections capture clients' experience in such a way that it becomes more vivid. There is some degree of going beyond following to help evoke an experience.

Using evocative language, metaphor, and imagery promotes reexperiencing via accessing episodic memory. Standard metaphors like "feeling like a motherless child" or spontaneously produced metaphors like "feeling stuck in the mud" to evoke a sense of being trapped can be used. Connotative and onomatopoetic words, like "squished," "slimy," "gritty," "velvety buzzing," and "splash," that convey the feeling and capture the sound of experience are helpful.

Empathic Exploration

Empathic exploration involves making explicit what is implicit, and understanding what is at the edge of the client's awareness. Here, in addition to following, the therapist is guiding attention to the client's internal track. This is based on a view of the mind as working by figure and background formation, or by a space with a center and boundaries where experience/ meaning can be at the edge of the mind. What is at the edge of awareness is brought to the center of awareness. By paying attention to something in the background, the mind begins to form a figure in the foreground. This is as opposed to a psychodynamic depth view of the mind in which material is buried in the unconscious—beneath a barrier that needs to be accessed by and interpreted by an observer because it is not available to awareness. Instead, empathic exploration helps clients become focally aware of the not-yet-aware feelings and to experience them.

Empathic Conjectures

These are tentative guesses of clients' immediate, implicit experience. Now, the proportion of leading increases. These responses come from the therapist's frame of reference and are more inferential than exploration. In exploration, the feelings come from the client's frame of reference and make explicit what the client may be feeling or thinking but has not yet said explicitly out loud. Here, the therapist adds a guess to something the client is not saying implicitly or explicitly. The guess comes from the therapist's understanding of the client and also the narrative and case formulation. It helps the client deepen or intensify their experiencing. An example is: "When you think of that, you feel a great sense of sadness and a real sense of loss. My hunch is that you still feel that, and it's still very much alive. Does that fit?"

Empathic Refocusing

Here, the therapist responds to something the client has said earlier that was poignant or seemed important even though the client has veered off in another direction. The therapist empathizes with what the client may be having difficulty facing to invite continued exploration of what seemed most salient. In this case, the therapist is leading by guiding the client to something that seemed poignant or important. When a client goes on a side narrative that takes the focus away from something that seemed meaning-ful or emotionally laden, the therapist may refocus the dialogue back to the earlier topic or experience. For example, the therapist might say, "So, it seems that what was most important is that feeling of being overlooked that you mentioned a while back."

In terms of the prevalence of the different types of responses in a general outpatient context, empathic exploration is seen as the fundamental mode of intervention. Exploratory empathy, however, is always balanced with empathic understanding to provide a framework of safety, acceptance, and validation. The therapist, thus, mixes roughly 50% understanding responses with at least 50% exploratory responses that focus more on articulating what is on the edge of a client's experience to get at what has not yet been said explicitly. When a therapist's exploratory response ends with a focus on what appears to be most alive in a client's statement, the client's attention is focused on this aspect of their experience. The client then is encouraged to focus on and differentiate the leading edges of their experience.

Exploratory empathy is exemplified in the following segment in which a depressed client explores her experience at the end of a romantic relationship:

CLIENT: I keep wondering if he will call.

THERAPIST: The image I have is of you is sitting there, waiting for the phone to ring, and even though there is only silence and emptiness, it is just so hard to get up and walk away [evocative empathy] . . . somehow feeling hopeful, hoping he will call. [exploratory empathic attunement]

CLIENT: I keep hoping he will come back (*weeps softly*).

THERAPIST: So, somehow hoping keeps the door open? [exploratory empathy]

CLIENT: Yes. I guess I have been reluctant to move on. . . . It makes me feel so sad, but I am beginning to realize there is no point in hanging around.

When the therapist's responses are structured in such a way that they end with a focus on what is felt, the client's attention is, in turn, focused on their feelings, and they are more likely to differentiate the feeling. This helps the client symbolize previously implicit experience consciously in awareness. In the next excerpt, the therapist consistently focuses on the client's emotional experience with exploratory responses and questions as well as with empathic conjectures. The client initially focuses externally, but the therapist's consistent focus internally guides the client inward:

CLIENT: My parents just expected me to work around the house. I didn't ever have the chance.

THERAPIST: It's sad that I don't have the freedom. It's sad that I'm trapped. I feel sad that my teens and early 20s, when I could be having fun . . . [conjecture]

CLIENT: There's no support at all. It just makes me feel locked up instead.

THERAPIST: What is it like to feel so trapped? [exploratory question]

CLIENT: Feels very depressing. You wake up every day, and it's just another day, here it goes again. You don't feel joy, you don't feel the hope for the future. You don't feel, you just feel dead. [external]

THERAPIST: Feel sad that there's nothing to look forward to but to earn money and pay the bills. I feel so sad. I used to want things, and now I don't. [internal focus]

CLIENT: And the future, it just doesn't—doesn't feel there's a future ahead of me, just feels there's a huge question mark in front of me. And then it's like growing up . . . you have to wonder through that question mark, like what's the next thing that's going to happen. I don't have a normal plan, a concrete plan of what I'm going to do. When I think I'm able to do this, it turns out . . . [reflexive]

THERAPIST: How are you feeling right now? I sense some sadness. [internal, exploratory]

CLIENT: Ya, just sadness only. The anger just gives way to sadness, I don't feel anger. The anger switches off, and it's sadness. [internal]

THERAPIST: How do you experience this sadness in your body sadness within? [exploratory question, internal]

CLIENT: I feel it on my shoulders. It's just like the only thing I can do is to smash it. [internal]

THERAPIST: I feel so heavy on my shoulders. I feel so burdened and tired, and I can't get it out. I can only harm. [internal]

CLIENT: Then, sometimes, you take the chisel, and you work on chipping everything off one by one, and it's so many things. [reflexive]

THERAPIST: I just feel so overwhelmed, so overloaded, feel like the weight is crushing me down. No choice but to keep going with this heavy weight upon my shoulders. [internal conjecture]

CLIENT: Ya, that's the only thing I can do. That's the only thing I can do for my mom also. [external]

It is important to remember that people's internal emotional signals might be so slight and may speak in a voice so soft that it may be hard for them to hear their own voice. Clients may need to be helped to pay attention to their soft, inner voice, and they may need to have therapists run the clients' experience through them, acting as a type of surrogate experiencer who is trying to find words to describe the experience. Therapists help clients make more attention available to listen to their internal voice. They do so first by providing safety and, second, by focusing on the leading edge of clients' experience. Safety helps clients increase the amount of attention available by reducing their interpersonal anxiety.

Earlier, I commented on the centrality of exploratory empathy for general outpatient populations, but I also have found that with more disorganized clients and with more alexithymic clients—those who do not have words for feelings—and for clients who are blocked, emotionally unskilled, or emotionally illiterate, that empathic conjectures often are the most helpful responses. Here, the therapist is more inferential and reaches in and speaks the unspoken, and symbolizes in words the probably not yet fully formed, not yet felt emotion. Therapists learning an emotion-based approach often find these the most challenging types of responses to include in their repertoire because they have been trained to be more nondirective, to not lead the witness or not put words in their client's mouth but, rather, to ask questions. Some therapists seem to be concerned that when they name a person's experience, it deprives that person of the opportunity to express it or name it themselves. I find that this is not really true; often it brings clients more into the present moment and helps them be in touch with themselves.

Psychotherapists are often taught to ask clients questions such as, "What did you experience?" Although standard therapeutic interviewing practice, asking questions about feeling when a client is not emotionally aroused often does little to further therapeutic exploration; such questions guide attention to provide more cognitive answers or to analyze what is going on. It is far better for therapists to notice what is actually unfolding in front of them in the present moment and to reflect what they see and hear. When therapists reflect the client's experience with compassion, curiosity, and transparency, people typically feel more understood and connected.

Trainees often fear that if they conjecture, they may not get it right or the client will feel intruded on or pushed, or both. The problem is that with clients who are emotionally blocked—like many clients who have eating disorders or a large proportion of men who avoid emotions—it is necessary to use a lot of emotion language to help them begin to identify emotions. Also, conjectures are offered, not from an expert stance of telling clients what they feel but in a collaborative, tentative, and exploratory fashion.

Some support for offering conjectures to help people symbolize what they feel comes from memory research, which shows that recall memory is much more demanding than recognition memory. Recalling something involves deeper processing and requires more time. If I ask what you had for breakfast this morning, it involves recall. If, instead, I say, "Did you have an egg for breakfast?" it involves recognition—that is, you have the word and check it against memory. Recall requires deeper processing than does recognition. Checking whether you had an egg for breakfast is a type of processing that occurs much more rapidly. When I offer the client a feeling— "I imagine you may have felt kind of humiliated or ashamed"—the client can check what I offered against what they felt and quickly either say, "Yes, exactly" or say, "No, not ashamed, just so afraid." In either case, it is much easier for the client to symbolize what was felt than if asked the question "What did you feel?"

Empathic Validation of Needs Versus Confrontation

In working empathically, the therapist adopts a nonexpert, validating stance. Confronting clients with discrepancies in what they say and do or suggesting that they are responsible for their problematic behaviors—when they themselves are not yet able to recognize this—is an intervention discussed in the literature (Adler & Myerson, 1973; Kernberg, 1984; Sachse, 2019) that automatically puts the therapist in the stance of a more challenging, knowing expert. To manage these situations empathically, the therapist first needs to talk about their own experience that they want to share with the client rather than about objective realities that define the client. Second, the therapist needs to validate the visible maladaptive behavior and emotions ("I understand how angry that made you feel") and recognize it as an important self-protective strategy from the past ("No wonder given how your father always criticized you"). Third, the therapist needs to try to go one level deeper and empathetically conjecture into the underlying vulnerable emotions ("But I guess you felt your efforts were so unrecognized"). Fourth, the therapist needs to link this to the unmet need ("And you have missed this all your life").

Most difficult interpersonal moments that arise in therapy can easily be bypassed without having to confront clients with counterproductive behavior or to contradict or challenge them. For example, imagine you have a client who frequently veers off topic into long monologues or stories rather than stays focused on the task at hand. Instead of saying, "You sometimes talk a lot, and I think you do this to avoid dealing with your own feelings," an empathic therapist would say something like the following:

> I really get that you need me to understand you, and when I miss meeting what you need, it leaves you feeling this terrible feeling of being unimportant and unseen, so you sometimes respond by telling a story or moving over to a topic you're interested in. And I really understand you missed the validation of your parents so much when you were a child, and it left you feeling sensitive to not feeling understood by people. But, somehow, right now, when you start off on a story or comment on current events, it doesn't really help me to grasp what is going on inside of you. And then, when I don't get you, it doesn't help you to get what you really need from me. So, I guess the thing we have to focus on is how to deal with this deep feeling of being unimportant in a way that helps you to get the validation you really need.

If you have a client who withdraws rather than fills the air with off-topic narrative, you can adjust your empathic response by saying, "When you stop talking, I am unable to understand your need, and, consequently, you aren't able to get what you need from me."

In sum, the steps of dealing with these difficult moments rather than confronting are:

1. Talk about the therapist's own experience.

2. Validate the client's need (what the client really yearns for).

3. Link the unmet need to the maladaptive emotion ("When your need for validation is not met, it leaves you feeling unimportant").

4. Link the maladaptive emotion to the secondary emotion or the reactive behavior ("And then, when you feel unimportant, you withdraw/talk a lot").

5. Emphasize and validate that the secondary emotion/behavior does not really help to get the need met ("But, somehow, withdrawing/talking a lot doesn't really help me to see you and for you to feel understood").

6. Guide the client's attention to the painful underlying maladaptive emotion that needs to be processed ("And, therefore, we have to help you deal with your feeling of being unimportant in a different way").

7. End by focusing again on the unmet need ("What you really need is validation").

Compassion

Another important aspect of the process of attunement to affect is the experience and expression of compassion. Rogers's (1957) unconditional regard is the closest to describing compassion. Therapists need to be present and have empathy to develop compassion. We (Geller & Greenberg, 2002) have proposed that therapeutic presence is a necessary foundation for the development of empathy. To empathy, compassion adds a deep caring and respect as well as a desire to reduce suffering. Compassion, empathy, and presence are all necessary for the development of a strong, effective therapeutic relationship and for emotional change in psychotherapy.

Compassion allows therapists to not focus on their own needs and issues but, rather, focus on the client's pain and suffering. Compassion does not have a distinct facial expression, but it does involve a look of intense interest in the other person (Davidson & Harrington, 2002). From a Buddhist perspective, *compassion* is defined as "the wish that all beings be free of suffering" (His Holiness the Dalai Lama, 2001, p. iv). From this perspective, compassion implies care for alleviation of the other's suffering but also implies engaging in some action to bring about that lessening in the other's suffering.

Compassion is not simply a sense of sympathy or caring for a person's suffering, and it is not simply warmth or the understanding of their needs and pains. Although compassion encompasses these, it also involves the sustained determination to do whatever is possible and necessary to help alleviate the other's suffering. One has the feeling of caring for another person and their suffering, and the desire to reduce that suffering, but also the taking of some action to help reduce the other's suffering. Compassion is not true compassion unless it involves action. Therapists need to be involved in engaging in whatever actions they can to alleviate their client's suffering, such as making calls, writing letters, coordinating with other helpers, and making referrals.

CASE FORMULATION

Empathic attunement is also aided by having a case formulation. Given that working with emotion focuses on accessing and transforming core painful emotions, and even though attunement is an automatic process coming out of being present in the moment to client's emotional states, it helps to have an understanding of what a client's core pain is. Goldman and Greenberg

(2015) elaborated on how to construct emotion-focused case formulations. These formulations have a unique dual focus privileging emotional process first but always understanding it in the context of narrative meaning-making. This supports the effort to build a picture of the case with the core emotion scheme at the center. Identifying the core painful emotion scheme is central to emotion-focused formulation.

Case formulation is helpful in facilitating the development of a focus. It is the client's presently felt experience that indicates what the difficulty is and indicates whether problem determinants are currently accessible and amenable to intervention. A collaborative focus and a coherent theme develop from a focus on current experience and an exploration of particular experiences to their edges within the context of the task-focused work at markers. It is by going deeply into experience in specific situations rather than by establishing patterns across situations that a focus is established. *Markers* are in-session states that reveal that the client is in a particular type of problem state that is an opportunity for a particular type of intervention (Greenberg, Rice, & Elliott, 1993). Formulations need to be coconstructions that emerge from joint understanding rather than formed by the therapist. In addition, all formulations are held tentatively and are repeatedly checked with the client for how well they fit and if they seem relevant to the client's aims. A client's moment-to-moment processing in the session, however, is the ultimate guide as to what the therapist does in the moment.

Therapists adopt the notion of a "pain compass" that guides formulation. The compass directs the therapist to the client's chronic enduring pain (Goldman & Greenberg, 2015; Greenberg, 2015; Greenberg & Paivio, 1997). The therapist follows what is most painful or poignant, which will lead to the client's core painful emotions. The goal of the treatment becomes to resolve this painful issue. Emotional pain is a strong cue that something for the client is feeling broken or shattered (Greenberg & Bolger, 2001). Using all of their sense mediums, therapists need to hear people's pain.

CONCLUSION

In this chapter, I attempted to highlight that empathic attunement to affect goes beyond empathy as generally understood to be the offering of understanding. Both empathic understanding and empathic attunement to affect are important, but affect attunement is more focused on emotion than meaning, and it is a more resonant, bodily mirroring of the client's affective contours. Creating an alliance to work on emotion is the entry point to attunement, whereas internal tracking is the key to maintaining an attuned connection.

Building on the ability to be present, and having as a first step letting go of personal distractions and any preformed ideas about clients, therapists need to engage in the following steps to be empathically attuned (Barrett-Lennard, 1993, 1997; Elliott et al., 2004). They need to enter the client's world, trying to become the client and attempting to see things as the client sees them rather than looking from an outside perspective. In supervision, I stop the supervisees' video recording and ask them, "Become your client. As your client, what is it you are feeling?" Then, therapists need to resonate with their client's experiencing by attending to what in them responds in kind (i.e., echoes, reverberates) to it. They need to identify in themselves what it might feel like to feel this. This is where the activation of mirror neurons and the brain's simulation of what it feels like to feel what they are imagining plays a role. Next, therapists need to search for, grasp, and capture what their client's core painful feelings are, aided by attending to their sense of what it might feel like for the client. Finally, therapists need to put words to their client's feelings. Symbolizing feelings in words helps clients externalize their feelings, look at them, and talk about and differentiate them to make new meaning.

Therapists using these steps always privilege affect over meaning, and responses are focused on attending to the client's core painful feeling. In focusing like this on core painful emotions, which clients find difficult to feel, therapists continually remind clients that they are in charge of the process and need go only as far as they can tolerate. They also remind them that it is the clients who are the experts on their own experience: They know best what hurts and that the therapist is searching with them to help them discover and experience their core painful feelings. In this regard, therapist curiosity and an inquiring attitude are important. Therapists need to adopt a not-knowing position, even when conjecturing about what the client feels. Therapists do not assume that they know but more are curious and work hard to understand the other, who remains somewhat of a delicate mystery. In addition, therapists convey the message to clients that, ultimately, the road to change lies within themselves and involves reclaiming disowned feelings, having new emotions to change old emotions, or both.

One of the things that was most helpful to me when I started off as a therapist in training, having come from South Africa to Canada and having changed my professional career from engineering to counseling, was that everything was completely novel: a new country, a new profession, the new activity of counseling. I experienced myself as something like a cultural anthropologist trying to learn about this new culture. My previous stereo-types, assumptions, and prejudices did not fit. I saw the Canadians and Americans (of whom there were many because of the Vietnam War), with whom I was in touch in and outside of counseling, as unusual creatures whom I had to learn about. This was incredibly helpful in being able to be nonjudgmental, accepting, and empathic, and in being able to simply listen carefully and try to understand.

In the next chapter, I elaborate more on the bodily experience of attune-ment. In the safe environment that empathic attunement makes possible, we therapists can invite clients to attend to, welcome, symbolize, and explore their more painful feelings.

6 FOCUSING ON BODILY FEELINGS

When Words Are Not Enough

In the ongoing practice of psychotherapy, a client and their therapist exchange many words in an attempt to make the therapeutic conversation come alive. In the midst of all the verbal communication, frequently missing is the sense of the client's experiencing what they are talking about at some depth and of both people's being emotionally engaged in the process. Therapy can too easily become reduced to *people-talking*: communicating with words but often ignoring the intense sense of life that can emerge if they tap into immediate emotional and body-centered experience. Becoming aware of bodily felt emotion is more important than awareness of thought.

In this chapter, I present different forms of guiding awareness to bodily felt experience with an emphasis on putting words to body experience. I look at the difference between experiencing and emotional arousal, and the importance of each in therapeutic change. I also delineate three general methods: awareness and symbolization of inner bodily feelings, expression of emotion, and observation of nonverbal behaviors. Finally, I present and illustrate through clinical examples methods of focusing on a bodily felt sense, promoting the vivid expression of emotions, and working on what the body expresses nonverbally.

https://doi.org/10.1037/0000248-007
Changing Emotion With Emotion: A Practitioner's Guide, by L. S. Greenberg

One of the key aspects of emotion-focused work is that it is experiential. Emotion-oriented therapists work actively to help clients become aware of their inner bodily felt experiences. It is new experience, not insight, that is viewed as changing the brain. The purpose of this work is to reclaim one's experience and action tendencies, and to reown emotions. Experiential work as opposed to insight-oriented psychotherapy teaches clients to work with their bodily felt experience and with emotional expression more than with understanding. The following example illustrates the difference between an experiential response and an understanding or insight-oriented one:

CLIENT: My boss really upset me this week. I did a huge project for him, spent the night working at home. It wasn't really even my job, and he didn't even say thank you. Then I heard yesterday that he talked about it in a meeting like he had done all the work.

SAMPLE UNDERSTANDING RESPONSE: Sounds like you are being taken advantage of. You're extending yourself and getting no appreciation. [This might include an additional insight-oriented component:] Does this remind you of your relationship with anyone?

SAMPLE EXPERIENTIAL RESPONSE: Let's try and slow down so you can stay with what is happening inside right now as you tell me this. [This might include a process-guiding component:] Maybe you can go inside to that place where you feel your feelings and see what you feel there right now.

The latter response differs from the more understanding/insight response, in which the therapist might adopt a following response, rather than a guiding one, that focuses more on the content of the story and possibly offers an interpretative aspect to help create meaning. The best way to be experiential in therapeutic work is to be present centered and to focus on bodily felt experience, In Chapter 5, I discussed the importance of empathic attunement to affect as a baseline skill for doing this. Another major method is to guide the client's attention to their bodily felt experience.

GUIDING ATTENTION TO PRESENT EXPERIENCE

Early on, William James (1890) pointed out, "My experience is what I choose to attend to" (pp. 403–404), adding that without selective interest, experience would be chaos. In the 1950s, Gestalt therapy, influenced by Zen Buddhist practice, introduced present-centered awareness exercises that helped people focus attention on their current body sensations and feelings (see Chapter 5, this volume, for a more detailed discussion of these exercises). Such awareness practices that link sensory awareness and thinking highlight the constructive nature of experience. Someone shuttling between inner or outer sensory awareness might say, "Now I'm aware of a tightening in my chest, and I imagine I am having a heart attack." This method of verbalizing present awareness is helpful in bringing awareness of bodily experience to the fore because body experience is always what is occurring in the present. One thus can suggest to clients—especially when they are unsure what emotions they feel or when they seem wrapped up in logistical details of a story—that they come into the present and, over the next few minutes, describe at each moment what they are aware of. The therapist can suggest the client begin every sentence with "Right now . . ." or "At this moment . . ." and complete it with their immediate experience.

Mindfulness

Mindfulness, in my clinical experience, is attending to present-moment experience with equanimity. This means maintaining a moment-by-moment awareness of thoughts, emotions, and bodily sensations with openness and curiosity. Mindfulness can be described as the practice of paying attention in the present moment and doing it intentionally and with nonjudgment. *Mindfulness meditation practices* refer to the deliberate acts of regulating attention through the observation of thoughts, emotions, and body states. Typical mindfulness activities include nonjudgmental awareness of breath, body, feelings, emotions, thoughts, or all of these in sitting meditation practice or throughout the day.

Mindfulness can be thought of a "state," a "trait," or a "practice." One can have a moment of mindfulness, which is a state of mind in the moment. One can also have a sustained experience that is more like a habit or strong tendency to be mindful—a trait. Or one can engage in a more intentional practice of mindfulness by using different forms, postures, and activities, such as seated mindfulness meditation, mindful walking, and mindful eating.

Focusing Approach

Gendlin (1981) in his focusing approach proposed a process of guiding attention to a different target: a bodily felt sense, the sensations in a person's body that provide information about situations, thoughts, and feelings. The felt sense differs from the more concrete-in-the-moment awareness of what one is. In focusing, therapists invite clients to go to that place inside where they feel their feelings, learn to "stay" with this felt sense, and follow where it goes once symbolized in awareness (Gendlin, 1969, 1991).

The intention in focusing is to deepen bodily felt experience, which might simply involve gently asking, "What is it inside?" and waiting for an answer. The client can then let words come from the bodily sensed feeling and maybe get a sense of the problem as a whole—and then let what is important about it come up from that bodily sensing. This is the focusing process and represents a basic style of engagement with internal experience that I am encouraging for working with emotion.

Focusing introduces a style of guiding and giving directions that goes beyond the relational aspect of therapy. The therapist is not only in dialogue with the client using empathic responses but is now guiding the client to engage in a new kind of relationship with themselves—to pay attention to their bodily felt sense. Focusing, then, is a powerful addition to the therapist's tool kit. It can be said that working with emotion stands on two legs: empathic attunement to affect and focus on the bodily felt sense. Therapists' empathic attunement to affect and exploratory empathic responses that focus on the leading edge of clients' experience have some of the effect of focusing by, to some degree, guiding attention to the implicit. Focusing as an intervention, however, does this more directly: It helps clients target their deeper "felt" sense of what they are talking about by guiding them to pause and stay with what they are feeling, to pay attention to their bodily felt sense, and to ask them how "all that" feels in their bodies. Only clients can know what they feel, and they can fully know only through paying attention to their own experiencing and finding ways to formulate it and carry it forward. Focusing is about clients' paying attention to their bodily felt sense.

How do therapists know when to use focusing as an intervention? Often therapists seamlessly guide their clients to focus on the felt sense in the ongoing interaction when, out of their own felt sense of what is needed, they slow the client down when some feeling is being expressed or simply ask the client to pay attention to what they feel inside. At other times, however, when there are specific indicators—what I have called "markers"—this is a time to use focusing. The classical markers for focusing are when the client refers to a vague or unclear felt sense or seems to be on the surface of something important but is unable to sink down into it. These are opportunities for a more major focusing intervention.

The Felt Sense

The notion of felt sense is important in understanding focusing, and I elaborate on it in this section. Focusing is neither getting in touch with feelings nor doing a rational analysis of a situation. Rather, it involves giving attention to the feel of the situation as a whole. For example, our sense of a situation as a whole might be that there is something "unfair" about it. We try that word out, and then it seems that it is not so much "unfair" as "diminishing." Our attention moves back and forth between the words we are trying out and something else. The "something else" is not exactly a thought or an emotion but a bodily feeling—the feeling of the whole situation. This is called a bodily felt sense and is similar to having a word on the tip of your tongue, but, this time, it is a feeling that is felt somewhere in the body. When people are eventually able to put words to it, it is often not a basic emotion like anger or sadness. Rather, it is a complex felt meaning of the whole situation, full of implications, such as feeling "over the hill," "all washed out," "fulfilled," or hurt, disappointed, small, or unsupported.

Focusing is a process of interacting with the felt sense of something. Suppose you look at a particular piece of art. You may think it was done by an impressionist, or it may evoke a feeling of sadness. As another option, you may focus on a felt sense of the whole picture and say, "It's filled with energy, unconstrained," or you might not even find *any* words, yet the felt sense is still there. The *felt sense*—the focused feel of the whole picture—is not a thought or an emotion, and it is also different from the initial unfocused experiencing of the picture.

Focusing involves moving back and forth between the bodily felt sense and words that symbolize it. Focusing is a way of helping to make the implicit explicit, and it helps to clarify what the process of "staying with" or "working through" actually entails. It is a matter of taking a bit of time to allow a felt sense to form and to then give it attention. Some people do this without having been taught to do so. Some clients do it naturally in therapy, and those who do tend to be more successful than those who do not. Research has provided evidence that clients who focus on the felt sense of their situation tend to make better progress than clients who do other things or talk in other ways (Hendricks, 2002).

Focusing shows that one's experiencing can be formulated in many ways but not in any old way (Purton, 2004). Someone who is focusing may first symbolize their experiencing as "feeling embarrassed." Then, they sense that this is not quite right. They go back to the felt sense of the situation that they are working with, and now it seems to them that it is not embarrassment they feel but humiliation. And then, with further focusing, an aspect of sadness comes to the fore. In the felt sense, all these formulations are implicit. It is not a matter of one of them being the truth and the others being mistaken. They each have their truth—at least at the time when they are felt. But that there are multiple formulations does not mean that the focuser could formulate their experience in any way they choose. Certainly, they are not feeling happy or jealous! And if their therapist tries out the suggestion that they are feeling regret, something in them will clearly say no. The felt sense determines precisely what can be said, and yet what is said may not be the only thing that can be said (Purton, 2004).

It is important to recognize that what people feel, in part, depends on how they describe it. Naming an emotion, however, is not simply discovering the right words to fit the feeling, like finding the right key to fit a lock. There is not only one correct word. Feelings are not sitting inside fully formed and articulated, and waiting to be named. People actively create what they feel by the way they describe the feeling. Helping a person articulate how they feel is more like the process of looking at the clouds and "seeing" a rabbit in the cloud than like the process involved in the seeing an actual rabbit hiding behind a tree. Emotional naming involves as much creation as it does discovery. This is all in line with the dialectical constructivist perspective discussed in Chapter 1.

Use of Focusing Techniques

A number of studies have been done in Japan, North America, and Europe on factors that enhance the effectiveness of focusing. For example, Morikawa (1997) factor analyzed questionnaires from focusing sessions and found that "clearing a space," "finding a right distance," and having a listener refer to their experiencing each helped clients focus. Iberg (1991) found that clients reported an increased impact of sessions in which therapists used focusing-type questions. Leijssen (1998) investigated whether focusing enhanced client-centered therapy. In an initial study, she took sessions with explicitly positive and negative evaluations by client or therapist and found that 75% of positive sessions contained focusing steps and 33% of negative sessions contained focusing. In a second study, Leijssen (1996–1997) looked at the video recorded therapies of eight clients who successfully terminated therapy in less than 20 sessions: Prominent use of focusing occurred in all eight cases; almost every session acquired an intense experience-oriented character in which the client discovered aspects of the problem that had formerly remained out of reach. All of these clients achieved contact with their bodily felt experience without being flooded by it.

Leijssen (1998) also investigated whether long-term clients deemed to be stagnating in their therapy could be taught to focus and to increase experiencing level. Of the four clients who were taught focusing, all returned to their regular therapy. She found that two of them who returned to their previous and less deep levels of experiencing in therapy expressed unhappiness with their regular therapists; they conveyed a wish to continue with the focusing trainer. For clients with initially low levels of experiencing, it appears that clients do not easily learn the skill; thus, for focusing to take place and be sustained, continued process direction is required (Leijssen et al., 2000).

In introducing focusing, the therapist might suggest to clients that it could be helpful to focus on the feeling that they had just talked about and then give some focusing instructions (Gendlin, 1981, 1996). The therapist might simply say, "Close your eyes and go inside to that place inside where you are feeling this feeling. Just stay with it and see what you feel now in your body, and let whatever comes come." The client then needs to stay very gently with the feeling, and the therapist needs to encourage them to welcome it, rather than try not to feel it. It can be helpful to tell the client to pay attention to any images that may come even before words.

The intervention might start with guiding the client to <u>clear a space in their mind</u> to pay attention inwardly to their body and see what comes there when they ask themselves, "What is the main thing for me right now?" Then, the therapist asks the client to put the concern aside, like pushing a piece of furniture to the side of a room to clear a space in the center. The client is then asked to select one personal problem to focus on and to pay attention to that place in their body where they usually feel things. There, they get a <u>felt sense</u> of what all of the problem feels like. The therapist guides the client to first get at the sensory quality of this unclear felt sense—like "tight" or "heavy" or "dark"—and then get to words or phrases or images to <u>describe in words</u> the felt sense. Next, they are given time to <u>check</u> that the words fit and to go back and forth between the felt sense and the words to see in their body that they feel the words fit. They then are guided to <u>ask</u> what is it about this whole problem that makes it feel this way and to see if there is a felt shift in the felt sense in the body. The last step is to <u>receive</u> and welcome whatever comes. It is helpful for the therapist to point out that whatever comes is just a step, and more steps will come, and no bad feeling is the last feeling. The therapist will probably continue after a little while but will stay here for a few moments.

A Clinical Example of Focusing and Experiencing an Emotional Shift

Let's look at a more specific example. Jonathan, a 59-year-old academic at a university, is feeling upset about not being awarded a grant he applied for. He found out this morning and has been busy since. He has felt tense and upset throughout the day, but this is the first time he is talking about it.

He says to his therapist, whom he has being seeing for a few months for anxiety and problems in living, that he is shocked because he was sure he would get the grant. After talking about it for a while and saying how upset he is, he says he does not really know what he feels.

The therapist suggests that Jonathan focus. The process of arriving at his feeling goes something like this: After focusing his attention on the unpleasant sensation in the center of his chest, Jonathan first says it is a tight knot and then a kind of sinking feeling. He then says, "I feel really disappointed." As he continues to focus inside on the feeling in his chest, he imagines the review committee sitting at a table criticizing his proposal. What comes for him is, "I feel like a failure. I'm also a bit ashamed." His body sense changes. New words come from this sense: "I'm unsure about what this means for the next steps of my life. Maybe I'm on the wrong path." His feeling develops slightly as he stays over time with his body sense of it. What comes next is, "I'm a bit embarrassed, but most of all, I'm tired and discouraged. I don't want to keep trying and repeatedly not have my efforts pay off. I feel powerless."

At this point, Jonathan stops, takes a breath, and says, "That's it! I feel so powerless. That's what is so disturbing." The tightness in his body now releases a bit. He feels something shift. The therapist encourages him to stay with whatever is new or fresh that comes from the feeling. Then, out of another place in his body, what emerges is: "I feel angry at the unfairness. A lot of it is politics and image management." His anger feels better than feeling powerless. What comes next is: "Maybe I was shooting too high. I didn't really want to do this; it's not really where my heart is. Maybe I need to reorganize my priorities." Notice how nonlinear this is; accessing his anger allows him to let go of, or reorganize, around the goal that has been frustrated. At this point, either this emerging sense—that it is not so important to him—feels right to him or doesn't. His bodily sense, if he really listens to it, will tell him if this meaning fits. If it does, he will again feel a shift in his body. The bad feeling will continue to open up and lighten. It will no longer be a tight knot. It will begin to move and become more fluid, spiraling into a different pattern, letting in more air and lightness. Something will have shifted.

This shift is quite different from what occurs when the meaning created is an excuse, a type of self-deception to save face or deceive himself. In the preceding example, Jonathan's saying "I didn't really want this" could be an excuse if, deep down in his heart, he was still set on doing this type of work and was trying to convince himself that he did not care anymore. Then, his inner bodily feeling might change but in quite a different way: It would become tighter. His shoulders might tense up, and his voice might become strained even if it is only the voice in his head. He will tense some part in his body in his efforts to distance himself from the disappointment to support the deception and to protect himself from some feeling he feels that he simply cannot bear.

The whole process in which the therapist has encouraged him to engage is not one of thinking about the issue in any effortful sense. Rather than rationally explaining, Jonathan is paying attention to his body. Words and pictures are coming from the felt sense. This is quite different from a reasoning process. Here, it is more like seeing than doing. It is a process in which he is more a recipient of impressions than an active problem-solver. This process has more in common with free association than reasoning, but it is highly body focused.

Whatever way he resolves it, it was feeling something new that led to change. He might begin to clarify: "Really, I don't want to keep working so hard. I've reached my ceiling. Maybe I will retire. I've always wanted to travel and read more. Maybe this is an opportunity in disguise." Or, he might say, "I'll change my focus. I really wasn't going with my strengths in that proposal. I need to reorient myself." Whichever solution emerges, it came about by a body-based feeling process that leads to the creation of new meaning.

MEASURING EXPERIENCING

To deepen bodily felt experience through a technique such as focusing, it can be helpful to use the depth of experiencing (EXP) Scale (Klein et al., 1969) to analyze video recorded sessions. Clinicians also can benefit by looking at the moment-by-moment impact on EXP of their empathic interventions or any intervention they may make to see if they deepen experience. Klein et al. (1969) developed the scale to measure EXP. The EXP Scale defines clients' involvement in inner referents of experience as moving from talking about things in impersonal way (Level 1), to describing one's experience at a superficial level (Level 2; e.g., "It's hard for people in close relationships to be angry at each other"), to expressing externalized or limited references to feelings and reactions (Level 3; e.g., "And then I got annoyed at what he said"), to a clear shift inward to directly focus on inner experiencing and feelings (Level 4; e.g., "I felt myself getting more and more upset, kind of like tightening up inside—inside, like wanting to explode, feeling, uh, both insulted and angry"). Level 4 is the point at which focusing on a felt sense is achieved. Now, the client's process shifts to questioning or propositioning about the self's internal feelings and personal experiences

(Level 5); to a synthesis of readily accessible and newly realized feelings and experiences to resolve personally-significant issues (Level 6; "Yeah, I realized that this feeling of anger and feeling insulted and wronged finally gave voice to what I have been carrying with me for a long time, and now there's no turning back"); to a point at which there is a full, easy presentation of experiencing. All elements are confidently integrated in an expansive, illuminating, confident, buoyant manner (Level 7).

When clients are processing at a low level of EXP, the therapist facilitates deeper experiencing sometimes by symbolizing feelings in words by empathically exploring or conjecturing as to what clients are presently experiencing. Or, the therapist may guide attention inward to focus directly on bodily felt experience. Promoting awareness of these bodily felt feelings involves engaging people in a real internal experiential search for what they are feeling. Here, the core feeling is often unclear or is initially even absent from awareness. There is something there—a felt meaning that can be sensed. It is in their bodies, but they do not yet know what it is.

Having just looked at how focusing works, let's now look at working with expressing emotions.

WORKING WITH EMOTIONAL AROUSAL AND EXPRESSION

The process of emotional arousal and expression also involves the body. Now, however, the process is not one of attending to the body but, rather, engaging the body in expressive action. It offers another way of working with emotion. It involves stimulating feelings, intensifying them so that they spontaneously break through the intellectual veil of words and express themselves in tears, in shakiness, or in anger. They are experienced in some visceral way in the body. In contrast to focusing on the bodily felt sense to create new felt meaning, in the arousal process, the emotion is evoked, and the client moves toward unrestricted expression. Instead of developing a form of knowing, the client develops a form of doing. In the focusing process, words bring out feelings not yet felt; in expression, felt feelings lead to words that make meanings. In focusing, the feeling does not rise up as readily as in the case of expression. Rather, the feeling is waiting in the felt sense to be formed into meaning, and the feeling is implicit in the person's body.

One could ask, Is it better or more therapeutic to work with emotional arousal or with the felt sense? I think that a strict focus on either alone can limit therapeutic possibilities. To be therapeutically effective in changing emotion with emotion, we therapists need to value both working with expressed emotion and the felt sense, and recognize that the way of working directly on emotional expression differs from the way of focusing on the felt sense. Each of these processes—attending to bodily experience and expressing aroused emotion—are central to emotion work, and both are important processes of change. Also important is this: In talking about emotional expression, we are talking about expressing previously unexpressed emotion in therapy. We are not encouraging unbridled expression of emotion in the real world, which can be highly counterproductive.

Emotion arousal involves the visceral experience of the emotion and a state of heightened physiological activity. It manifests itself in some form of heightened overt and covert bodily activities that create a readiness for action. Arousal, then, is a state of heightened activity in both body and mind that makes us more alert and acts along a spectrum from low to high. One can be slightly aroused, or one can be extremely highly aroused. Acute states of arousal characterize all vital emotions, and the subjective experience of these acute states is part and parcel of all strong feelings. Emotional arousal is consequently an essential component of such experiences as sadness and happiness, love and hate, despair and elation, grief and joy, anger and calm, pleasure and displeasure, and so on.

Stimulation

Arousal is the result of stimulation. When people are stimulated appropriately, then we become aroused. With greater stimulation, we become more aroused. Arousal in an emotion-focused view typically happens when the body releases chemicals into the brain that act to stimulate emotions, reduce cortical functioning and hence conscious control, and create physical activation and readiness for action. Arousal starts in the primitive brain stem, proceeds through different parts of the brain, and engages the endocrine system. It increases oxygen and glucose flow; dilates the pupils (so one can see better); and suppresses nonurgent systems, such as digestion and the immune system. Arousal is spread through the sympathetic nervous system with effects, such as increasing the heart rate and breathing to enable physical action and perspiration to cool the body. Clearly, it involves a change in experiential state. Expressing how one feels is not always easy to do.

When emotional arousal and expression occur in therapy, a strong feeling rises up for the client, washes over them, and takes over what they say. There is no need for the person to go looking for this emotion; it comes to the person very clearly. People, who have words for emotions, describe them easily with such words as "I feel angry, sad, or afraid." Expressing the feeling promotes the experience of it. A person might then say, "I miss him" and burst into tears or say, "I hate you" to an imagined other in an empty chair and feel the anger. When expressed, the emotions become readily available and intensely felt. As people express these clearly felt emotions, they begin to speak from them, and more meaning emerges. People then begin to speak from the strong feeling and say, "I feel so empty without him, like I don't quite have my bearings" or "I can never forgive him for what he did." This is the process, of expressing aroused emotion in words.

Emotion can be expressed at differing degrees of arousal in different ways: verbally in conversation, in writing (e.g., a diary), or in movement. Sometimes it helps to use more nonverbal means to express emotion. Asking people to paint what they feel, sculpt it, or play it in music can offer release through creativity, but then, in therapy, it is usually advantageous to try and help them put what they have expressed nonverbally into words.

Once people have words, it is easier to work with their emotions. For example, say a client has difficult feelings regarding her father's abandonment of her as a child. The therapist helps her to attend to and explore her bad feeling. The client feels many emotions: feelings of sadness, anger at the father, pain and fear of being left alone in the world, grief and anger at her mother for not being there for her, and fear that an expression of anger would result in the loss of her father's and mother's love. At some point in a session, the therapist, sensing that the client's fear interrupts her expression of anger at her father, helps her to access her anger rather than interrupt it by expressing her anger at him in an empty chair. The client, in imagination, becomes the 4-year-old child and expresses to the imagined father of her childhood the sadness of her unmet longings for comfort and protection. After expressing her unmet need, the anger comes to her—the anger that he had been blind to her pain.

As the process continues, having expressed her sadness, her need, and her anger, the client's sense that her father abandoned her begins to change and becomes a sense that he actually was not able to support her and that he would have responded to her if he had known how. In this way, by accessing and expressing emotion, she was able to work through and transform her sadness and anger toward him, and grieve fully for her losses. This is a different process from focusing. It spans a larger period of time than the moment-by-moment process of finding words to express feelings along the way. This process of stimulating arousal and expression also uses both empathic attunement to affect and focus at moments in the process. However, the aim of the whole process goes beyond conveying empathic understanding and beyond focusing on a bodily felt sense to help the client put words to feelings.

Exploration to Activate Emotion

In addition to expressive stimulation, therapists also promote exploration to access emotion. They ask exploratory questions, such as: "How does this emotion make you feel?" "Where do you feel it on your body?" "Where is it coming from, and what triggered it?" and "How do you feel afterward?" They are a sort of cross between asking the person to express to stimulate and focusing on the body felt sense to stimulate. The aim of exploratory questions is not to gain information but to activate by helping people attend to and express what they feel.

But focusing is alive and well in the stimulation process described earlier. First, the client is working with her whole sense of her relationship with her father—a holistic feeling that cannot be divided into distinct emotions. At times, she focuses, or the therapist guides her to focus, to get at the idio-syncratic flavor of the whole experience of her relationship with her father, such as her anger about her father's being blind to her pain. Here is a piece of focusing in action to capture this felt meaning. She is not just expressing anger; she is also differentiating it by focusing on it and finding words to make sense of it. However, her arousal and expression of it comes from stimulation by imagining her father in an empty chair and from the evoking of emotion schematic memories. Her image of herself as a small child that needed protection is not separate from her memory of that time nor from her emotion of longing to be protected. Here, the therapist, in stimulating arousal and expression, is not working just with the client's emotional arousal but with the client's total response to her situation. In the final analysis, work on expressing of aroused emotion and work on focusing are integrated in a seamless fashion.

MEASURING CLIENT EMOTIONAL AROUSAL

As with measurement of a client's EXP, it can be clinically useful to quantify emotional arousal. Clinicians can benefit from analyzing video recordings of their sessions to see which interventions aid and which hinder emotional arousal in their clients. To capture the difference between EXP and arousal, two overlapping but different processes, Warwar and I (Warwar & Greenberg, 1999) developed the Client Emotional Arousal Scale-III-R (see Exhibit 6.1), which rates the degree of arousal in expression as opposed to attention to a bodily felt sense. In this scale, what is being rated is clients' intensity in voice and body, degree of overflow, and degree of restriction of experience and expression. At Level 1, the person does not express emotions and voice,

EXHIBIT 6.1. Client Emotional Arousal Scale-III-R

1 Person does not express emotions
   Voice or gestures **do not** disclose any emotional arousal

2 Person may allow some emotion, but there is **very little** arousal in voice or body
   - There is no disruption of usual speech patterns
   - Any arousal is almost **completely restricted**

3 At this level of arousal as well as higher levels, the person allows emotions
   Arousal is **mild** in voice and body
   - There is very little emotional overflow
   - Any arousal is still **very restricted**
   - Usual speech patterns are only **mildly disrupted**

4 Arousal is **moderate** in voice and body
   - Emotional voice is present: Ordinary speech patterns are **moderately** disrupted by emotional overflow as represented by changes in accentuation patterns, unevenness of pace, changes in pitch
   - Although there is some freedom from control and restraints, arousal may still be **somewhat restricted**

5 Arousal is **fairly intense and full** in voice and body
   - Emotion overflows into speech pattern to a great extent: Speech patterns deviate **markedly** from the client's baseline and are fragmented or broken
   - There is elevated loudness and volume
   - Arousal seems only slightly restricted

6 Arousal is **very intense and extremely full** as the person is freely expressing emotion with voice and body
   - Usual speech patterns are **extremely disrupted** as indicated by changes in accentuation patterns, unevenness of pace, changes in pitch, and volume or force of voice
   - There is spontaneous expression of emotion and there is **almost no sense of restriction**

7* Arousal is **extremely intense and full** in voice and body
   - Usual speech patterns are **completely disrupted** by emotional overflow
   - The expression is completely dysregulated and unrestricted
   - Arousal appears uncontrollable and enduring
   - There is a falling apart quality: Although arousal can be a completely unrestricted therapeutic experience, it may also be a disruptive negative experience in which the clients feels like they are falling apart

   Note: control = containment in contrast to control = restriction

   *The distinguishing feature between Level 6 and Level 7 is that in Level 6, there is the sense that although a person's expression may be fairly unrestricted, this individual would be able to contain or control their arousal, whereas in Level 7, a person's expression is completely unrestricted and there is the sense that emotional arousal would not be within this person's control.

From *Client Emotional Arousal Scale-III-R* [Unpublished manuscript], by S. Warwar and L. S. Greenberg, 1999, York Psychotherapy Research Clinic, York University. Copyright 1999 by Serine Warwar and Leslie S. Greenberg. Adapted with permission.

or gestures do not display any emotional arousal. At Level 2, there is a little arousal in voice or body with no disruption of usual speech patterns. At Level 3, the person allows emotions, but the expression is mild in voice and body, there is little emotional overflow, and any arousal is still very restricted. At Level 4, one gets a noticeable level of arousal that is now moderate in voice and body. There is some freedom from control and restraint, but arousal is still somewhat restricted. At Level 5, arousal is now fairly intense and full in voice and body, and arousal seems only slightly restricted. At Level 6, arousal is intense and extremely full because the person is freely expressing emotion; there is almost no sense of restriction. Level 7 takes a turn in that it represents dysregulation.

This is not a linear scale. Levels 1 to 6 are viewed as increasing step by step, so the more, the better. However, Level 7 represents too much of a good thing because it produces an undesirable state. At Level 7, arousal is extremely intense and full, the expression is completely dysregulated and unrestricted, and arousal appears uncontrollable and enduring. The distinguishing feature between Level 6 and Level 7 is that, at Level 6, there is the sense that although a person's expression may be fairly unrestricted, this individual would be able to make cognitive sense of their emotion, which is still sufficiently contained or under control. At Level 7, on the other hand, a person's expression is completely unrestricted. There is the sense that emotional arousal is not in this person's control, and cognition cannot be brought to bear on it to make sense of it.

Using this scale (see Exhibit 6.1), an emotional response is indicated when a person acknowledges having experienced an emotion (e.g., "I feel afraid") or demonstrates an emotion action tendency (e.g., covering one's head in shame or shrinking back in fear). Warwar and I (Warwar & Greenberg, 1999) found 15 emotion categories most relevant to psychotherapy sessions. Before a segment can be rated on arousal, it first must be categorized according to the following emotion list. If the segment does not fit into any of the categories, it is considered unclassifiable and cannot be rated using the Client Emotional Arousal Scale-III-R (Warwar & Greenberg, 1999):

1. Pain/Hurt
2. Sadness
3. Hopelessness/Helplessness
4. Loneliness
5. Anger/Resentment
6. Contempt/Disgust
7. Fear/Anxiety
8. Love

9. Joy/Excitement
10. Contentment/Calm/Relief
11. Shame/Guilt
12. Pride/Self-confidence
13. Anger and Sadness (both present simultaneously)
14. Pride (Self-Assertion) and Anger (both present simultaneously)
15. Surprise/Shock

PRACTICING BODY WORK: OBSERVING NONVERBAL BEHAVIOR

There are a number of different ways of working even more directly with the body as a carrier of feeling and meaning. Body work is a relatively newer, less-investigated area of clinical practice in emotion work (Totton, 2003). The first step toward working with the body in therapy usually involves therapists' noticing and guiding attention to outward signs of internal experience. This form of working with the body involves taking an observational stance and giving the client feedback or guiding their attention to observable expressions. Bodywork most generally focuses on drawing attention to the client's gestures or body positioning.

A therapist, for example, might ask the client to bring attention to a gesture, ask what those gestures feel like, and then facilitate further discussion about these feelings. This form of intervention is based on the idea that inner states and implicit models of the world express themselves through nonverbal expressions, such as gestures, postures, pace, tension, or relaxation of muscles and other subtle somatic communications. Working with bodily expressions moves therapy from focusing on verbal consciousness and narrative description to deepening into the body. For example, if a client seems to be tightening their jaw when talking about their job, therapists might contact their feeling states by saying, "Your jaw seems like it is clenching." This is to help immerse people in the experience. The therapist might then say, "Just let yourself stay with that and invite that feeling in."

One good way therapists can help themselves develop or enhance this skill is to keep asking themselves, "What is the client doing right now?" For instance, the person could be looking down, looking away, moving in their seat, or perhaps frozen. Each indicates an internal experience that underlies the person's behavior. The therapist also listens to the voice: How much or how little emotion is contained in somebody's voice? Is the tone of their voice weak, loud, quiet, or strong? What is the verbal pace and tonal quality? Is the person's speech pace fast, slow, or does it vary? Is the tone of their voice harsh, even, melodic, monotone, or soft?

The therapist observes the body: What's the body's position? How is the body in relationship to gravity? What images does the body evoke? Is the body grounded? Is it constricted, flaccid, or tight? What are the movements? Are the person's movements relaxed or active? Are their movements jerky or smooth, controlled or spontaneous? What are the gestures? Does the person move or gesture? Is their gesture repetitive? What is the quality of the gesture? Is it gentle, aggressive, or abrupt? What are the postures? Is the posture rigid, collapsed, threatening, overgrounded, ready to spring into action, or expressive? What do the eyes say? Do the eyes look glazed? Do they lack luster or liveliness? Do they look scared, defiant, or threatening? What about muscle tension and relaxation? Notice the patterns of tension and when the client changes. Is the client in touch with their breathing? Does the client feel the ground beneath them, or is most of their awareness above the neck? Much of the unconscious is present on the surface.

How people walk, talk, shake hands, or move are all holographic fragments of how they are psychologically organized in the larger arena of their lives. Through the process of awareness, therapists help the person stop what is an automatic habit pattern and start to be aware of themselves. This allows a more intimate understanding of how their body is organized and what is going on below ordinary consciousness. Interventions may involve experiments, such as having clients change a position or posture and experience what that is like, or working with gesture and asking clients to repeat or even exaggerate them. A study published in 2009 (Levy Berg et al., 2009) demonstrated greater improvement in participants who received affect-focused body psychotherapy than in those who received the standard treatment.

Body-focused work also incorporates working with touch, breathing, and movement. Working with movement and increasing the sensorimotor awareness help people learn to modulate their traumatic experience and increase their capacity for self-regulation. Ogden (2015) developed a sensorimotor approach that helps individuals in therapy reexperience traumatic events in a safe environment and carry out any previously unfulfilled actions to achieve feelings of completion and closure. Here, clients complete the movement that was truncated in the original situation, thus giving them an experience of triumph that they can savor and integrate into their nervous system. Levine (2010) developed an approach to body work called *somatic experiencing*, which is partially based on the similarities between the regulatory systems of animals and humans in dealing with traumatic events. It teaches people how to slowly and safely complete survival actions, interrupted at the time of trauma, as they learn to renegotiate their traumas rather than relive them. These approaches all privilege body movement over talk as crucial in change in psychotherapy.

In working with the body, once the therapist has noticed the physical aspects of an individual's experience and drawn attention to it, the next step in body-centered process is to allow the experience to move or unfold toward core painful emotions that organize these expressions. When clients are immersed in their actual experience, they have the opportunity to bypass usual responses and protective defenses. They can now explore, in a more visceral fashion, what underlies their perceptions, behaviors, and feelings.

CONCLUSION

In this chapter, I presented how to go beyond words to gather information from the body that only later is put into words. This is done by attending to the felt sense both through expressive arousal and observation of nonverbal behaviors. In line with the importance of new experience as the key change process, the body is the seat of experience, and therapists need to pay attention to the information in the body. As mentioned, the brain talks in two languages: (a) the verbal conceptual language of the prefrontal cortex and (b) emotion in which the brain speaks through the body with a sensory motor tongue. Therapists, therefore, need to listen to the body if we are to access the brain's intelligent emotion system.

7

BLOCKS TO EMOTION

At times, some clients stop themselves—deliberately or automatically—from having certain feelings. They might say something like, "I can feel the tears coming up, but I just tighten and suck them back in. No way am I going to cry." What is occurring in clients who have difficulties accessing emotion, who cannot locate feelings in their body or simply do not allow themselves to feel or express emotion? In this chapter, I discuss how to understand what is happening internally in people who lack emotional awareness or, more specifically, have difficulty identifying and describing feelings or experiencing the bodily sensations associated with emotions, or both.

Two possible processes are involved in the nonawareness or lack of expression of emotion: The first is a deficit in learning; the second, defense or inhibition. *Deficits* refers to clients who have never learned to pay attention to or to label emotions. They simply have no words for emotion possibly because they were brought up in environments where emotions were disregarded and never learned to pay attention to, or talk about, emotion. *Defense* assumes that emotional experiences are kept out of awareness through intentional (e.g., suppression) or unintentional (e.g., repression) mechanisms because of their threatening nature.

https://doi.org/10.1037/0000248-008
Changing Emotion With Emotion: A Practitioner's Guide, by L. S. Greenberg

Therapeutic work with clients who have no words for emotion differs from work with clients who are inhibiting and blocking emotion. Some clients have difficulties with identifying, naming, or expressing—or all three—emotions that are deemed socially appropriate, such as happiness on a joyous occasion. Treatment involves skill training, which starts with being aware of physiological responses and journaling about emotions, and involves concentrating on building a foundation for naming emotions and appreciating a range of feelings. The process likely includes both consideration of the experiences of other people and self-reflection. Although this may seem basic, it is difficult for some people, such as those with *alexithymia*, a term that describes people who have difficulty finding words to express their emotions.

Other clients have the ability to name their emotions, but they inhibit them and do not allow themselves to experience or express them. They know they have them, but they disown them as "not me" and disclaim the action tendencies in their emotions. In this chapter, I describe *inhibition* as a process by which people interrupt or block emotion, and I view this process as involving action by the self on the self to prevent the experiencing of emotion. Seeing interruptive processes as clients blocking their emotions highlights that clients are active agents in the process of not being aware of emotions. They are not passive recipients, as implied in statements like, "I just went blank" or "My sadness suddenly disappeared." In therapy, clients are helped to see themselves as agents who do things to interrupt their experience and block their expression of emotion, and to see that they cut themselves off from the adaptive information associated with the emotions.

In this discussion, I stress the therapeutic importance of seeing interruptions and blocks as self-protection, and as a means of coping rather than as the avoidance of pain. In this way, blocks to emotion, which are often referred to in the literature as "avoidance" or "defense," are revisioned as coping strategies coming out of people's attempts to prevent falling apart. Blocking emotions are thus seen as survival efforts and attempts to enhance coping. Therefore, it is important that, as clinicians, we help people approach dreaded emotions by first validating their fear that allowing the emotion will result in falling apart.

First, I discuss psychoeducative forms of intervention for people with emotion learning deficits. After that, to more deeply understand the clients in-session process and internal experience of blocking, I engage in an in-depth discussion of the results of task analyses and grounded theory qualitative analyses of the process of interruption. Understanding these processes is key to informing the therapist how to best facilitate the unblocking of dreaded emotions.

HAVING NO WORDS FOR EMOTION

When clients first enter therapy, it often is surprisingly difficult for them to answer, "How are you feeling?" Answering that question can be even more of a challenge for clients who have alexithymia, which may appear as a clinical feature in clients with autism spectrum disorder, depression, eating disorders, posttraumatic stress disorder, or other diagnoses. These clients present behaviorally or cognitively, are external and intellectualizing, or are somatizing and have psychosomatic symptoms or are anorexic and have little or no access to feeling and have no capacity to focus internally. They are organized characterologically to not show any emotions. They differ from people who have emotions that they are aware of having but suppress them or actively block them. People who are alexithymic have difficulty finding words to describe their emotions, are often imaginally constricted, and have an externally oriented cognitive style (Bagby et al., 1994). These clients seem to have little access to emotion, and therapists often end up feeling unable to work with them in an emotion-focused way. But all people have emotions, so it is not a matter of absence of emotion but a lack of emotional competence in describing emotion.

When a supervisee says something to me like, "My client has difficulty getting in touch with his emotions. I've tried to get him to focus on his feelings, but he just doesn't seem to have any, maybe I should do something else?" my response is usually to ask, "What is your relationship like?" As therapists, we deal with clients talking to *us* about their emotions. They are in relationships with us, so it is not a simple matter of the client's characteristics alone. It is also an issue of what the therapist is like, the nature of the relationship, and whether an alliance between client and therapist to work on emotion has been established.

Establishing an alliance to work on emotion means therapists must understand that most people feel vulnerable expressing emotions. This is probably because society has deemphasized emotions and has cast emotions as weak, needing to be controlled, irrational, and potentially dysfunctional such that people do not feel safe talking about emotions. In addition, if their life experience included growing up in emotion-unfriendly environments at home or in school, they learned languages other than talking feelings. If you do not speak an emotion language at home, how can you suddenly come into therapy and speak about emotion? It is like expecting someone to suddenly be conversant in Mandarin having never been exposed to it or taught it. What is needed first to help people who lack words for emotion to speak the language of emotion is an emotion-friendly and permission-giving environment. Therapists need to explicitly give people permission to be emotional by saying, "This is a place where your feelings are welcome. Even more, they are desirable."

When my supervisees or trainees ask how to work with people who do not have emotion, my first answer is to ask about the nature of the therapeutic relationship to highlight that it is not simply an intrapsychic issue but an interpersonal one. Clients need to feel safe and trust the therapist before they will attend to their emotions. I then suggest that they focus on clients' sensory and motor experience—not on feelings but on sensations because those are more easily accessible, especially to men—and be attentive to nonverbal communication. I often say, "Don't think about what's coming out of people's mouths but think about what's going on in their stomachs. What is their visceral experience?"

How does one work with clients who are alexithymic? Empathic attunement to affect, present-centered awareness, and focus on instructions covered in Chapters 5 and 6 are helpful as baseline skills. However, given that the difficulty is a lack of emotional competence, and the problem is, to some degree, a deficit in learning, guiding clients toward their feelings is insufficient. The first form of intervention I suggest is experientially oriented psychoeducation.

TEACHING CLIENTS WORDS FOR EMOTION

At the most basic level, the client has to be aware of any emotion they may have and attend to it. Clients often are unaware of their emotional experience and responses. For example, they might nonverbally express emotions without being aware that they are doing so. A client, while talking about his abusive mother, for instance, may clench his jaw or speak with an angry tone, but when he is asked by his therapist what he is feeling, he responds that he feels nothing. Although the client may be visibly distressed or angry, he is unaware of what he is feeling. In situations of this nature, therapists can help clients increase awareness of their emotion by focusing attention to their nonverbal actions (e.g., "I'm aware of you clenching your jaw. What's that feel like?" "I hear some anger in your voice. Are you aware of feeling angry?"). Attention is guided to nonverbal expression, to bodily experience, and to internal physical sensations.

Therapists need to focus on a client's sensations and the bodily felt sense, inquiring into internal experience and asking them to describe what it is like inside. Nonverbal aspects of expression, especially facial expression, quivering lip, and sagging cheeks as well as general posture, need to be attended to and the experience invited to come more fully. Sighs need to be noticed; they are important expressions of core experience and often indicate either an underlying unacknowledged sadness or a sense of having touched on it. Ask clients to sigh again and to take a breath because doing so allows the feeling to intensify. Ask them to put some words to the sigh to help them symbolize the feeling behind it. Evocative language and metaphor, such as "It's like wanting to cry out but being afraid that no one will hear me," can help evoke the feeling. Memories of situations in which this feeling was felt can be evoked by using imagery to make the feelings as concrete and vivid as possible.

Once an experience is felt in awareness, it has to be symbolized (i.e., generally in words but it could be in painting, movement, and so on) to be able to fully use it as information. Naming emotional responses and describing what they feel like enables clients to use the informational value inherent in their primary emotions. Exact labeling of emotional experience is not what is needed; rather, clients need to be engaged in a process of trying to symbolize what they are experiencing. Description of emotion can be promoted in dialogue with the therapist or in homework, such as writing about the emotion in a diary. Using more nonverbal means, such as asking people to paint what they feel, to sculpt it, or to play it in music, also can be helpful. Later, clients can put these expressions into words. The ability to label and describe emotions helps clients to be able to work with their emotions to solve problems. The goal of describing feelings in words is to help people speak them rather simply act them out. A parent coaches a child in naming emotions, first by giving words to the child's experience by saying, for example, "Johnny is angry" when Johnny yells and grabs his toy from another child.

Being a Surrogate for Others' Personal Experience

Through empathic attunement to affect, therapists try to help clients enter the highly subjective domain of their unformulated personal experience. For example, the therapist here offers words to help the client symbolize what he might be feeling:

CLIENT: I don't know what I feel. It wasn't good, though.

THERAPIST: Something like "it was like a loss." Maybe you felt sad or disappointed.

CLIENT: Yeah, I guess that is what it is. It just wasn't what I expected.

Therapists serve as surrogate information processors and are constantly engaged in helping clients to put words to what they feel. In the dialectical constructivist view I propose for emotion work, meaning is created in the process of symbolizing the emotion. In other words, emotion is not sitting fully formed inside a person. However, there is an emotional experience there, and that emotional experience constrains but does not fully determine how it can be symbolized. Thus, how emotions are symbolized influence what they become.

Using Structured Homework for Identifying Emotions

Often the best place to go next is the use of structured homework exercises: keeping an emotion log or a diary. Homework exercises can be helpful to clients to track their emotions during the day (see, e.g., Greenberg, 2015). The first way is by keeping an emotion log. The therapist might suggest that at three appointed times during the day, the client write down the last emotion they experienced and describe anything it led them to think or do. Keeping an emotion log may be easier for some people than keeping a diary because the log is more structured; in addition, rather than logging emotion three times a day, the therapist can ask clients to keep the log at the end of the day or before bed. On a sheet, the therapist provides a list of emotion words to the client and asks the client to check if they felt this feeling during the day and when. The client also marks on the sheet what feeling they are feeling at the moment. This begins a training in emotion labeling, which itself has been shown to lead to beneficial emotional processing (Kircanski et al., 2012).

The therapist can ask the client to write down a name for the emotion and suggest that, rather than writing frequently used words like "frustrated" or "happy," the client try to find more varied and differentiated words like "annoyed," "angry," or "furious." The client also can be asked to describe any body sensations they may have had that accompanied the emotion. Then, the following week, the therapist can ask the client to add comments on whether it was a sudden-onset emotion or a more enduring mood, and how long it lasted.

In the session, the therapist can ask the client to describe the last time they felt one of the following emotions: anger, sadness, fear, or shame. The therapist then describes this feeling to the client to help them understand the situation, how the client reacted, what happened in their bodies, how they felt, and what they did. The client can also be asked to consider how long the feeling lasted, how intense it was on a scale from 1 (*not at all*) to 10 (*very high*), how frequently they experienced this emotion, and whether the emotion was generally helpful or was a problem for them.

Slowing Down

To enter states of feeling, which are quite different from states of thinking or acting, people need to be able to slow down to smell the coffee or to feel the feeling. To feel is a slow process. Feelings cannot be felt when clients are talking rapidly, concentrating on content, or even trying to communicate to the therapist. It, therefore, is important in sessions to help clients to stay with a feeling they may be beginning to have by guiding them through the following four steps. Creating a space for feeling is one of the most basic processes in working with emotion. It is simple but crucial. Therapists can help clients create a space for an emotion by saying phrases like:

1. Stay very gently with what you are feeling.
2. Make a space for it in your body and just feel it. Put some words to it.
3. Receive and welcome the feeling.
4. Feel it fully.

If clients enter their emotional states but then interrupt the experience, the therapist needs to guide them to become aware of how they do this interruption. Maybe they think of something else; get scared; or say, "I can't handle this." Help them become aware that they are interrupting and then guide them to choose to attend to their experience.

ENGAGING IN SELF-INTERRUPTION

For those clients who have words for emotions but find allowing emotional experience so difficult that they quell their primary emotions and any asso-ciated tendencies, psychoeducation as suggested for alexithymic clients is not the intervention of choice. This form of inhibition in which emotional experience is interrupted and prevented from blossoming into full emotional experience and expression then becomes an important focus in therapy and needs to be worked with in a way more suited to it.

Self-interruption of emotion (SIE) has been described as the client's engage-ment in action against the self (Greenberg, 2002; Greenberg, Rice, & Elliott, 1993). Actions against the self-involve such things as physiological control over visceral experience, muscular tightening against the expression of emotion, negative beliefs and thoughts that serve to quash emotion, or avoidant behaviors like laughing or joking to ward off painful emotion (see, e.g., Perls et al., 1951). In addition, secondary emotion often can prevent experience and expression of an initial primary emotional experience, such as when fear of sadness obscures the sadness.

The process of interruption of emotion has possible roots in early relational experience in which attempts to express feelings and needs as a child were consistently met with disapproval, humiliation, or abuse. The individual then began to function as a "divided self": One part of the self engaged in activity to control the expressive action of another experiencing part of the self. The end result is that the person develops processes of self-control to guard against vulnerability or painful experience. This process may result either in awareness of the inhibitory process itself, such as choking back tears, or in awareness of a lack of feeling, muscular tension, or psychosomatic symptoms without any awareness of the self-interruptive processes. From a transdiagnostic perspective, limited emotional awareness is a major underlying determinant of many major disorders, including posttraumatic stress disorder, anxiety, depression, eating disorders, addictions, and personality disorders. Therefore, it is vital that the self-interruptive process is brought front and center in the case formulation and treatment plan for many clients.

HELPING CLIENTS SEE HOW THEY SELF-INTERRUPT

Therapists can help clients overcome blocks to emotion by making the interruptive activity against the self more explicit. First, the therapist helps the client become aware that they are interrupting. Next, and most importantly, the therapist demonstrates how the client is interrupting (not why). Once the client understands this, only then do they truly experience what they are interrupting. Helping clients experience a sense that "it is me doing this to myself" leads to the possibility of choice to not do it any longer. The recognition of personal agency in the interruptive process—that is, the experience that it is me doing this to myself—is a primary aim.

After becoming aware of how they interrupt themselves, clients develop the capacity to undo the interruption or at least develop some tolerance of the vulnerable emotion rather than completely suppress it. Undoing interruption ultimately leads to experiencing the blocked emotion. For example, clients can be helped to become aware that they are blocking whenever they talk, for example, about their mother and become aware of their muscular tightening or breathing constrictions as a means of interrupting their experience. Once aware of how they are blocking and experiencing what they are doing to themselves, they then can stop doing these things and have the option to let the feeling emerge.

Process of Self-Interruption and Blocking of Emotion

In this section, I discuss what we have learned about clients' observable processes and subjective experiences of the blocking of emotion. This discussion informs when and how to intervene. At York University, over the past 20 years, my students and I have engaged in a number of grounded theory and task analytic studies of both the blocking and allowing of emotion (Bolger, 1999; Vrana, 2020; Weston, 2018). *Grounded theory* (Glaser & Strauss, 1967) is a qualitative method of discovering emerging patterns in data. People are interviewed about their experience, and a rigorous analysis of the client self-reports of their experience leads to the building of a set of descriptive categories and ultimately a grounded theory of the phenomena or process of interest. In contrast, a *task analysis* (Greenberg, 2007) studies clients' actual performance in sessions and, by a similar method of building descriptive categories, constructs a model comprising the components of resolution of the phenomena under study. Measurements of the components are developed, and the model is later tested and validated.

In these studies, the first step involves defining a marker of self-interruption by observing therapy video recordings and interviewing people about the experience of self-interruption (Greenberg, Rice, & Elliott, 1993). An *in-session marker of self-interruption* is a statement made by the client or therapist indicating the client's opposition toward allowing themselves to fully experience or express an emotion. This opposition may either be automatic or deliberate. Two possible aspects of what is blocked are (a) the internal experience of emotion with its subjective sense of arousal or (b) the outward expression of emotion in words or expressive actions.

SIE is viewed as involving two parts of the self in which the one part limits the experience or expression of a feeling, and experiences distress as a result (Greenberg, 2011; Greenberg, Rice, & Elliott, 1993). Individuals interrupt their emotional experience in many different ways: The client can constrict, stop, or distance the self from the experience or expression of a feeling. When a primary emotional experience (e.g., anger, sadness, vulnerability) is emerging, it may be abruptly followed by a client's inhibition of the experience via some secondary emotion (e.g., anger to cover fear or shame). Emotions also can be interrupted via client cognition, including injunctions against feelings (e.g., "Anger is a sin," "Crying is feeling sorry for oneself"). Catastrophic expectations about emotional experience and expression (e.g., "If I start crying, I will never stop") block emotions. Some clients also may believe that they have no right to feel angry or sad. Moreover, automatic physical and physiological processes like squeezing, holding one's breath, and deflecting attention are often ways of interrupting without any awareness.

When clients make statements in sessions opposing, fighting against, or stopping the initial feeling or expression of emotion—or both—or make statements indicating physiological changes that serve to restrict or constrain the emotion, such as swallowing or squeezing down feelings, the clients are seen as engaging in an interruption of their emotions. Their statements also need to include paralinguistic communication (i.e., sighing or silence, which indicate the effort in stopping emotion) as well as indications that the initial experience of emotion has disappeared. For example, a marker of SIE might involve acknowledging an experience of emotion that quickly is followed by the action of "sucking it in" or a desire to not allow the emotion, which is followed by an awareness of the absence of feeling. The following are examples of markers of SIE:

CLIENT: Ooh, very sad!

THERAPIST: Very! Sad, uh-huh. (*Client sighs.*) Can you let yourself feel the sadness?

CLIENT: (*Is silent for about 6 seconds*)

THERAPIST: Let the tears flow if you need to?

CLIENT: (*Is silent for about 6 seconds*) Oh, a part of me is fighting it, too. [Another client interrupts; anger]

THERAPIST: What's happening inside now?

CLIENT: Ooh! I'm just (*sighs*)—I'm, oh! I want to scream at him so badly.

THERAPIST: What do you want to scream at him?

CLIENT: Ooh! He just—oh, I can't even express it, I'm just so! Furious with him (*gives a big sigh*). I can't tell him that. I can feel my— I am just sucking it all in.

Here is an example of the blocking of tears:

THERAPIST: So, what's happening for you now as you speak?

CLIENT: Um (*pauses*). I'm feeling kind of tearful.

THERAPIST: Can you stay with that, see what words come? Tearful? Sad?

CLIENT: I don't want to feel tearful.

Protection From Dangerous Emotions

In a study, one of my doctoral students (Weston, 2018) observed a number of client video recordings in which self-interruption occurred and interviewed some of these clients using *interpersonal process recall*. This is a method in which clients are asked to look at a video recorded session involving their process of SIE and talk about their internal experience at the time of interruption. My student titled her dissertation *Protection from Dangerous Emotions: Interruption of Emotional Experience in Psychotherapy*. This investigation supported that SIE was a process of providing self-protection initiated at moments in a therapy session during which clients experienced a sense of threat or danger from their own emotional experience or expression. Findings showed that client's awareness of the self as vulnerable was a central feature of the interruptive process. This awareness of vulnerability was followed by self-protective secondary emotional reactions like fear, self-protective acts of control or avoidance, or both.

Weston (2018) found that clients' process of SIE in therapy sessions involved six steps. Self-interruption begins with the *activation* of emotional experience, expression that is soon followed by the client's *awareness/ expression of an emotionally vulnerable* sense of self. This awareness of vulnerability then gives rise to *opposition* to emotional experience, which is the marker indicating the presence of SIE. The process of opposition to emotion involves the client's experiencing *secondary reactive emotions, controlling or avoidant inhibitory behaviors*, or both. That is, the experience of an emotion is interrupted either by the experience of another emotional reaction to the first emotion or by some active process of blocking. The process of SIE culminates in the client's *awareness of limited emotional experience*.

Self-interruption, then, involves some initial awareness/expression of an emotionally vulnerable sense of self, followed by the enactment of an interruptive process, and a final recognition of having limited or no emotion.

Feeling vulnerable to an emerging emotion evokes a variety of secondary emotional reactions with fear being the most predominant one. Clients fear physiological arousal and falling apart, and it is often the intensity of feelings that leads the clients to fear them. They fear that if they fully acknowledge these dreaded negative feelings, these emotions will be bottomless and engulfing, and the clients will lose control and be overwhelmed by these emotions.

Activation of Emotional Experience

Self-interruptive process can be seen as starting with the rising awareness of some emotional experience. The client may only vaguely sense the emotion and may express a vague or limited awareness of undifferentiated, meaningless bodily sensations or a general sense of physiological arousal. For example, one client cried and then asked, "Why do I do this?" in reference to crying and some limited awareness of what she called "that feeling." One client described awareness that she was teary and "choked up," and then said, "I don't know why." She differentiated this inchoate experience first as feeling "upset" and then as feeling "very sad."

Other clients, however, may be consciously aware of their emotional experience. For example, one therapist asked a client how she felt as she described how her parents were critical and unaffectionate toward her. The client reported clearly, "I feel sad." There may be descriptions of an increase in arousal that is defined by physiological correlates of a particular emotion, such as fear and related changes in breathing patterns; anger and a roiling, churning sense in the stomach; hurt and a feeling of bodily pain; sadness; and a physical sense of loss.

Clients' emotional experience generally is activated or "triggered" in the therapy session in response to their own thoughts, perception, or memories. Memories related to loss or to traumatic experiences in childhood or adulthood are major precipitators of emotion. Specific types of therapist interventions also evoke emotion: empathically reflecting: "My sense is that there's a kind of sadness that you still feel"; paying close attention to and inquiring about feelings: "What does it physically feel like in your body?"; directing the client's attention inward to emotional experience or outward to the expression of emotion: "There's a sadness there. Somehow, we need to find words to put to that. I'm sad that . . ."; or offering an image to capture emotional experience: "It's as if he took a knife and just slashed through all you had had together." All can evoke an emotion. Emotion might also be activated in connection with clients' subjective sense of contact with the therapist: "He was just going close to me with his words, and I felt sad."

Clients often say feelings were just suddenly "triggered" in their bodies; for example: "When my therapist said what is so undeserving about me, I suddenly got really sad."

Emotions are experienced as dangerous, and this is what produces the sense of vulnerability. Clients used metaphors to describe emotion, such as a "monster," "alien," or a "wave" of tidal proportions felt inside the body. Self-interruption is a self-protective act; it protects against dangerous emotions. Fear, other secondary emotions, or both, and suppressive behaviors are engaged in to help protect against the emotions. Behind the self-protection is not so much the pain of the emotion that the client is avoiding but the feared consequences of falling apart and being unable to cope.

The following are clients' reports of their experience of the dangers (Weston, 2018). Some participants described how the experience of emotion earlier in life was dangerous because it rendered them vulnerable to harsh consequences: "I wasn't allowed to cry, so, obviously, emotion must be a bad thing to feel. But I also equated feeling emotion with getting beaten." One participant described his adolescent experience of emotion as one of being trapped in a "black hole of despair":

> It's terrible. It's a feeling of your worst nightmare and a tremendous amount of fear. You can't control the situation, and you just want to get the hell out of there. And it's a very terrifying place because you feel physically sick, your stomach gets into knots. I can feel the nausea.

Another reported, "When my mother was hitting me, I wasn't allowed to cry, and if I held my breath really hard, I could never cry." One woman described how she used to distract herself from feeling sad or bad by singing when she was a child. She explained that, as an adult, she only likes pursuing the issue of how she is feeling "intellectually." Another participant described how she avoided the danger of showing sadness in public by habitually not paying attention to sad feelings. She explained, "Rarely do I address it even when I'm alone . . . I don't want to make it a pattern. I don't want to be like that . . . I don't want it to become a part of something I'm gonna do whenever I feel sad is show it."

Vulnerability

This danger of emotions produces a sense of vulnerability to the self often associated with awareness of the visceral experience of emotion (Weston, 2018). Clients may make explicit statements about a sense of vulnerability associated with the emotional experience. One client, in her recall interview, described her sense of sorrow as "vulnerability, loss. I would say something at the very core." She recalled "how deep the emotion is, and how vulnerable I feel." Another client recalled how she felt "very vulnerable" when she was sad. Other clients described awareness of feeling exposed, unprotected, or at the mercy of a powerful force they might not be able to survive. Overall, the experience of vulnerability in the context of emerging emotional experience involved a sense or a clear feeling of a threat to physical self-integrity, to psychological self-cohesion, to existence, or all three.

Some participants recalled awareness of how they felt an extreme sense of hurt. One man recalled how he felt a "strong, strong hurt" while recalling a childhood incident in which he was bullied. Looking at the video recording, he explained, "This is where I really started getting into the body. I'm getting into the feelings of what's happening . . . I heard all the laughter around me in my head . . . I hurt so much." Anger was also described in terms of awareness of intense feeling. One man recalled, "I'm aware of having those angry feelings. . . . It's high intensity." Some also recalled extreme feelings of fear. One woman described a "sense of fear or threat" that was "slightly less than panic." She explained, "It feels very frightening" Another woman recalled, "The feeling I had there was a total feeling of fear." The preceding examples demonstrate that it is an awareness of the intensity of feeling emotion that is so threatening and produces the sense of vulnerability.

Vulnerable feelings are threatening partly because they are experienced as happening to us. They are experienced as rising up in our bodies. One person, for example, reported, "There I was, feeling it in my chest coming up to my brain." Anger was described in terms of the qualities of a powerful and aggressive force in motion. One participant described how an "unknown sense of it" was "coming up in my face." There was a sense of the emotion rising up. One woman recalled awareness of hurt and how she "felt it coming up" from her "gut" to her throat, and she was "ready to sob [her] heart out." Another woman explained that when she was emotionally "upset," she "sort of feels a wave of that coming on. It kind of rushes up." And one woman recalled awareness of the increasing intensity of the emotional pain of aloneness: "It was so explosive. I remember that feeling of it coming . . . this feeling that was growing in me."

The sense of an all-encompassing vulnerability in the emotional self seems pivotal in the process of SIE because it sets the stage for the next phase of opposition to emotion. So, as clients allow the experience of, or expression of, the emotion, a sense of vulnerability to harm emerges explicitly or implicitly. This sense of self as unsafe in the face of emotion promotes opposition to allowing the feeling, expressing it, or both. The opposition includes secondary reactive emotions and behaviors that serve to interrupt the initial emotional experience.

Intensity of feeling across a wide range of emotional experience is the visceral experience that is associated with a vulnerable sense of self. Some people's descriptions also included the quality of a surfacing or fast-moving sensation that rushed upward in the body. It is this experience of the self as emotionally vulnerable to dangerous emotions that leads people to protect themselves. In the context of an experience of self as emotionally vulnerable, participants described an explicit or implicit need for self-protection that was met by engagement in three main processes: addressing reactive emotions, controlling emotional vulnerability, and avoiding emotional vulnerability (Weston, 2018). The next two sections discuss these three processes.

Reactive Emotions

Secondary reactive emotions, such as fear, serve to protect against the dangers and sense of threat posed by continuing the initial experience of emotion. In some cases, the client is aware of this function. As one client explained, she was aware in the session that her reactive anger protected against her sadness, and she thought to herself, "This is the protector." Often, however, there is a more automatic quality to the onset of reactive emotion. Reactive emotions interfere with experiencing the initial emotion as shown in the excerpts that follow.

In this excerpt from Weston (2018), a 28-year-old, African American, female client presents with anxiety and depression as well as unresolved trauma:

CLIENT: It hurts too much. I'm afraid if I go there, I may end up hurting myself physically.

THERAPIST: Afraid that somehow if you stay with the hurt . . .

CLIENT: If I stay with that, physically, I will hurt myself.

In the next example from Weston (2018), another client, a 47-year-old, European man with work-related interpersonal difficulties, is afraid of and embarrassed about his anger:

THERAPIST: You don't want to express that rage in here.

CLIENT: No. I think I'm really afraid of it.

THERAPIST: What'll happen if you express it?

CLIENT: I don't know. Well, oh! I do. I'll be embarrassed, or I'll lose control. . . . Even small angers . . . I don't feel safe when the feelings of anger start coming up.

In the following excerpt from Weston (2018), a 32-year-old, Caucasian, female client who suffers from social anxiety describes her fear of allowing crying because her therapist might judge her:

THERAPIST: What are you feeling right now?

CLIENT: (*Sniffs*) Well, looking at your face, you're sympathetic, and you're encouraging me to let go, and I feel like I'm going to lose it (*cries*).

THERAPIST: Okay, and you're scared?

CLIENT: (*Blows nose*) Yeah. Scared, and I think you'll think less of me. . . . I'm almost afraid to look at you [therapist] because it's going to bring it (*cries*) on again.

The four main fears that clients appear to feel are the fear of losing control, fear of expression of emotion, fear of the unknown, and fear of dying (Weston, 2018). In the Weston study, participants recalled the visceral qualities of an extremely intense, deep, or painful (or all three) feeling and then a sense or feeling of fear that, in some cases, also included catastrophic beliefs. Participants described specific fears such as losing their sanity, losing control of an explosive force or strong impulse, or ending up trapped in a "black hole." In some instances, participants described a fear of losing their mind in the face of deep, intense emotion. Some participants described how fear involved either a visceral sense or "underlying feeling," whereas for others, reactive fear involved beliefs and thoughts about the catastrophic consequences of allowing emotion to flow unabated.

In expressing her fear of emotion, one woman described her awareness of deep, intense anger in her "belly" followed by a fear that it would be unleashed in an explosion at the expense of her sanity. Another woman described a nervous reaction to a "really sad" feeling in her body. She recalled feeling "really anxious" in her stomach and that she had a "big lump" in her throat. One man recalled that when he felt anger "coming on," he felt "threatened, a lot of apprehension, and a lot of anxiety" in his "solar plexus." A third participant described awareness of reactive fear when she focused on inchoate emotional experience. She reported, "It feels frightening . . . I feel that kind of fear or threat."

Some more verbatim accounts of reports of the fear of emotion captured the intensity of the fear:

It's so deep, so like a monster. It's scary . . . I felt it several times. What's the use of going on with this and then the fear that "Oh my God, it's gonna explode right here in this room, and they're going to have to take me away in a white jacket."

Another participant said,

> I'm scared to let it come. . . . I'm really scared to do that. . . . I felt scared right there. . . . My biggest fear is that if I let all my emotion, I'll become catatonic. I won't be able to face all that is in there. It'll be just too overwhelming for me.

For other participants, fear was a reaction to the unknown qualities, meaning, or course of intense and overwhelming emotional experience, or all of these—essentially a fear of the unknown. One man reported,

> It's an unknown thing that I'm having a hard time dealing with. What is it? Can't define it. . . . And for me, it's sort of a scary thing because I want to know what it is. This fear, it makes me, yeah, it scares me. I don't know what "it" is, so how can I deal with it? "It" is unknown. . . . How can I deal with it if I don't know what it is, yet it keeps coming up in my face.

For other participants, existential fear was central. There was a fear of dying. Here, participants recalled a wordless, visceral sense that should emotional experience be allowed or expressed, they could die. Fear was rooted in a profound sense of aloneness or abandonment as they grappled with seemingly life-threatening emotional experience. One woman viewed a segment of the therapy video recording in which she had told the therapist, "I'm frightened" and recalled that she was experiencing a feeling of "preverbal fear" in response to awareness of a wordless "wave" of "really deep . . . really sad feeling." She explained that she had a sense that she could die. She likened her experience to the fear she has felt when she senses that she is going to have a seizure, a symptom of her potentially life-threatening seizure disorder, and no one is going to help her manage it. Another participant described her reactive fear as a strong sense that allowing an unsafe painful, overwhelming feeling of aloneness, and expressing it in tears, was "dangerous." She likened the experience to an old familiar "feeling of dying."

Some participants described only one type of fear, whereas others described more than one type. For example, one man recalled an initial reaction of fear of losing control that followed awareness of the feeling of intense, deep, and painful anger. At a later point, he was afraid to express anger by raising his voice because of its unpredictable, unknown course.

Controlling and Avoidant Behaviors
At this point, when the self feels vulnerable and has possibly reacted with a secondary feeling, the process of interruption unfolds more actively. Clients' needs for self-protection now lead to controlling or avoidant behavior (Weston, 2018). Whereas earlier in the process there was a sense of a struggle between two opposing parts of self (allow/express emotion vs. do not allow/express), now the force opposing experience is dominant, and

clients engage in behaviors to inhibit emotion by either actively avoiding their emotional experience or trying to control it. Avoidance is characterized by flight or escape behaviors that serve to move away and disengage from the emotion, whereas acts of self-control involve moving toward emotional experience with the intention of controlling it (Weston, 2018).

Avoidance may take the form of an explicit expression of a general desire to avoid internal experience as well as specific desires to hide or flee. Avoidant behavior takes a variety of forms, including an urge to flee the session or hide, joking, laughter, worry, distraction or dissociation, disconnection from the perception of emotion, a pushing away of emotional experience, and expressions of hopelessness or helplessness.

Behaviors of physical control include constricting muscles, posture (e.g., hunches over, folds arms), swallowing, breath control (e.g., holds, sighs), or silence that serves to contain or suppress the visceral experience or expression of emotion. Acts of cognitive control include invalidation of emotion and self-criticism (e.g., attacks, questions), as well as negative beliefs or prohibitions about emotion (e.g., hopelessness, negative consequences to self, relationships, or both), all of which serve to suppress emotional experience.

Clients thus consciously and actively engage in behaviors that inhibit the feeling or expression of an initial emotional experience. The following (Weston, 2018) is an example of a 45-year-old Middle Eastern woman in a session who "sucks the emotion in," which is accompanied by nonverbal behaviors that serve to oppose continuation of an initial feeling, expression of the emotion (e.g., physical constriction, sigh, body posture, shaking of head), or both:

CLIENT: He abandoned me (*sighs*), but I can't tell him that I'm angry. I can feel my—I'm sucking it all in . . . (*slumps over*).

THERAPIST: What does it feel like as you suck it all in?

CLIENT: Ordinary. I do it all the time . . . (*physically constricts her jaw, shakes her head*).

THERAPIST: What else?

CLIENT: Ooh! I can feel it's . . . tingling at the edge of every muscle trying to get out.

In his interview (Weston, 2018), one man reported that despite his desire to feel and express emotion, "I completely close off. I have a long history of blocking my emotional experience with various hurdles . . . barriers . . .

doors." Clients control through complex protective meanings as shown in the following statement by another client:

> I'm stopping by saying that if I cry about it, even though they aren't here, I will be somehow or another allowing them to have some kind of gratification out of my pain. And by not letting the pain out, I keep them from influencing and having some kind of control over my life.

Another client expressed awareness that she was "choking down a lot of anger." Another gave voice to a choking feeling that controlled the expression of anger: "I'm the choker, and I'm holding my breath so I can't speak."

The following example from Weston's (2018) study illustrates a process in which a depressed, 43-year-old Chinese American, female client, an engineer who lost her father when she was 12, is working on how she interrupts sadness in the session. The therapist has suggested the use of a two-chair enactment (explained briefly later and in more depth in Chapter 8). In this segment, the therapist guides the client to enact the suppression of sadness. Through this enactment, the client becomes aware of how she "squelched" sadness and that it was related to fear of embarrassment of showing her feelings to others.

CLIENT: I was sad.

THERAPIST: You were sad just before you cut off?

CLIENT: Just before, yeah . . . I feel nothing until it just escapes, whatever it is that's being squelched, and then I just feel really, really bad until I pack it down again.

At this point, the therapist guides her into the enactment of squelching sadness by packing down her cleansing tissues into a box to bring the interruptive process into an active form of "doing":

THERAPIST: Let's see if we can just pack it in. Can you try? . . . Just pack it in the way you do. You're the squelcher. Just pack in those feelings.

CLIENT: (*Folds the tissue. Can hear sounds of the client "packing" the tissue.*)

THERAPIST: What's happening to you now?

CLIENT: I think I need to keep things all tidy and in their place. I don't want to make a mess or something.

THERAPIST: Mm-hmm. So, what are you doing with the Kleenex now? You're packing it in.

CLIENT: (*Laughs*) I guess I'm almost trying to pack the Kleenex into the shape of a rectangle.

THERAPIST: Do you have the sense as you're doing that of being the squelcher, the packer-in, to pack in these feelings?

CLIENT: It kind of feels like trying to keep everything together to prevent it from spilling out.

THERAPIST: I see. But if you weren't there doing that, what might happen?

CLIENT: Maybe embarrass myself. Maybe let on to other people that I'm unhappy or that other things that they do bother me.

As the sense of vulnerability in the self is regulated, the behaviors the client engages in to avoid or control the underlying emotion become the focus of therapy. The process moves to engagement with how the person interrupts the emotion and, if possible, helps develop a sense of being an agent in the interruptive process and of the possibility of not interrupting. Then, processing of the initial emotional experience can take place. If a client has had an experience of "surviving" emotion at a visceral level, this new experience of safety will serve to circumvent the activation of protective secondary reactive emotion and related avoidant and controlling actions, and will promote taking the risk of working on fully allowing and processing emotional experience.

WORKING WITH SELF-INTERRUPTION: THERAPEUTIC CAVEATS

In the case of a client's difficulty tolerating the sudden awareness of intense, deep, or painful (or all three) feelings, the therapist can work with the client to stay focused on bodily based, concrete sensation rather than emotion. Here, the therapist guides the client to describe the body feeling at a working distance rather than going into the feeling itself. If, however, arousal is experienced as unbearably high and threatening, the client can be instructed to use coping self-soothing methods, such as regulated breathing, calming imagery, and self-empathy or validation, to promote tolerance and acceptance of this distressing emotional experience (Greenberg, 2015). The function of instruction to self-soothe at these junctures is to help people cope with highly overwhelming feelings and to help them calm down and cope better. This generally involves regulating secondary reactive feelings. It also fundamentally involves psychoeducation to teach the client to deliberately perform and to practice efforts to down-regulate emotion by soothing self-talk or by evoking a safe place to get a positive or calming feeling. However, it is also important at this point to assess if self-soothing has become another means of interruption because the ultimate goal is for the client to be able to allow emotion with the reassuring understanding that they have the ability to step in and out of it rather than be overwhelmed by it.

Recognizing Precursors to Vulnerability

It also is helpful for therapists to early on identify client moments of emotional vulnerability because they are precursors to subsequent interruptions of the dreaded experience. Recognition that the client is experiencing emotional vulnerability thus is an essential first step toward intervening in the interruptive process to prevent it by heading it off at the pass. Therapists need to pay close attention to how clients are handling visceral experience; there is more going on internally than the client may be saying. One client reported that long before the interruption became apparent, she was aware her therapist was trying to take her to her feelings, and she was actively trying to deflect his efforts.

In addition, there is typically a personal history to the client's difficulty of allowing and expressing emotion. Historical experience of emotional experience may include dangerous consequences to allowing or expressing emotion, such as being physically abused by a caregiver, suffering verbal attack by another, losing control (e.g., vomiting up feelings, lashing out in anger resulting in physical or interpersonal injury), or feeling depressed. Given the historical origins of self-interruption, it may, at some time, be important to work on these origins. Secondary emotions serve a protective function as they interrupt and, in some cases, override the initial feeling and expression of emotion. For example, secondary reactive fear stops the emotionally vulnerable client from experiencing and expressing sadness, shame, or anger and related needs. In some instances, the feeling of reactive sadness may calm and soothe an intense feeling of anger in the vulnerable self, or anger may protect against sadness.

Addressing Secondary Reactive Emotions

How should the therapist address secondary reactive emotions in response to vulnerability? Deepening the experience of secondary emotion is inadvisable given that it interferes with the processing of adaptive emotion that is more central to well-being (Greenberg & Paivio, 1997; Greenberg & Pascual-Leone, 2006). Instead, therapists need to recognize and validate secondary emotions in the moment but then bypass them by shifting the focus to underlying feelings and needs.

Secondary reactive fear is the most common reaction to the initial emotion. Other secondary reactive emotions include secondary reactive shame, which arises from a feeling that allowing or expressing emotion will have negative social consequences, or personal values will be violated. Secondary reactive guilt thwarts the expression of emotion and the associated need. Reactive sadness occurs in response to experience and expression of intense anger, whereas secondary anger follows awareness of the experience of sadness and a weakened sense of self.

Therapists need to validate secondary fear or shame by saying,

> So it's so scary [embarrassing] to acknowledge this emotion. It even feels like it could destroy you or you'll never get over it, but you're saying as much as "I am terrified and don't want to feel it. It is there, I do feel sad [angry], and I really did need comfort [recognition] of what was happening for me."

It is important for therapists to validate clients' fear of emotion and to acknowledge its protective function and its intensity, but at the same time not allow that fear to prevent focusing on the process of emotion awareness and ultimately on the self-interruptive process itself. A therapist might say, "It's so frightening to go into this painful sadness. I understand you are afraid of being overwhelmed by it. So, somehow you manage to step away from it to protect yourself, but it's still there waiting to be heard." This is then followed by an invitation to explore how the client steps away from their sadness.

The therapist needs to adopt a focusing stance toward the secondary fear. The attitude is one of validating and accepting the fear. The therapist's response to the client's fear of emotion might be:

> It's all right. We will just take it slowly. Don't force yourself to go where you don't want to go. If you're afraid of that feeling, keep your distance. Let's stay right here and see what the fear is. What does this "fear" feel like from here? If you don't want to go into it, don't. But don't back off either. Just stay right here and see what is this feeling of not wanting to.

Or the therapist might more simply say, "Scared. Let's just stay right here with this 'scared.' What is this 'scared'? What kind of 'scared' is it? What is the whole feel of it?"

During an interpersonal process recall interview (Weston, 2018), one woman, while watching her self-interruption in the session, was asked by the interviewer, "How are you feeling right now?" She replied, "Overwhelmed" and added,

> A very deep sense of pain and grief. I remember stopping and crying. She [therapist] was telling me to keep going. . . . She kept saying, "Let it go and

really cry. It's okay. Let it go." . . . And I couldn't remember what I was crying about, but I remember stopping it because I had a feeling at that time if I let this feeling go and I really cry, I will break, I will just break because I might die because I won't be able to stand it—the pain. . . . When I explode and all at once, I have this sinking feeling like I'm dying or just drowning or sinking, and I have to stop it. . . . This is dangerous.

Her sense of fear about allowing herself to keep crying served to interrupt the initial experience of emotional pain. However, this secondary reactive fear of intensely painful feeling was not apparent to the therapist, nor was the client expressing it overtly. The end result here was that the client could not "let it go" because she felt overwhelmed and unsafe in the face of intense, deep feeling. So, she ultimately stopped feeling altogether. It is important for therapists to not only encourage facing the emotion but also to validate the fear of the emotion.

Seeing the Self as an Agent of the Shutting-Down Process

Intervention involves both exploring the interruptive process—the internalized messages, beliefs, fears, physiology and their impact—and accessing the interrupted experience. Self-interruption involves a conflict between the feeling part of the self and the part of self that prevents its expression. One strategy for addressing self-interruption of internal experience is to use a two-chair enactment, a technique elaborated in the next chapter but described here briefly because this chapter offers examples of it. In the two-chair enactment, the interrupting part of the self is often enacted to make explicit both that it is an active process and how it is done. Clients become aware of how they interrupt and are guided to enact the ways they do it, whether verbally by telling themselves to shut up or to not feel; by frightening themselves that it is too dangerous; by physically squeezing muscles; or, metaphorically, by, say, trapping or caging themselves. This helps them experience themselves as an agent in the process of shutting down and then they can react to and challenge the interrupting part of the self. Resolution involves expression of the previously blocked experience.

UNDERSTANDING THE EFFECTS OF INTERRUPTION: LIMITED EMOTIONAL EXPERIENCE

The main effect of interruption, as the Weston (2018) study found, was the limiting of emotional experience and awareness. The most frequent effect was a sense of feeling depleted or drained. Many participants described how engagement in protective behavior(s) that served to limit emotional experience ultimately had a negative effect because interruption of emotion left them with an encompassing sense of depletion or that they were drained of energy. Some recalled how physical control over intense, overwhelming, and dangerous feeling or expression, or both, left them with an internal sense of emptiness. One woman described how "squashing down" the angry "monster" that she felt in her body left her feeling "kind of empty . . . like a void . . . not a good feeling." Some participants described how the suppression or avoidance of angry or hurt and painful feelings left them feeling depressed or sad. One man recalled that the effect of dissociation from intensely painful feelings of hurt was that he felt numb and "depressed even more. I wanted to give up." One woman explained,

> Physically, to hold back tears and such pain, it doesn't hurt . . . and I'm not tired after I finish, but . . . it takes a lot of strength to hold it back. It's a lot of effort and energy . . . to hold this back for the amount of pain that I have . . . and I'm not tired after this.

Another client reported that, after interrupting, she felt

> nothing. To be honest, I walk out of there, and I don't remember half the things that went on in there two seconds after I've left there. I get in the car and drive off. Just a depression. Just that total depression . . . nothingness.

Some participants described how avoiding emotional experience by dissociation from the perception or physical experience of it left them in a disembodied or alienated self-state. As one woman recalled that after she reacted to awareness of sadness with shame and anger, "a foggy feeling [came] in. It's like I don't exist. I'm oblivious." Another woman described the effect of avoiding an overwhelming feeling of "distressing" inchoate emotion by withdrawing from contact with the therapist: "Mainly, it's a feeling of being disconnected with her." One man explained, "As you can see, I'm just sort of saying what I see [inside], but I don't feel it . . . I kept getting number and number [increasingly numb] as we went along. Especially in the end there."

In addition to the uncomfortable effects of protection by avoidance of emotional experience, some participants described the physically uncomfortable outcome of control over it. They recalled how the physical "constriction" of or "resistance" to feelings of sadness or anger left them feeling like their body was squeezed in a vise and often with painful consequences. One woman described how she felt a constriction of sadness that left her with a sore throat Another participant described the effects of physically controlling feared anger as

> a lot of tension through my whole body . . . I've been noticing what I call a tingling in my extremities, my hands, my arms, usually from my elbow down,

and my leg, usually from my knee to my feet. I think the only part that is free from it is my head somehow.

In contrast to the negative effect of protection, the positive effect of the avoidance or control of emotional experience was feeling less vulnerable. One woman described how she felt safe and protected following avoidance of the dangerous sense of intense, painful, and overwhelming sadness that also served to stop her tears:

> It's gone. There's nothing. It's like, all of a sudden, it's like total peace. Like being wrapped in cotton and totally protected. There is nothing that can penetrate that. . . . It's relief. I'm okay now. My whole body is different now.

Other participants recalled how various means of control over emotional experience left them with a strengthened sense self that was more "in control." One woman explained how cognitive control over her emotional experience of profound sorrow involved a shift from a sense of self as vulnerable, "a victim," to more of an active agent "somewhat in control of my emotions." Another participant described how he controlled the intense and overwhelming feeling of emotion that evoked reactive fear by sighing at various points. In turn, he recalled, "The tightness is gone. The flush is gone from the face. All the physical stuff is dissipated. [I am] uncomfortable but not emotionally overwrought. The emotions are not in control." He also explained that although protection against vulnerability brought relief, he had come to realize the high long-term cost to his sense of well-being because he remained depressed. Sometimes the sense of protection that was gained by control over emotion, however, was transient. One woman described how reactive anger about sadness left her feeling "in total control." However, the feeling of control was fleeting, and she was left in a state of "hopelessness" that she described as "resignation. It doesn't really matter. Nothing matters."

Overall, the effect of self-protection was to limit awareness of threatening emotion. Participants in the Weston (2018) study described how emotional experience was diminished, controlled, avoided, or stopped altogether. Moreover, many participants described how, subsequent to various means of protection that served to limit emotional awareness, they were left with an overall negative sense of self characterized by numbness, detachment, alienation, sadness, confusion, physical tension or pain, emptiness, depression, uncertainty, or an overall bad feeling. In contrast, a smaller number of participants recalled a more positive effect whereby they felt protected and less vulnerable. This shift to a less vulnerable state was characterized by a sense of relief and a feeling that they were now "in control" of emotion as opposed to an earlier experience of self as emotionally vulnerable. Some reported that the positive sense of protection was transient.

CONCLUSION

From my clinical research on emotion work, I have learned that the client's experience of protecting against threatening emotion in a therapy session is nested within a historical context of the difficulty of allowing or expressing emotion, or doing both. Phenomenological findings show that the process of protection begins with awareness of feeling that is initiated in the body by specific emotion triggers, and a subjective sense of vulnerability soon follows. The profound sense of self as vulnerable is the catalyst for a related implicit or explicit need for protection.

In this chapter, I outlined the steps by which self-protection is provided. In the majority of cases, the activation of an emotion leads to awareness of an emotionally vulnerable sense of self that is interrupted by secondary reactive emotions and behaviors of avoidance, or control, or both, that serve to stop or shut down the initial emotional experience. These reactive emotions and behaviors serve to protect against the experience of an emotionally vulnerable sense of self. Reactive emotions include fear, shame, anger, guilt, or sadness. Four specific classes of fear are fear of losing control, fear of expression of emotion, fear of the unknown, and fear of dying.

Awareness of vulnerability is also followed by avoidant or controlling behavior that serves to protect against the experience, the expression of emotion, or both. The effect of self-protection is either negative for those who are left with a "bad" or "drained" sense of self or, to a lesser extent, positive for others who feel less vulnerable and more in control. Overall, the process of providing protection leaves clients with limited emotional awareness.

In the next chapter, I explore the process of reversing emotional suppression and how this contributes to a positive therapeutic outcome. As alluded to in the discussion and examples shared thus far, it begins with helping clients be aware of their aversion to emotion in the moment.

8

UNBLOCKING EMOTION

A recent study showed that pretreatment suppression of emotion was the strongest predictor of poor therapeutic outcomes (Scherer et al., 2017), a finding that supports the importance of unblocking emotion suppression. In this chapter, and continuing the line of study on the experience of blocking of emotion reported in Chapter 7, one of my doctoral students and I engaged in a task analysis of the self-interruption of emotion (Vrana, 2020). We looked at the undoing of interruption in a sample of nine clients who started with markers of self-interruption of emotion and resolved their interruption. We then compared them with nine clients who started with markers of self-interruption but did not resolve to see what differed in the in-session performance between the two samples. In all cases, therapists attempted to guide the clients to approach a dreaded emotion.

Task analysis is a two-phase method of intensive analysis of therapy transcripts for identifying change processes in psychotherapy (Greenberg, 2007). The first phase is discovery oriented. To develop an initial model of task resolution, an intensive qualitative analysis is done of a relatively small number of pure gold examples (usually three) of a change process. Cases are added progressively to help refine the model until no new information is

https://doi.org/10.1037/0000248-009
Changing Emotion With Emotion: A Practitioner's Guide, by L. S. Greenberg

added and saturation is achieved. The second phase of a task analysis involves quantitative validation-oriented studies on a large number of participants to statistically validate the model (Greenberg, 2007). In this chapter, I discuss the model built in the discovery-oriented phase. To my knowledge, this is the first study in the literature of the unblocking of emotion in psychotherapy and represents the first step in a research program.

The method involves a number of steps:

Step 1. Specify the marker.

Step 2. Explicate the researcher's cognitive map. The theoretical and clinical assumptions are spelled out to specify a framework because no observations are theory free.

Step 3. Specify the task environment. The therapist's intervention framework is defined.

Step 4. Construct a rational model. The researcher's rational understanding of the resolution performance—informed by clinical experience, case observation, and a review of the literature on the process under study—is spelled out. This acts as a type of hypothetical framework to be modified by what is discovered.

Step 5. Conduct an empirical analysis. Observed client affective/cognitive/behavioral processes in task resolvers and nonresolvers are analyzed, and a model of the identified steps to resolution is constructed.

Step 6. Synthesize a rational-empirical model. After the first empirical models have been established, the rational and empirical models are compared. The rational models are modified or elaborated based on observations made during the construction of the empirical models.

Step 7. Conduct a preliminary validation of the model. New sets of clients with the same marker are studied to further validate the rational-empirical model until no new discoveries emerge and saturation is achieved.

Step 8. Explain the model: Theoretical analysis. In this last step, the researcher moves from a descriptive level to a causal level by considering the psychological processes that allow the client to progress from one component to another to complete the tasks.

Further step: The validation phase involves constructing measures to evaluate the degree to which components of the model of resolution are predictive of in-session resolution and, ultimately, final therapy outcome.

OVERCOMING SELF-INTERRUPTION OF EMOTION: THE COMPONENTS

In the Vrana (2020) study, the factors that appeared most important in unblocking the interruption were (a) clients' experience of the negative effects resulting from their self-protective acts of interrupting combined with (b) support and encouragement by the therapist to allow their emotions. Together, these factors motivated clients to cross the bridge, face their fears of disintegration, and allow their emotion. It seemed that when clients came to experience that the harm of the interruptions outweighed the benefit, they were ready to face the difficult emotion.

Vrana (2020) identified the following components as important in overcoming interruption of emotion: First, clients had to become *aware of their own aversion* to emotion in the moment—that they had experienced a conflict between having an emotion and blocking it. They then needed to become aware of *how they interrupt their emotion and the purpose of the interruption*. When clients experienced that they were agents of the interruption and that they were doing it to themselves, it helped them *realize the negative impact of the interruption* by feeling the pain it caused. This realization plus a *reduction of fear of emotion* helped them develop a *desire to*, and the *motivation to, allow the emotion*. This desire to allow was aided by the provision of *support and encouragement by therapists*, which reduced the threat of allowing the emotion. The clients then *allowed the emotion and integrated opposing sides*. They expressed and stayed with the motion, processing it in productive ways either in the session or sometimes outside the session in situations in which they had previously blocked the expression. Many clients along the way revisited a memory that triggered the emotion that had been interrupted—either a memory of recent interaction in the context of a current relationship or a memory from the past with a significant other.

Therapists' support and encouragement helped clients progress through the later stages of the model. In these stages, therapists worked to reduce their clients' fears of their emotions in a number of ways. They were seen as validating their clients' emotional experience and associated needs. They related to their clients with compassion and encouraged them to face their feared emotional experience in the same way. Moreover, therapists conveyed support by reassuring their clients that they were safe, that they were not alone, and that the therapist was there to guide and help them through the process of allowing their emotions. In addition, therapists were observed to explicitly encourage their clients to allow and express the emotion. They directed their clients' attention toward their internal experience, emphasized its importance, and encouraged them to stay with it and symbolize it. Therapists also used evocative empathy to heighten clients' experience of the feared emotion.

A model of the resolution process is shown in Figure 8.1. The components in the rational-empirical model that were found to facilitate the process of resolution are represented by the series of light gray boxes in the middle of the flowchart. In contrast, the components represented by the boxes with dotted lines—*secondary emotions and reluctance to allow the emotion*—signify the states in which unresolved clients tended to become stuck. The component represented by the darker gray box at the top right highlights the importance of the therapists' support and encouragement to clients as they progress through later stages in the model. Later sections in this chapter describe the components of resolution in more detail.

The clients' acknowledgment of the negative impact of the interruption—an acknowledgment that resulted from their experience of the emotional cost of interrupting—was important in developing the motivation to overcome the blocking. In addition, once clients saw the cost and the suffering of constriction, those who overcame the blocks felt compassion for, and acceptance of, the constricted emotional self. All these factors combined led to the development of the motivation in the client to want to allow the previously blocked emotion.

Once clients reached a state of wanting to allow their emotions, they were guided to attend to and symbolize their blocked bodily felt emotional experience and to symbolize, in words, the emotional impact of past injury, trauma, or neglect. Direct attention to internal or bodily experience was important at this point because of possible reentry into past memory/scene of emotional trauma. Clients expressed the previously blocked emotions, and resolution involved reduction of opposition to allowing emotion and processing emotion in a productive way by being able to stay with the experience of the previously blocked emotion (e.g., pain/hurt/sadness, anger) rather than deflect from it. At times, there might have been a gradual, small, step-by-step approach toward experiencing and expressing the previously blocked emotion to keep it in the clients' zone of tolerance.

Therapists reduced the barrier to accessing emotion by having clients attend to and express their fear of experiencing or expressing the blocked emotion, and by reducing clients' sense of vulnerability to the emotion. These two processes were achieved mostly by the therapists' provision of safety through empathy and validation, and by encouraging the clients that they could do it and would not be so overwhelmed that they would not survive having the feeling. Relational support was an important ingredient of

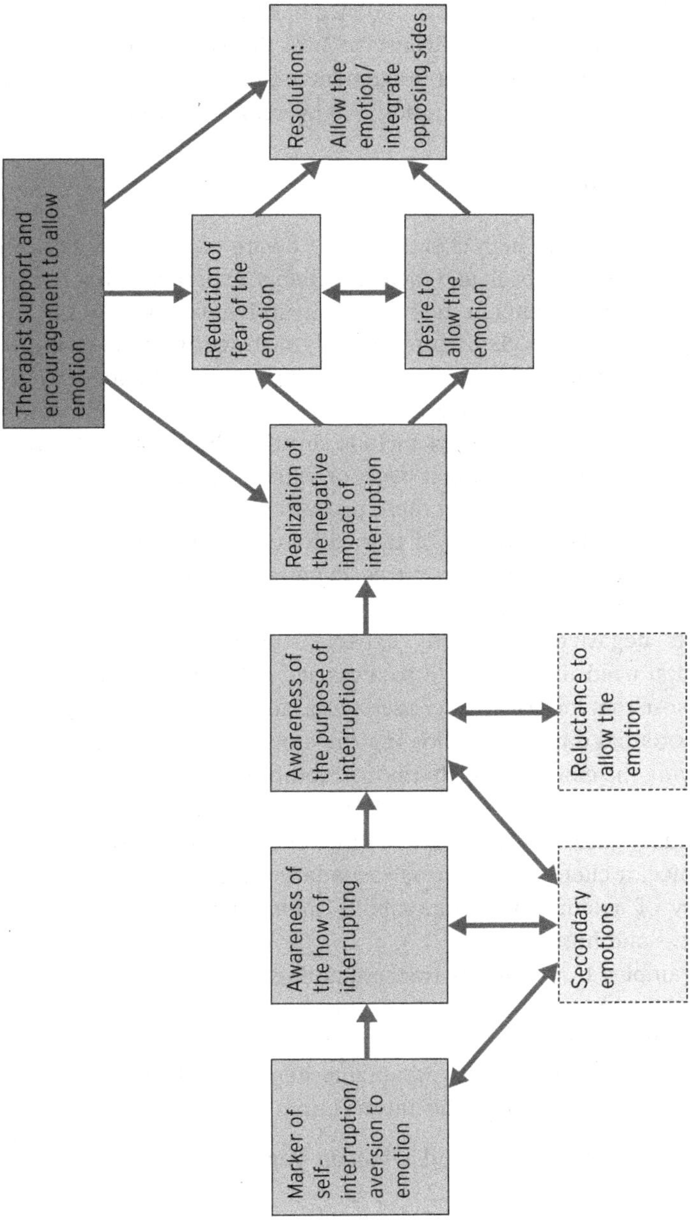

FIGURE 8.1. Resolution of Self-Interruption/Aversion to Emotion

reducing fear and vulnerability. Therapists provided this support by helping clients have a sense of control (e.g., "You can come out of this process at any time") and by engendering confidence in clients in their ability to deal with the emotions (e.g., "You will survive"). As this study (Vrana, 2020) showed, therapists' support and encouragement are important ingredients in helping people face their fear of emotion and overcome their blocking of it.

Awareness of the How of Interrupting

Therapists need to help clients become aware of, or enact, how their interrupter holds them back and facilitate clients' experience that it is they themselves who are agents in their self-interruptive process. Clients interrupt or escape from emotions by intentionally distracting themselves, deflecting, becoming numb, or losing contact with the emotion. In addition, they physically (muscularly or physiologically) control, restrict, or constrict the emotion in various ways. These ways include shutting the emotion down, holding it back, squeezing it, sucking it back, or making it smaller.

Therapists need to bring these processes to awareness; they also need to bring to clients awareness of their different means of cognitive control in the form of self-injunctions against experiencing or expressing the emotion. Self-injunctions that produce guilt/shame, anxiety, or hopelessness and clients' negative evaluations, expectations, or beliefs about allowing the emotion need to be brought to awareness. Additional types of injunctions are those that induce anxiety or hopelessness by either scaring the self about the potential dangers of allowing the emotion or warning of the futility of allowing the emotion. Furthermore, therapists need to recognize that clients can stop or prevent the blocked emotion by experiencing and expressing secondary emotions that are less threatening than the primary emotion. For instance, a client may express secondary anger toward another person as a way of avoiding the vulnerability inherent in expressing their primary sadness and hurt.

Examples from various transcripts illustrate bringing awareness to this self-interruptive process. In the first example, during a two-chair enactment of an interruption, the client enacts how she physically holds herself back (physical control) from experiencing her anger. The enactment brings to awareness how she does this interrupting:

THERAPIST: Mm-hmm, and what do you do to her? Do you squish her down or what?

CLIENT [as interrupter]:   Yeah, that's exactly what I do—squish her (*Therapist: Mm-hmm.*) into the wood.

THERAPIST: With your hands like this (*presses hands together*)?

CLIENT [as interrupter]: No, with my feet.

THERAPIST: With your feet. Can you do it?

CLIENT [as interrupter]: (*Noises of feet pushing down on ground*) Push down, down, down.

Another client describes how she distracts herself and takes a deep breath [physical control] to stop herself from attending to her sadness. Her self-injunctions [cognitive control] against allowing the sadness leave her feeling hopeless:

THERAPIST: Yeah, but since it's there and it kind of always—it won't go— I mean, it won't go away, how do you do that? I want you to do that here: Push it away.

CLIENT [as interrupter]: Well, I just tell myself to think of something else and take a deep breath, and (*Therapist: Mm-hmm.*) then it's just gone.

THERAPIST: Tell her—tell her what she should do.

CLIENT [as interrupter]: Well, I—I guess you don't—don't—don't think about it. (*Therapist: Mm-hmm.*) It makes you feel bad and, um, you won't be able to do anything. Might as well just, and not really . . . you can't really do anything about it, can't change anything, so . . .

THERAPIST: Mm-hmm . . . So don't feel—don't go into it.

CLIENT [as interrupter]: Right.

Awareness of the Purpose of Interruption: Protection Against Feared Consequences

For this component, therapists help clients become aware of and articulate their motivation for interrupting the emotion. Clients need to be helped to realize that the interruption serves to protect them against feared consequences of fully experiencing or expressing the emotion. These feared consequences are generally either (a) fear of damage to identity, attachment, or both—they fear being embarrassed, humiliated, criticized, judged, or rejected by others for expressing the emotion or an associated need—or (b) fear of being overwhelmed by the emotion—they fear that the emotion will be too intense or unending.

It is important for a therapist's clients to explore the origins of their feared consequences. These origins often involve clients' previous experiences with the emotion, including how others in their lives have expressed the emotion in question (e.g., parents who never argued, a caregiver with explosive anger), how others responded to them for expressing the emotion (e.g., punishment, rejection, invalidation), or the internal and external resources they had at the time to help cope with the emotion (e.g., a child left to cope with an overwhelming emotion without adequate support from caregivers). Historical origins also often reflect socially or culturally prescribed rules and expectations about emotional expression (e.g., "Children should always respect and obey their parents").

The client in the following excerpt interrupts her anger during interactions with her husband because she is afraid that he will abandon her if she expresses herself (i.e., damage to attachment):

THERAPIST: Wh—what are you afraid? What do you think is going (*Client sniffs.*)—going to happen? Can you tell me?

CLIENT: (*Sighs*) I'm afraid that if I give him an ultimatum, it might end up being a separation, and, at this point, I feel like I've put in so much, you know, the last 20 years (*Therapist: Um-hum. Client sniffs.*), that maybe what I'm complaining about is too trivial. (*Therapist: Um-hum, um-hum.*)

Another client reports fear of losing control and harming his father if he were to express his anger toward him:

THERAPIST: What—what do you say—what would happen to you if you express the anger? What's your feeling? [inaudible]

CLIENT: That I'm doing wrong, that's not the right thing to do. . . . You don't put your father down, you don't—and because I don't want to hurt him . . . because when I lash out, I go for the jugular verbally.

Realization of the Negative Impact of Interruption

Therapists need to help clients realize that their self-interruptions have a negative impact on them. Negative impacts fall into one of two categories: (a) physical discomfort and painful emotions experienced by clients during the session or (b) long-term consequences of continued self-interruption. Clients need to become aware of how interruption leaves them feeling tired, resigned, depleted, trapped, tense, squeezed, or experiencing physical pain, such as a headache. The negative long-term consequences of continued interruption include maintaining the status quo of feeling depressed and stuck, being unable to move forward from their unfinished business, or remaining unable to form close relationships or have their needs met by others. Although some clients can self-generate these negative long-term consequences, many clients come to this with explication by their therapists.

In the next excerpt, the therapist explains how the client's interruption of her sadness leaves her feeling resigned and unhappy. The client's responses indicate that she has internalized this understanding:

THERAPIST: But it's also important to be kind to yourself, you know, not just to sort of push that sadness away, 'cause then I think it leaves you feeling kind of resigned, you know, not as happy as you can be.

CLIENT: Yeah, that makes sense.

THERAPIST: One way is to try to just put [the sadness] aside and say it's— you know, I don't wanna pay attention to it, but somehow it keeps knocking on your door.

CLIENT: Yes, it does.

In the following excerpt during a two-chair intervention, another client describes the physical discomfort she experiences as the result of being controlled and constricted by her interrupter:

THERAPIST: Tell her what it does to you.

CLIENT [Self, speaking to interrupter]: When you block me, it feels impossible. . . . It feels painful—my head and my heart. It's almost like I can feel. Imagine walls coming up around me.

Reduction of Fear of Emotion

Clients' fears associated with allowing the emotion are reduced as they internalize the validity of their feelings and needs as well as experience a sense of safety in relation to allowing the emotion. They come to see that their emotions are justified and understandable, or they accept these messages about their emotions from their therapists. Therapists need to help clients view themselves as being entitled to their emotions and associated needs as well as to believe that they can cope with allowing the emotion.

This excerpt illustrates the client's validation of his sadness:

CLIENT: Well, I don't know. Right now, I'm just telling myself that it's okay to be sad.

THERAPIST: Yeah, mm-hmm. It's okay to be sad. You deserve, I mean, you're entitled to feel that way given what happened to you. (*Client: Yeah.*)

The following client was able to internalize support from her therapist, which increased her sense of safety:

THERAPIST: Do you want to sort of stay with the anger and see? What comes from there and . . .? (*Client: Yeah.*) But if there's any other stuff that comes up, I'll try to guide you through it, and you can just tell me if it's not comfortable.

CLIENT: Yeah, I think so. I'll try.

Desire to Allow the Emotion

In this step, clients indicate that they want to allow the emotion or that they make attempts to approach or stay with the emotion. In the following excerpt, the client expresses excitement about getting to know the interrupted emotion that he has kept hidden. He refers to the season of spring as a metaphor to describe a feeling of hope for positive change and growth:

CLIENT: You know, I don't know if it's the fog in my head. You know, all week, I've been feeling like, uh, there's something inside me, a feeling that's waiting to come out, and sometimes I get so excited, I can hardly even breathe (*sighs*).

THERAPIST: So, it's like something that's waiting to be born.

CLIENT: Mm, yeah, probably. I, uh, like someone I'm looking forward to meeting, too, I would think. Sometimes it's hard to know why all the—why all the—yeah, anytime, it's funny all the things are happening. It's—it's almost like spring—it's almost like the garden's running a bloom, all sorts of little things that seem to want to grow up all over the place.

UNDERSTANDING THE COMPONENTS OF UNRESOLVED SELF-INTERRUPTION OF EMOTION

In the unresolved group in the Vrana (2020) study, the clients did not experience a realization of the negative impact of interruption, the desire to allow the emotion, or the reduction of fear of the emotion. Unresolved clients were especially observed to be prone to relying on cognitive control to interrupt their emotions by inducing anxiety and fear of the potential dangers of allowing the emotion or in the form of criticism and invalidation. As a result, they often became stuck in unproductive secondary emotions of shame or guilt about having the emotion. Cognitive control via hopeless beliefs and expectations about allowing the emotion was more prominent.

Despite therapists' efforts to have them see the negative impact of the interruption, clients in the unresolved group tended to view the protective benefits of their interruption as greater than the negative impact of their interruption. They were more likely to minimize, rationalize, or dismiss the extent of the negative impact of interrupting their emotions compared with the resolved group. This tendency, along with their aforementioned lack of agency, further deterred them from developing a desire to allow the emotion.

Unresolved clients, therefore, maintained the view that the potential negative consequences of allowing the emotion outweighed the negative consequences of interrupting the emotion as well as the potential positive benefits of allowing the emotion. In these cases, more therapeutic work is needed to both validate their fear as a way of supporting them but continue to work on how they block their emotions to help them realize the negative impact and cost of this self-protective strategy.

INTERVENING USING TWO-CHAIR ENACTMENTS

A particularly helpful intervention for working with blocks to emotion is one in which therapists have clients enact the process of interruption in a dialogue between two sides of the personality (Elliott et al., 2004; Greenberg, Rice, & Elliott, 1993). In this *two-chair enactment*, clients are encouraged to act out how they stop themselves from feeling, verbalize the particular injunctions used, and exaggerate the muscular constrictions involved in the interruption (Greenberg, Rice, & Elliott, 1993; Greenberg & Watson, 2006). Eventually, this intervention provokes a response from the suppressed aspect—often a rebellion against the suppression—and the interrupted self challenges the injunctions by restraining thoughts or muscular blocks of the interrupter. Then, the suppressed emotion bursts through the constrictions, thus undoing the block.

This intervention is meant to turn the passive, automatic process of interruption into an active one and to heighten clients' awareness of how they interrupt themselves. The aim is to help undo these interruptive processes so that clients can access and process emotions.

Markers

Interruptions often appear during a client's narrative while they are addressing vulnerable experiences from the past or in narratives about the fear of feeling certain emotions. Self-interruption is essentially giving oneself this instruction: "Don't feel. Don't need." Self-interruptive splits typically have a nonverbal, bodily aspect—and are sometimes purely nonverbal, such as a headache or tightness in the chest—and may be completely automatic. Nonverbal markers of interruption are abrupt changes or even the disappearance of the emotion that was about to emerge. These markers involve changes in respiratory rhythm, facial expression, and body tension that are accompanied by shifts in emotional processing. All are signs of self-interruption and may arise in conjunction with other nonverbal markers, such as body posture that reflects giving up; shy and weak voices; and, in extreme cases, dissociation.

Interruption involves complex physiological, muscular, emotional, and cognitive processes that inhibit experience and expression. Resignation and hopelessness experienced by some clients in the face of their core emotional needs not being met is another important marker of interruption. Resignation and deadness often are the result of squashing and suppressing anger or sadness. "What's the use" frequently captures this feeling. "I don't care" often is an expression of cynical resignation. People express resignation through their bodies by sighing or shrugging their shoulders and then saying things like, "What's the point? Why even bother?"

Intervention

Two-chair enactment is an unusual task involving talking to oneself in an empty chair; therefore, the therapist needs to provide a lot of structure. To begin this intervention, the therapist encourages the client to enact how a part of the self is stopping, blocking, interrupting, or constricting the expression of the emotion. The therapist invites the client to begin the dialogue in the chair:

THERAPIST: So, let's set up an experiment to explore how this blocking takes place. In this chair in front of you, you will be the side that does stop you from expressing your emotion. The chair where you are sitting now will be your feeling that is blocked. Can you come and sit in this chair and be the part of you that stops you from getting angry? Be the part that stops you. How does this part not let you feel angry? What do you do to yourself?

Providing some form of psychoeducation before entering the intervention is important, and it's best to give it at the moment the client blocks, thus promoting experiential learning. By doing this psychoeducation when the block occurs, the therapist promotes an experiential as opposed to a conceptual understanding of how the block is affecting clients. Pointing out nonverbal behaviors can also bring the experience alive. When, for example, sadness is blocked, the therapist might draw the client's attention to how their breathing changed. When it is anger that is blocked, the therapist might point out how clients tighten their neck muscles and clutch their hands. The therapist might then say that it is important to feel sad after a loss, similarly with unexpressed anger, and that, if not processed, these emotions can lead to depression. The therapist then checks with the client if this all make sense, saying things like, "It's as if you were talking to yourself . . . I can't be angry. I have to swallow my feelings for the rest of my life? Does that make sense to you?"

The two-chair enactment task requires three essential steps on the part of the therapist:

1. Bring the client's attention to the fact that he or she is interrupting or suppressing (i.e., by noting that the client looks away whenever mentioning certain things, or changes the topic, or smiles).

2. Turn the passive to active and the automatic to deliberate by inquiring and ascribing personal agency to the client in the interruptive process (e.g., "How do you stop yourself or interrupt yourself?"). This is an awareness task that the therapist can use to elaborate conscious experience and specify what the interrupters are (e.g., "What do you say to yourself?" "What do you do muscularly?" "How would you do it to me?").

3. Access what is being suppressed or integrate the two sides of the struggle, or both.

Therapists need to help clients discover first *that* they interrupt and then *how* they interrupt. They also need to acknowledge the protective function of the interruption, help clients experience the fear that drives the self-protective interruption, and ultimately allow what has been interrupted. It is really important for therapists to validate clients' fears of the emotion being interrupted and acknowledge its protective function. Clients, on the other hand, need to develop a sense of themselves as agents who interrupt as opposed to being victims of interruption.

Two important aspects of the blocking process need to be attended to by the therapist. The first is the verbal cognitive aspect, which essentially is what people say to themselves—the words that appear in the client's narrative. The therapist then asks the client to verbally express the content linked to the restriction on feeling emotions. The second is the nonverbal aspect of blocking; with this aspect, the interruption of emotion has a body component. For example, clients may block themselves by increasing muscle tension and breathing rate. The therapist assists the client in locating muscular tension and blocking points, and discovering how they are produced. The therapist asks the client to enact the experience of blocking emotions, highlighting how it is that the client has produced the block through their motor activity. Once clients realize they are the ones producing the block, they are inclined to choose to stop doing so.

The following clinical example shows how Desh, a 29-year-old, South Asian man, a computer analyst with generalized anxiety disorder, both verbally and nonverbally blocks:

THERAPIST [with client already sitting on the "interrupter chair" representing the interruptive self]:   I want you to block, to stop this side of you. What do you say to make him stop feeling? What do you say to this part of you?

CLIENT: You can't be angry at your father. You must respect him! How the hell can you feel that about your own father?

The therapist then advises this client to return to the experiential self. Again, what matters is that the dialogue is not a logical or rational reflection on the importance of expressing emotions. The focus is now on how the client is impacted by the emotional block. The therapist tries to make the client perceive this impact, articulating it through language and expressing it:

THERAPIST: (*Points to the chair of the experiential self*) Sit here. What happens inside you when you hear this? Talk to him (*points to the interrupter chair*).

CLIENT: I don't know . . . I think that's right . . . I should just let it be.

THERAPIST: I understand. But what is it like, this experience of feeling and not being able to express it? Not being able to respond to your own feelings? How does this affect you in your daily life?

CLIENT: I don't know . . .

Once clients have experienced the process of interrupting emotions, the therapist helps them overcome the blocks and get in touch with the disconnected emotions, thus recovering their information and healing power.

This is done by guiding the client to further intensify the self-interruptive activity so that a self-preservation reaction emerges in the experiential self. The therapist continues to support and follow the painful experience in the experiential self until the client achieves some reaction and empowerment of that self.

The following is an example of work using two chairs for interruption with a 31-year-old, male, French Canadian client who presented with depression and anxiety disorders:

CLIENT: I'm so angry at him [referring to the imagined father in the empty chair].

THERAPIST: Tell him.

CLIENT: I couldn't do that. I just hold it all in.

THERAPIST: Come over here and stop him from being angry.

CLIENT: (*Sits in the chair that, up to this point, represented his father*) Who am I here?

THERAPIST: Be a part of yourself that stops him.

CLIENT: Well, my father just seems so superior, so powerful. I just retreat.

THERAPIST: Okay, but as yourself, not your father, make yourself retreat. How do you do that? What does this voice inside you say?

CLIENT: It says, "Well, you have no legitimacy. Don't get angry. I get scared. It's not okay; it's dangerous."

THERAPIST: Make him scared. What do you say?

CLIENT: "Watch out. You won't be able to speak."

THERAPIST: Make him not able to speak.

CLIENT: "Well, you're stupid. You don't have what it takes. Also, you'll get too emotional and you'll cry or you'll damage the relationship. So just retreat."

THERAPIST: Yeah, tell him this again.

CLIENT: "Retreat, just shrink away, disappear."

THERAPIST: Change chairs now. What do you say to that?

CLIENT: (*Sits in the interrupter chair*) I feel sort of hopeless, resigned— like it's been such a long time always feeling like, weak, never supported. But I do feel like I have a valid point of view. I have a right to be me. I was never supported. I do deserve it; I didn't do anything wrong,

THERAPIST: What's that like in your body?

CLIENT: I just feel so angry that, well, I sort of feel my back straighten, kind of like feeling taller.

THERAPIST: (*Redirects to the father*) Good. Put your father there. Tell him, "I'm angry at you."

As shown in this example, after working on a self-interruption of resignation, once the client gets to the point of feeling more deserving and says, "I do deserve it; I didn't do anything wrong," the therapist then directs the newly accessed feelings and needs back toward the father.

HELPING CLIENTS ACCESS THEIR ABILITY TO TOLERATE BLOCKED EMOTIONS

It is essential to ensure that clients have sufficient internal support for making contact with emotions before the blocks are undone and emotions are evoked and experienced. Some clients become tense at the prospect of encountering their feelings. At these times, the therapist has to empathize with the fear, understand that the block is a protection, and provide more support. On the one hand, more relational support in the form of validation and trust building is indicated. On the other hand, the building of internal support by a slower approach to emotion—in small steps—helps clients deal with their anxiety. A type of graded exposure or desensitization process is most useful in helping clients to approach and tolerate their emotions. The therapist also helps clients mobilize internal support by suggesting, for example, that clients breathe, put their feet on the ground, and describe what they are experiencing to increase contact with sensory reality.

The next example illustrates one client's progression toward symbolizing her emotion progressing from unsymbolized affect/feeling to the differentiation and expression of her emotional experience. The client, a 52-year-old, married, Caucasian woman of Slovakian origin, was a highly successful business executive in her second marriage of 12 years and had three children, two from her first marriage. She began the first session by explaining to the therapist what brought her to therapy: She had been suffering from depression and a chronic skin problem (hives) that she was told was related to stress. As she acknowledged a need to "deal with what's really bothering me," she began to cry. She further explained that she cries often and feels like she has "no control" over it. As illustrated in the following passage, she worked with her therapist to differentiate her blocked unsymbolized feeling:

CLIENT: Part of me wants to sort of let it all out . . . but I don't know what it is that I'm supposed to let out (*cries*).

THERAPIST: Mm-hmm. So, there's a lot in there, but you're not quite sure how to let it out.

CLIENT: Mm-hmm.

THERAPIST: Okay. Well, what do you feel like right now? 'Cause I can see the tears and I can see you trying really hard to push them back, but . . .

CLIENT: 'Cause you see right now, I don't know why I'm crying . . . I can't, you know, put my finger on it. Like, what is it about this? I'm talking about something that's not that difficult. Why am I crying (*sniffs*)?

THERAPIST: Okay, well instead of wondering about the why, why don't we just look at what it is you're feeling right now. (*Client: Mm-hmm.*) Since that seems to be very alive, what's happening inside here?

CLIENT: (*Sighs and pauses*) I feel like an ache inside all the time, like I'm not really happy. (*Therapist: Mm-hmm. Client pauses.*) Um, I'm very close to my sons, and I miss them a lot 'cause they're not here. (*Therapist: Mm-hmm.*) And I'd like to spend more time with them, and that's not, you know, feasible.

THERAPIST: Mm-hmm. Tell me about the ache that you feel.

CLIENT: I dunno, it's almost like a physical, you know (*Therapist: Mm-hmm.*) hurting. (*Therapist: Mm-hmm.*) And it's almost always with me.

THERAPIST: That must be draining to have it always.

CLIENT: I guess that's why I'm so tired and exhausted all the time.

In the final stage of overcoming the block, clients feel more empowered, regaining the adaptive and informative role of emotions. They are able to contact painful emotions and themes, recognizing unmet emotional needs, and to start to reclaim them. Unblocking allows the accomplishment of other therapeutic tasks that might present themselves in therapy as well as the creation of new meaning.

Sometimes interruption is caused by protective anxiety, and unblocking involves standing up to and reassuring the catastrophizer. For example, in the following excerpt, the therapist works to help the client, Susan, a 33-year-old European business executive, stand up to the part that is silencing her by worrying she will make a mistake. Susan tells the worrying side that the worrying makes her tense and that she needs to relax. However, the worrier responds that she is scared and cannot stop worrying in case she cannot protect her.

CLIENT: *(Speaks to the worrying side)* Stop telling me to be careful. I feel so exhausted trying to ensure I don't make a mistake.

THERAPIST: So, from this side, what do you need? Tell her.

CLIENT: I need you to stop worrying. Stop telling me that "things will go wrong." I need you to calm down.

THERAPIST: Come over here *(points to the interrupter chair, where the client now sits)*. So how do you respond to her? She [in the self chair] says, "I need you to calm down. I am so tired and exhausted."

CLIENT: *(Speaks from interrupter chair)* I can't stop. I'm scared [that] without me, you might get into trouble—make mistakes, and you'll be rejected.

After reprocessing some memories of always being corrected by her mother, the client from the self chair says the following to the interrupter:

CLIENT: I am capable. I don't need you always on my shoulder. And even if I sometimes make mistakes, I can fix them, and I will survive. I want you to back off and give me space . . .

THERAPIST: So, you are reassuring her that you will be able to manage without her constant monitoring and that you are capable and can manage.

CLIENT: *(Sighs with tears in her eyes)* Oh, that's it. . . . That's what I need. That feels so good.

After this, Susan's anxiety lifted, and she feels more joyful and less fearful. Next, we turn to a full example of a two-chair enactment for unblocking. Interspersed with the transcript are interpretive notes that indicate the different components of the model of change.

EATING THE SADNESS: UNBLOCKING ANGER AND SADNESS

In this example, Jeanne, a 38-year-old Caucasian woman, client came to therapy suffering from depression and anxiety, and had concerns about an eating disorder plus her addiction to marijuana. This client, as illustrated in the following excerpt, is working through her interrupted anger and sadness after the breakup of a more than 14-year relationship (with John), which led to an exacerbation of her eating and marijuana problems. In the first part of the session transcript, she talks about spending the weekend at a vacation home with a new partner (Yarrow):

THERAPIST: So, it's really hard for you to accept these—these feelings, this emotional part of you?

CLIENT: I think so (*nods*). I think so (*nods*). Because I did notice that there was a real gap. (*Therapist: Uh-huh.*) When I was— particularly when I was talking about feeling angry with John. And I realized that these—there's a real gap 'cause I don't like to think of myself as a person who just, you know, dislikes or— I mean throws spears or anything like that. And yet—I am. (*Therapist: You do.*) Yeah, and that's—and that's—I'm getting more comfortable with that when I realized that I'm obviously not very—well even now because I can feel myself struggling to talk—in—in first person. To talk in the first person. I'm— I'm, uh . . . [awareness of aversion to anger]

THERAPIST: It's really hard for you to kind of express yourself sort of that one—that other—that passive intellectual, knowing part.

CLIENT: Well, because there's an ideal me (*giggles*) and there's me, and I'm finding it—I've been very careful building up this ideal me, and the gaps are troublesome.

THERAPIST: (*Points to the interrupter chair*) Would you want to split them apart? Talk to each other?

CLIENT: I'm not sure—I'm not quite—I don't think I'm fighting against it (*holds her throat*)—I'm not sure I—I'll be able to because I'm sort of watching it. If that makes sense—I'm in a real . . . I don't know I can try—who's supposed to be (*giggles*) there?

THERAPIST: Are you more in touch with the ideal self? The kind one who wants to keep everything cool, collected?

CLIENT: The other in actually—the entire, um, I'm on pure—sort of, ugh (*sighs*), for lack of a better term—left brain right now, I mean it's very intellectual, I'm very—watching it, I'm, you know . . .

THERAPIST: So, this your cerebral, analytical, yeah. (*Client nods head; therapist points to the interrupter chair.*) This is the cool, collected, rational side. Okay, stop the emotional side—tell her you shouldn't express yourself? How do you stop yourself from expressing itself, its emotions?

CLIENT: I'll try and (*covers her eyes and takes a deep breath*)—no, because intellectually, I think I should be expressing those emotions more clearly. I know I should be expressing those emotions more clearly—it would just simplify my life.

THERAPIST: Uh-huh. Stop her from expressing her emotions.

CLIENT: I don't know—I do know how I do it, but I do it . . . by pauses like this. When I can feel myself getting emotional.

THERAPIST: So . . . what are you doing? (*Client: Yeah.*) And then what happens inside—do you go blank?

CLIENT: No, I—I sigh. I mean that's where I kind of give myself a breathing space and, well (*sighs*), okay, just kind of—um—it's—I can only think in metaphors—but I eat the emotion, this is really what I do. [awareness of self-protective function of self-interruption]

THERAPIST: So, you stop yourself by eating your emotions?

CLIENT: Uh-huh. I don't know—I think you were for asking how I—how—why I stop myself?

THERAPIST: Uh, looking at how you stop yourself—you eat them? (*Client: Uh-huh.*) Swallow them back down.

CLIENT: Uh-huh (*nods*). (*Therapist: Okay.*) I save—or I save them for later.

THERAPIST: Okay (*nods; therapist mimics swallowing something*). What does it feel like—swallowing it down?

CLIENT: Um, fine. I feel—I mean, in some ways—in some ways, I feel better. I mean, I could feel sort of tension happening through my spine and through my shoulders (*points to the back of her neck and shoulders*). [awareness of self-protective function of self-interruption]

THERAPIST: Is there any indigestion? (*Client: But—no. No [laughs]. Therapist laughs.*)

CLIENT: No—I'm kind of very good at it (*continues to laugh*). Very used to it. Um . . .

THERAPIST: Tense in here. Can you speak from your tension? (*Client sighs. Therapist whispers.*) What does your tension say?

CLIENT: Yeah. I—I—I mean, I can feel a sort of lodging in my throat (*points to neck*).

THERAPIST: (*Points to own neck*) Sitting here?

CLIENT: I'm swallowing things right now (*takes a deep breath and covers her face*). I know I'm getting all tense about going up to the cottage this weekend—so that's one of the things I am getting tense about.

THERAPIST: What does it feel like?

CLIENT: Um, I don't know. I've been trying to work that out. And (*sighs*), no.

THERAPIST: Stay with the tension. (*Client nods.*) Um-hmm. (*Therapist whispers.*) Can you focus on the tension? (*Client sighs.*) Put words to that tension?

CLIENT: Now it's my space is disappearing again. That's what it feels like.

THERAPIST: Somehow, you're feeling more what? You're feeling a bit . . . ?

CLIENT: Um, yeah. Because up there at the cottage, it's not—I feel like it's not my space. And (*sighs*) yes, so the idea—ugh—and this is intellectualizing it again, but—I feel like there's going to be—I'm going to have to sit in my ideal self a lot more than trying to find out what my natural self is. I mean, those are sort of . . .

THERAPIST: Feel you're going to have to be what? On your best behavior? Is that it? Well, not to be you?

CLIENT: Yes, because—not because (*sighs*) me is particularly bad, but I think right now—what I'm trying to work or what I'm trying to find out how I express (*sighs*) things is—is a lot of negative emotions. There's a lot of anger, there's a lot of, um, frustration, um, that—that type of emotion.

THERAPIST: What's the anger and frustration about? (*Client sighs.*) Lots of things all at once. Um, I'll try and split them up (*sighs*). Yarrow [new partner] encroaches upon space, or I feel like he encroaches upon my space—that I'm trying to—that I'm really working hard to sort of define—but more than that, I know that the anger has a lot to do with John [former partner]. I still haven't worked out that.

THERAPIST: So, you're feeling angry?

CLIENT: Uh-huh.

THERAPIST: And frustrated? You're not quite sure how to express it?

CLIENT: Uh-huh.

THERAPIST: You're still really angry at John?

CLIENT: I can feel my tone is very (*Therapist: Uh-huh.*)—but I am—oh, I'm furious at him! I'm furious at him. And every time—well I had to call him, too, so that he had to take care of my cats and my birds for the weekend. And it's infuriating, it's—we get—we got along—we do get along so well on certain levels. And yet—he complete—I mean he just—he just walked out on all of that, and I'm furious. There! I'm keeping it nice and cool. I'm just (*sighs*) . . .

THERAPIST: Swallowing now?

CLIENT: Uh-huh.

THERAPIST: Swallowing it down?

CLIENT: Uh-huh. It just doesn't feel so pleasant. I can just—I can feel it sort of poisoning—I mean it's poisoning everything. [realization of negative impact of interruption]

THERAPIST: What does it feel like as you swallow? So, it goes inside, and you, it poisons.

CLIENT: And it does—it poisons—it does—it poisons my relationship with Yarrow.

THERAPIST: It corrodes your insides.

CLIENT: I mean, I could feel that all the time because when I'm angry, I confuse their names. I mean it's awful. I'm always calling Yarrow "John" when I'm angry with him. So, I'm really sad— I know that somewhere along the line (*lifts her arms up*) . . .

THERAPIST: What's happening over there? (*Therapist points to the client's arms moving.*)

CLIENT: (*Closes her eyes and shakes her head*) Oh, I want just (*sigh*)— I am (*covers her face with her hands*). Oh, I want to scream at him so badly.

THERAPIST: Well, why don't you scream at him (*points to the other chair now representing John, her ex*)? Scream at him (*brings the chair closer to the client*).

CLIENT: Oh! He just—oh, I can't even express that I'm just so furious with him (*covers her eyes, voice trembling, and takes a deep breath*).

THERAPIST: What do you want to scream at him? (*Therapist speaks quietly.*) Try it out. [support and encouragement from the therapist]

CLIENT: He just (*takes deep breath*)——he walked out—I mean he just walked out on everything, and now it's (*takes a deep breath*) . . .

THERAPIST: It doesn't sound angry yet.

CLIENT: I know it doesn't sound angry. It's (*takes deep breath*) . . .

THERAPIST: (*Slaps the chair*) "How dare you walk away? How dare you!" [approach to emotion with support and encouragement from the therapist]

CLIENT: And without even—I mean it wasn't—it didn't even mean anything to him. It was just it was going to be . . .

THERAPIST: "You just abandoned—you just turned your back on us!"

CLIENT: Completely! (*The client covers her face with her hands and takes a deep breath.*)

THERAPIST: Can you tell him that?

CLIENT: Ugh, ugh, no! (*She puts her face in her hands.*) No—that's the problem, I can't tell him. I can feel my—I'm just sucking it all in.

THERAPIST: Okay, then swallow it some more. (*Client takes a deep breath.*) More. Take it right in. (*Client takes a deep breath.*) Don't want any of it—take it right in (*points to the other chair*). How do you do that?

CLIENT: I squeeze my stomach. Hold my breath. [articulation/enactment of self-protective function of self-interruption]

THERAPIST: Yes, do that. Do it with your hands to the pillow. (*Client squeezes the pillow.*) Just tighten up. Hold it in. . . . Come over here.

CLIENT: (*Sits on the self chair and takes a deep breath*)

THERAPIST: What is it like—to take it right in? What does it feel like inside as you swallow it down? What it is doing to you?

CLIENT: (*Takes a deep breath*) Oh it's—it is—it (*covers her eyes*)—it—corroding is the right word. It's—it's destroying me. [realization of negative impact of interruption]

THERAPIST: Can you speak from it? This feeling—that it's destroying you? Eating away like a cancer?

CLIENT: No. It's more like I'm fraying around the edges. I'm just breaking up.

THERAPIST: Feel like you're slowly falling apart, disintegrating?

CLIENT: (*Client nods. Therapist: Uh-huh [sighs].*)

THERAPIST: So, you can't go there?

CLIENT: (*Shakes her head and takes a deep breath*) And every time I talk to him—oh—I want to—a part of me wants to stay angry long enough to—[desire to allow]—but every time I talk to him, I remember why I really wanted everything to work. And, so, it's all of that (*sighs and covers her eyes*).

THERAPIST: (*Points to the self chair*)

CLIENT: (*Moves onto the self chair*)

THERAPIST: Tell me what you miss about your relationship? It's special?

CLIENT: (*Covers her eyes*) Oh, how . . .

THERAPIST: Something special?

CLIENT: How bright it was and how (*sighs*), oh, it was (*sighs*)—it was so quick and so bright, and we could talk about anything, and,

I mean, the steps between ideas were like infinitesimal, and it was wonderful, and it was exciting, and, oh, and what's worst is that he betrayed all of that even while we were living together (*voice trembles*). I did prize that. And at the—I mean that's what was so horrible—at the same time, he was undermining me at every step (*covers her eyes*), and I was like—it was—but, at the same time, he undermined me, but I was protecting what we had protecting myself. I was afraid to be angry. [awareness of self-protective function of self-interruption]

THERAPIST: "I really prized that." How did he undermine you?

At this point, the client elaborates on how John undermined her intellectually and on her resulting feelings of self-doubt. The transcript picks up again a few minutes later with the therapist asking the client how she feels now after she has enacted her ex putting her down:

THERAPIST: What happens inside when you hear him say, "Ugh, you're very bright—but you know, really, these ideas, are just corrupt. They're just . . ."

CLIENT: (*Takes a deep breath*) Now or then or both? (*Therapist: Now.*) Um (*sighs*), I get so—not angry, I get so sad (*Therapist: Uh-huh.*) (*Client eyes tear, and she covers them up.*) because all I remember was how I kept trying to run to catch up—so it was sort of—like, well, okay, this isn't a good idea, so I'll do this—and it was never a good—none of it was ever . . .

THERAPIST: Can you stay with the sadness? (*Client nods.*) Can you let it flow? (*Therapist whispers.*) So, just let it out.

CLIENT: Nope (*shakes head*). I can't. [awareness of aversion of sadness]

THERAPIST: Can you suck in the sadness? (*Client takes a deep breath.*) Suck it right in.

CLIENT: (*Nods*) I'm sucking it in right away (*sighs, then takes a deep breath, then sighs*). Yeah, that I'm good at (*grabs a tissue and nods*)—I'm sucking it in right away (*sighs and takes a deep breath*), then I'm safe. [awareness of self-protective function of self-interruption]

THERAPIST: What did it feel like inside? Did you suck it in? (*Client sighs and wipes her face with a tissue.*) Can you exaggerate that "sucking in"? Uhh (*makes sucking in sound*) . . . (*Client mimics the sucking sound.*) Uhh . . . Can you exaggerate them some more? Some more (*Client takes a breath.*)? What does it feel like as you suck it all in?

CLIENT: (*Takes a breath*) Ordinary. I do it all the time. It stops me from having to feel it. [awareness of self-protective function of self-interruption]

THERAPIST: What does it feel like? It's familiar? (*Client: Uh-huh. It does.*)

CLIENT: (*Takes a breath*) Oh, I can feel it's tingling at the edge of every muscle, trying to get out.

THERAPIST: Uh-huh. Something struggling to get out?

CLIENT: (*Sighs*) And it does—it's like this dark cloud that I'm sort of carrying around (*sighs*). I have images of wanting to take a knife to him and slash him up because I'm so angry with him. (*Therapist: Uh-huh.*) And I don't really—but I—I know that I want to slash him and that's the way I feel—that he's slashed me open (*tears up and covers her face*). [desire to allow]

THERAPIST: So, you kind of feel slashed open, wounded? (*Client nods.*) Uh-huh. (*Client: Yup.*) You'd like to wound him somehow, make him feel as painful?

CLIENT: Yup. And I can't—I mean, that's the thing—I can't get to him at all (*sighs*).

THERAPIST: So, you feel very powerless? (*Client: Yes [nods, then sighs and covers her eyes].*) You don't want—you don't want do it in here? . . . You don't want to express that rage on him?

CLIENT: No—I think I'm really afraid of it. [awareness of self-protective function of self-interruption]

THERAPIST: What would happen if you express it?

CLIENT: I don't know. Well—oh, I do. I'll be embarrassed or I'll be, you know, I'll lose control.

THERAPIST: It doesn't feel like it's safe to be angry here?

CLIENT: No (*shakes her head*). It doesn't feel (*sighs*)—I don't think I ever felt very safe, but that's the one—this sounds so intellectual, but it's not—I know that that's the one thing that he really managed (*sighs*) to really reinforce was—I don't feel safe at all. And I mean, it's not . . .

THERAPIST: You don't feel safe, anywhere?

CLIENT: (*Shakes her head*) No, no, he was always managing to pull the rug out from under me. I mean, every time I thought I'd created little edifices, I was safe—it was, um, it was destroyed. And I mean, he was never (*sighs*) . . .

THERAPIST: So, if you let your guard down in here (*Client: Yeah.*) and feel those strong feelings of anger and sadness . . .What? He might kind of use it again you? (*Client sighs.*) Would get some power over you? (*Client: Uh-huh.*) You scared to argue it out in here?

CLIENT: Um (*sighs*), I don't feel that there are many ways that I can— I can feel it . . . I mean, it's not a thought that I have but I know—I know I must have it because I don't feel safe, up to a—ugh, a fairly small limit, and I mean, well, hell—I'm sure you've seen it. . . . Every time I try to express anger, I can't do it. I completely close off (*Therapist: Uh-huh [sighs].*). Even (*swallows*)—I mean, it's like protection (*shakes her head and sighs*). [awareness of self-protective function of self-interruption]

THERAPIST: It just seems to me that it might actually be useful to you— to express it. [reduction of fear of the emotion through reassurance from self or therapist]

CLIENT: It would be.

THERAPIST: If you could, to get some of that anger out because I think it could provide a shift for you, in so many ways . . .

CLIENT: Oh, I know. And I mean, I know that's . . . (*sighs*)—I know (*takes a deep breath*) [desire to allow]. Oh, I don't know how to—I don't know how to do it. I mean, I don't know how to do it (*voice trembles; sighs*).

THERAPIST: (*Whispers*) It's so stuck. (*Client nods.*) There's no formula.

CLIENT: (*Shakes her head*) No, I mean, I'm (*sighs and covers her face, starts to sniffle*) . . . And then, of course, it just starts to get into feeling badly because it's not that I don't trust you, it's just that something—I can't get past it. [awareness of aversion/interruption]

THERAPIST: Uh-huh. So, it's not just me personally.

CLIENT: No. It's just a terrible sense of—even with you, I don't feel safe when I—when the feelings of anger start coming up.

THERAPIST: What do you think it'll do? Break a chair? Hurt me?

CLIENT: No—not hurt you. Um . . .

THERAPIST: Break a hole through the wall?

CLIENT: Yeah (*sniffles and exhales*). Yeah, I've had—I've had two (*sighs*), I mean, I know, I think I know intellectually what's happened. I've had two models of—of anger. I've had my mother's model where it's just—and that's the one I end up using—where you don't (*Therapist: Uh-huh.*) express, you sort of—it sort of—yeah. But it ends, oh, yeah, all over the place. (*Therapist: Um.*) It ends up all over the place. Or, my father, who did throw chairs around. (*Therapist: Uh-huh.*) I mean, he never—he never touched any of us. He was always very careful about that, but I mean, there would be these huge, explosive, destructive . . .

THERAPIST: So, I think that's very scary for you, knowing how to express— you don't how—how is it kind of, um—you have these two extremes? And, somehow, it's hard to kind of trust yourself to be able to express anger in a way that is—is not as kind of explosive (*Client: Uh-huh.*) and out of control as your dad. (*Client: Yeah.*) Almost corrosive to you, as your mom. You need to find a way beyond—express that anger. [therapist support and encouragement to allow emotion]

CLIENT: Yeah. And I don't know how to do it because I've just got— I mean, when I think of expressing anger—I mean, it really is— it is throwing chairs through windows and—and (*sighs*) . . .

THERAPIST: Can you hit the chair? You can do it, and you won't be destructive.

CLIENT: No. No, because I feel embarrassed about it. I mean—there's that, too. I just—I'm (*sighs*).

THERAPIST: Can you give words to the anger? (*Client sighs.*) That's another way of expressing it. (*Whispers*) And I'm here to support you. [safety: reduction of fear through support and encouragement from therapist]

CLIENT: (*Shakes her head*) Oh, it's so hard. I mean that—I should be able to do that—but I don't—well, I know, I don't have any angry words. I have all these lovely, passive—you know, "I'm upset," "It upsets me." I mean those—those are—those aren't angry words. Those are just ways of avoiding, but I want to be able to be angry. I deserved better. [desire to allow]

THERAPIST: Tell him what he did to you.

CLIENT: (*Sighs and covers her eyes*) Because I'm not (*sniffles*)—I go over and over what he did to me, but what I'm furious about is the fact that he did it (*sniffles*) . . .

THERAPIST: Yes, you have a right to be furious.

CLIENT: I do [reduction of fear through validation of self]. I am— I really am furious at him and how he treated me. He's an arrogant, selfish person, and I hate him for what he did. I'm also sad—sad I didn't stand up for myself and sad I have lost all the good parts. [allow emotion]

The client and therapist then continue for the next 14 minutes of the session. In this period, the client stays with the emotion, processing her feelings in productive ways to differentiate complex aspects of the client's relationship with John—both the good and the bad. A new narrative begins to develop that helps her understand why she, for fear of losing the good parts, did not stand up to him. She ends with talking about how she now needs to let go and move on but that she needs time to both grieve the loss and support herself. In the excerpt, we see how with the therapist's support and encouragement, she approaches the feared emotion and articulates the self-protective function of self-interruption, and by enacting it, comes to experience its negative impact. This leads to a desire to accept and express the emotion, which she goes on to do.

CONCLUSION

The perspective offered in this chapter is that, to heal their troubled souls and minds, clients need to experience the emotions that go with their stories. It is, however, understandable that clients protect themselves from feeling their dreaded, painful emotions. They fear that if they allow these emotions, they will fall apart, disintegrate, and be unable to cope, so they do all in their power to not feel. However, what they resist persists, so blocking is not an effective solution. Protection or avoidance is not always deliberate and intentional; it's just how the mind habitually protects itself from falling apart. Clients, therefore, often need assistance connecting to their emotions.

In this chapter, I outlined the steps involved in unblocking emotion and highlighted the importance of the client's realizing the negative impact of the blocking. Several examples illustrated how a therapist's encouragement helps clients to face the emotion; the therapist reassures clients that they can undo the protection and will survive. In addition, I discussed how two-chair enactments that focus on how interruption works are a good intervention for helping clients overcome their blocking; examples demonstrated what that can look like.

In the next chapters, I turn to the processes and skills needed to facilitate the leaving of emotions by creating more adaptive emotional responses to their life circumstances.

PART **III** LEAVING
EMOTION

9

WORKING WITH NEEDS

In a therapy focused on emotional change, the aim is to change painful, maladaptive emotions like fear of abandonment or of annihilation from past childhood maltreatment. Once these emotions are aroused in the present, as described in Chapters 5 to 8, they can be transformed by the activation of more empowering emotions. How do we therapists help clients access more empowering emotions? My colleagues and I (Greenberg & Malcolm, 2002; Greenberg & Paivio, 1997; A. Pascual-Leone & Greenberg, 2007) found that mobilizing the unmet need in the emotion is one of the most helpful ways of activating an adaptive emotion. For example, maladaptive shame, which is internalized from the contempt of others, can be transformed by accessing the need for validation. When the client acknowledges that they need and, in fact, deserve validation, the accessing of this need activates adaptive emotions, such as anger at invalidation, grief for all the losses involved, and possibly self-compassion. What ensues is a sense of pride and self-worth.

Every emotion people experience involves a specific set of needs. When these needs are met, the cycle of experience flows normally, and the emotion is fast and fleeting. If we feel shame, but, at the same time, our needs for validation by someone meaningful are fulfilled, we feel reassured and again

https://doi.org/10.1037/0000248-010
Changing Emotion With Emotion: A Practitioner's Guide, by L. S. Greenberg

feel comfortable and confident within ourselves and in our interactions with the outside world. However, if these needs are not met, discomfort, pain, and suffering persist. In an attempt to deal with this suffering, people form emotion schematic memories of the unmet need and the emotional pain to act as a warning system to protect themselves. This system can then be triggered in different situations, alerting us to danger whenever a situation resembles the original cause of the pain. The emotion scheme acts as a sort of exaggerated warning system. People also may protect themselves from the suffering with secondary emotions that disguise primary emotions; these secondary emotions involve a sort of paralysis or imprisonment in bad feelings, such as hopelessness, anxiety, or reactive anger.

We have found that focusing on reowning previously unmet emotional needs helps mobilize primary adaptive emotions (Greenberg, 2015; A. Pascual-Leone & Greenberg, 2007), and that is a powerful driver of change. These new, adaptive emotions that help modify old, maladaptive emotions are precisely those the client was never able to experience in the past. And, focusing on adaptive primary emotions moves people even further toward having other emotional needs met because these emotions guide us in the direction of actions and problem-solving to get the needs met. The newly experienced primary adaptive emotions present new possibilities that people can now access, thus undoing the existing problematic affective and cognitive responses. The adaptive sadness of grief helps douse the pangs of loneliness and unworthiness; it also helps people let go of the unmet need for closeness that they never received from a parent. Accessing needs and new emotions helps people change old beliefs not by disputing them rationally but by having vivid emotional experience that disconfirms the beliefs. People cannot believe that they are unlovable while they experience themselves as deserving of love; likewise, they cannot shrink away in fear while thrusting forward in assertion.

WHAT ARE NEEDS?

A key way of activating a new emotion is by focusing on what is needed (Greenberg, 2002, 2015; A. Pascual-Leone & Greenberg, 2007). The essence of this process is this: When clients access core painful maladaptive emotions of fear, shame, or sadness, accessed core needs for connection, safety, and validation embedded within them are mobilized. If clients can be helped to feel deserving of these previously unmet needs, they are able to generate more adaptive emotions related to their unmet needs. Thus, when clients feel that they deserve to be loved or valued, a need is brought to central awareness. The emotion system then appraises that the need was not met and automatically generates an emotional reaction, usually healthy anger or sadness, or compassion for the self's pain.

Given the crucial role of accessing unmet needs for changing emotion, therapists need to discuss what needs are, where they originate, and whether they precede or come from emotion. Also, how do we know whether something is a need? Are people born with certain intrinsic needs, or do our emotions provide us with a template for the development of our needs? Assumptions that basic drives or motivations are a fundamental, innate, part of our nature are so deeply embedded in our theoretical preconceptions that it often takes a great deal of thought to recognize that life might not necessarily be governed by predetermined motivational systems. I suggest that psychological needs are not simply inborn. They are not similar to biologically based drives like hunger or thirst, or the fundamental motivation to survive and thrive; rather, they develop from emotions.

Motivation and Needs

Motivation refers to what a person needs, wants, wants to do, desires, or intends. Derived from the word *motivus*, it means "to move." Motivation is hypothesized to have evolved from many different human imperatives, including survival needs, attachment, self-actualizing, belonging, mastery, power, and self-esteem (Bowlby, 1988; Maslow, 1968; Murray, 1938; Rogers, 1959; White, 1959). While not denying the importance of these motivations, I believe that it is actually emotions that we are born with—emotions are the "givens"—and that motives, needs, wishes, and desires develop from basic emotions and the fundamental processes of affect regulation and meaning creation.

Human psychological needs, then, rather than being givens like instincts or reflexes, are emergent phenomena constructed in a complex process of development. Human needs emerge out of affect, and they represent basic likes and dislikes, things that the organism desires to preserve a state of well-being. We desire things because they are good for us and promote survival. These needs or desires are constructed in interaction with the environment by the operation of two fundamental inborn processes: affect regulation and meaning construction. Basically, we come to desire that which helped achieve the survival aim of the emotion and thereby felt good. Emotions evolved because they promoted survival, and we come to develop needs for what promotes our survival. The aim in anger, for example, is one of protecting boundaries or overcoming hurdles; in fear, the aim is to flee from danger. In both examples, when the aim is achieved, organisms relax and develop a desire or need to protect or flee because it is good for them. In sadness, the aim is reaching or crying out for contact or comfort; in disgust, the aim is to dispel what is noxious and tastes bad. All evolved as action-oriented systems to aid survival and lead to feeling good when the aim is reached and then wanting more of this feeling to achieve this aim. Thereafter, organisms develop needs or desires for boundaries, safety, comfort, and expulsion of noxious substances because these things are good for them.

In my view, the motive to survive and grow is the only inborn motive common across species. This innate motivation works in conjunction with two major inborn operating processes: (a) *affect regulation*, the effort to physiologically stabilize the organism to regulate the sympathetic and parasympathetic nervous systems; affect regulation manifests functionally as trying to have the feelings we want and not have the feelings we do not want; and (b) *meaning creation*, the effort to make sense of emotions and more broadly make sense of ourselves, our lives, and our world; meaning creation manifests functionally in narrative construction. These are general purpose operating processes and not specific content motives.

However, the attempt to identify specific content motives, such as attachment, autonomy, achievement, or power, is so strong in Western thinking that it is hard for people to see these content motivations as derivatives of emotion. For example, *attachment*, the need to be connected and protected, has been postulated to be the master motive. It clearly is an extremely important and powerful force, especially in infants and toddlers, but to attribute specific content to it, or any other motive, beyond survival and claim that attachment is an inborn drive is, I believe, a mistake. Rather than postulating that attachment is an inborn motivation, the question to ask is, What is the mechanism by which attachment works? We need an explanation of what produces it rather than postulating a motive as an abstraction. The same applies to other postulated motives, such as the need for mastery or self-esteem, or the motivation to form a coherent identity.

The problem here is exemplified by the fact that 16th century doctors, in observing that all human beings—all mammals—slept, postulated a dormitive motivation (in Latin, *dormio* is to sleep). This is not an explanation of what produces sleep. To name something a motivation is to create a fictional phenomenon by confusing explanation and description. Human beings clearly do attach and do strive for power, status, achievement, and mastery (Bowlby, 1998; White, 1959), but these strivings are better explained by complex underlying processes rather than postulating inborn motives as an answer. Love and power are important in understanding human experience (Gilbert, 1992). The need for security and interest or stimulation as well as mastery also appears to be important (Greenberg & Goldman, 2008). Our ancestors probably survived if they belonged to a group because the group provided protection and comfort. Survival also was aided by their curiosity and interest in novelty because they learned about things ahead of time before the necessities of survival demanded. All of this helped people be safe and master their situations but not because they had inborn motives to do these things. Rather, those whose emotion systems oriented them toward attaining attachment and mastery survived better than those who lacked this emotional makeup. What was inborn were emotions with differentiated goals to promote survival.

How, then, do people come to develop an attachment motive that is so strong and leads to needing and seeking comfort and closeness if it is not inborn? When softness, contact, and comfort have been experienced as regulating infants' physiology and have thus felt satisfying, the infants develop a desire for it because it is good for the infant and feels good. The organism's feeling of being thus regulated is automatically sought after, and, over time, as this experience becomes reinforced, it becomes consciously articulated and is called a need or a desire for whatever was found to be good for one and thus satisfying. People come to desire and want this particular person; or they desire and want to listen to opera or rock; or they want to do an activity, such as skiing or reading. These desires are experienced as psychological needs of different degrees of intensity. This process of desiring also leads to its opposite, feelings of need deprivation, when the want or need cannot be satisfied, which can become a source of great psychological distress.

The Role of Affect Regulation and Meaning Creation

In the view I present here, affect regulation and meaning creation are the important processes that are involved in the development of needs. These two major human processes act to serve the basic macromotive of survival and help create needs. Thus, rather than postulate a set of basic motivations, such as attachment, mastery, or control, I see psychological needs as arising from a process of construction from an interaction between four elements: basic inborn biases, preferences and affective values of what is good and bad for us, lived experience, and affect regulation and meaning creation.

People are born with a motivation to survive, a set of basic evolutionary developed emotions plus affect regulating and meaning creation systems to achieve the aim of survival. All psychological needs emerge from these fundamentals. Infants, for example, are prewired through the affect system to favor warmth, familiar smell, softness, smiling faces, high-pitched voices, and shared gaze. These all produce neurochemical reaction, action tendencies, and positive affect that support life. Once experienced, these favored experiences begin to be sought after. Similarly, infants have negative reactions to restraint, loud noises, interoceptive discomfort, and overstimulation, and they move away from these. Experience leads to the development of emotion schematic memories with expectancies of what feels good and bad. As cognition develops, likes and dislikes are further consolidated in awareness and become conscious needs and desires.

Need or desire is created from the seeking or avoiding of those things that helped one survive and made one feel good or bad. Need or desire also is created from the coding of it in memory and in narrative meaning. Feelings that this is good for us are the rewards or punishments that lead to desiring more or less of something. We come to desire what we have experienced and know will help us survive. Being physiologically balanced and maintaining a sense of coherence is signaled to us by feeling good and by our experience making sense to us and to our culture. This, then, leads to adaptive action.

In addition, needs are situationally evoked rather than being inner drives. They are pulled from us rather than pushing us. Witness that even the sexual drive in primates, for example, in male apes, is aroused by a new female in heat even if the males have recently engaged in copulation. Human psychological needs are stimulus activated. A desire for the fresh-baked bread we smell coming from the kitchen or for the touch of the other when we see them is evoked by the stimulus rather than by a drive from within. And these needs or desires are not inborn but developed from having tasted bread and having been touched.

Neural Circuits

Research in affective neuroscience is beginning to inform our understanding of needs as physical entities that exist in the brain, namely, neural circuits. As a result of experience guided by a relatively small set of affectively based biases and preferences—manifested in early organisms initially as action tendencies (to move toward or away from) and later experienced as feelings—there is a selective strengthening and weakening of populations of synapses. This carves out circuits that become needs (Damasio, 1999); the circuits that are developed are organized based on lived experience.

Emotions are viewed as being generated psychologically by appraisal of situations in relation to needs. This view, however, seems to imply, semantically, that need may preexist emotion. Isn't there a circularity here? If emotion is generated by needs being met, then don't needs have to exist before emotion can be generated? A type of chicken or egg question arises. Essentially, there is a circular relation between emotion and need but only once needs have been developed to help satisfy emotional aims. Buck (2014), for example, suggested that emotions and needs are two sides of a coin, and offered use of the term *emotivation* to describe the interdependence of emotion and motivation. But as I have proposed, once needs are developed from basic emotions, they become barometers of what the organism has found aids survival and has felt good in the past, and, thus, guides the organism's current strivings. So, as Harlow (1960) found, a need for contact/comfort developed from the good feeling of the cloth covering the wire mother because the cloth felt good. A child looks at the mother's face seeking to experience the joy that was produced by the smile on the mother's face. What was wired in were basic action patterns like rooting, sucking, grasping, crying, and smiling as well as a system of preference for the pleasant feelings that come from softness, warmth and smiles. It is only once needs have been developed that their satisfaction or frustration becomes the activator of emotion. That does not mean they were inborn or preceded emotion, however, because emotion was initially activated by inborn cues like faces, touch, and sounds. It is only once needs are developed from basic emotions and lived experience that they become involved in the generation of emotion.

The organism thus possesses two general purpose systems beyond the emotion system itself: A presymbolic, affect regulation process of seeking what feels good for its well-being and avoiding what feels bad, and a later developed symbolic, narrative construction process that creates meaning. These are the two systems we work with in therapy. What do you feel, and what does experience mean? Therapists do not look for motives or needs as explanatory to produce insight, but we work with reowning disowned needs. Accessing and reowning those unmet needs for which action tendencies have been disclaimed are vital to psychological health. The reclaimed needs provide a sense of direction and promote access to new emotions and, ultimately, to change.

In this view, then, human beings are seen as wired to seek emotions because how the emotions make them feel aids survival, and they come to desire what is good for them. This is not a simple hedonistic view in which people seek pleasure and avoid pain. Rather, people seek to attain and achieve the survival-related needs, goals, and concerns embedded in their emotions: goals, such as closeness and proximity, the lack of which is signaled by sadness; safety, the lack of which is signaled by fear; agency, the lack of which is signaled by shame. Those with feelings like these fare better than those who do not. I hope this explanation puts to rest the apparent chicken and egg paradox.

Most important for practice, then, is the knowledge that emotions provide evaluations of whether needs are being met or not and also help generate new emotions. Emotions, therefore, are not just emotions. They contain needs, and it is therapeutically important to access the needs implied in the emotion to provide clients with a sense of direction. Emotion work requires that therapists work to access previously disowned needs and validate them as health giving. In addition, when unmet needs are reclaimed and brought to awareness, the brain automatically generates new emotions based on its automatic appraisal of whether the need was met or not. This leads to the generation of new emotions to cope with the situation as it is now perceived. Thus, for example, a person will feel sad for the loss of closeness they needed, or angry at the deprivation of what they deserved, or compassionate to themselves for the pain they experienced.

Need Satisfaction and Frustration

I now focus on one last important aspect of the topic of needs: the process of need satisfaction and frustration, which is essential to the development of the ability to regulate emotion. Emotion results from appraisals of situations in relation to need. Emotion dysregulation results from people's ways of reacting to need deprivation. So, it is people's responses, often emotional, to need frustration and deprivation, not their needs themselves, that are problematic (Greenberg & Goldman, 2008; Greenberg & Johnson, 1988). Need satisfaction is seen as leading potentially to completion of the need and moving on to other concerns (Perls et al., 1951). Maslow (1954) argued that once a need is satisfied, the person moves on to pursuing higher needs based on his hierarchy. It seems fairly self-evident, for example, that controlling for other factors, if you are suffering from danger or cold and hunger, then safety, food, and warmth are a priority. You just do not have the time or energy to pursue self-esteem needs until other needs are met. On the other hand, Perls et al. (1951) proposed that, rather than a hierarchy, people had thousands of psychological needs but that present awareness led to the most urgent need arising. That action led to need satisfaction, which led to the need fading into the background and the next need arising and becoming figural in governing striving. These hypotheses represent the idea that human beings are propelled into action by psychological needs and goals, and that satisfaction of one set of needs/goals leads to the pursuit of other needs/goals.

By contrast, a simple learning theory approach, explicitly or implicitly adopted by many therapists, would suggest that encouraging and responding to the painful emotion could be viewed as positive reinforcement that would lead to an increase in frequency of these behaviors. In this view, people are seen as stimulus-driven organisms governed either by stimulus–response links or stimulus–organism–response links formed by association or reinforcement. Learning and reinforcement explanations suggest exposure treatments to extinguish associations. An affective view of functioning, by contrast, works with that aspect of human functioning that is purposive and goal driven; the brain is automatically comparing where they are with where they want to be. The brain works by predicting and reducing discrepancy between present and desired states in addition to associative learning. Need satisfaction by reduction of discrepancy between desired and achieved states is seen as leading to a reduction in feelings and need. It also leads the experience of a sense of greater security or confidence rather than a strengthening of the bad feelings of deprivation. Moreover, need satisfaction produces a reduction of preoccupation with getting the need met based on positive expectations of its satisfaction.

Need satisfaction, thus, leads to the abatement of the need. For example, satisfaction of the need for closeness leads to the person's moving on to explore and meet other needs. When the need to achieve is satisfied, the person relaxes and moves on to meet other needs. This is important for therapy in which accessing previously unresolved feelings and unmet needs is seen as necessary in satisfying or changing them. Rather than leading to a reinforcement of the activated feelings and needs, activation makes them amenable to new input. If, in therapy, a person is able to access the sadness of the loss of security suffered in childhood by a distant parent or access the fear of violence by an abusive parent, that, rather than lead to reinforcement of the sadness or fear, will lead to its reduction. When the sadness and fear are empathized with and soothed by the therapist's attunement, and the unmet needs for security or protection are met in therapy, they are transformed by this corrective emotional experience. In addition, the experience of resolution and need validation in the present leads to positive expectations of future need satisfaction and less overall future anxiety or concern about need satisfaction.

CLIENTS DESERVE TO HAVE NEEDS MET

Therapists work to access feelings, but it is not just acceptance of emotion and their symbolization in words that is important. All emotions carry within them needs, met or unmet, and it is these needs that have to be reclaimed to get the emotion's message and action tendency. Therapists need to help clients get to their needs. Psychological suffering and emotional pain are indicators of unmet needs; thus, considering what needs are unmet is a crucial part of the therapist's work. When activated in therapy, previously disclaimed emotions can be used to reclaim unwanted self-experience, therefore giving the person information about needs met or not met, one's response to situations, and action tendencies to cope with them.

The psychological needs most commonly violated or not responded to, which, thus, bring an experience of emotional suffering, are:

- the need to be connected and understood, the lack of which produces a sad loneliness and the basic anxiety of insecurity
- the need to be respected, acknowledged as valuable, appreciated, and validated in what the person does and who they are, the lack of which produces shame
- the need for safety and security, the lack of which produces fear

Once emotions are accessed, they inform people about their wants or needs; emotion work involves accessing emotion schemes to get at the needs inherent in them. An important distinction when working with needs is that of accessing a heartfelt need versus facilitation of the cognitive articulation of a need. It is the heartfelt need that helps facilitate transformation. The *heartfelt need* is one that comes out of experiencing the painful primary emotion when emotion schematic processing is activated. It is the activation of the scheme that gives access to the unmet need. Now, the need is felt as opposed to merely talking about the need in a more conceptual manner. By analogy, if someone has a dagger sticking in their side and is asked what they need, the experienced pain lets them know that they need the dagger removed and relief from the pain. This is experiential knowing, not conceptual knowing. The body knows what it needs to survive. This is not existential pondering but organismic necessity. So, in this discussion of needs, I mean heartfelt needs that are made obviously clear and accessible by the felt pain of the emotion schematic activated experience.

In working with emotion to achieve change, we therapists are not trying to understand and promote understanding of people's motives by analyzing the content of their lives and interactions and looking for patterns or explanations of why they do certain things. Rather, we let the emotions reveal their motivations and action tendencies. We do not see dysfunction as arising from neurotic needs or their denial, nor do we see dysfunction as occurring because of interpersonal patterns based on unfulfilled wishes or on internal working models related to attachment. Rather, therapists see problems arising from (a) the disclaiming of emotion, (b) the perseveration of certain past emotional responses in the present, (c) emotion dysregulation, and (d) narrative construction. Therapeutic work involves keeping our finger on the emotional pulse of our clients rather than figuring out their conscious or unconscious motivated patterns or errors in thinking. Emotions are the royal road to needs.

In therapy, unmet needs often arise in the context of past situations of abandonment, neglect, and abuse. The learning from those past experiences, when it was impossible to get the need met, was that it was too painful to feel and to need, so people shut down to avoid feeling the excruciating loneliness of isolation, the fear of abuse, and the shame of invalidation. As a result, they do not need and do not feel, which impacts their current life because they are unable to, from meaningful relations, connect with others and experience love or joy. Therapeutic work often involves the client's letting go of trying to get the need met by the people who so disappointed them. It requires separation of the need from the particular other in question. Therapists promote reowning the need and validating it but also help clients redirect their efforts at need satisfaction to alternative sources. In doing so, therapists are attempting to mobilize the disowned, unmet needs from the past but, at the same time, help clients let go of trying to get the need met by the people who so disappointed them.

After having helped the client process the painful feeling and access the unmet need, therapists ask, "Who else could meet this need?" Ultimately, the client must accept that the need is valid and healthy, and that they are deserving of having it met but that the particular relationship, which originally never met the need, was inadequate. Therefore, they need to let go of trying to get the need met by the depriving person.

Evaluating the Worth of One's Needs

A further important aspect of working with needs is to recognize people's ability to evaluate the value of their own desires, feelings, and needs (Taylor, 1990). Thus, in determining the self one wishes to be, people have the ability either to desire or not desire their first-order feelings and desires. In this second, higher order, more conscious evaluation, the worth of a desire is evaluated against some ideal or aspired-to standard. Being a self involves being self-evaluatively reflective and developing and acting according to higher order values or desires. Essentially, this means developing feelings and desires about feelings and desires. For the emotion system, the evaluation is simply, "Is it good or bad for me?" whereas in the stronger, self-reflective evaluation, there is also a judgment of the value of the emotion and its accompanying desire. People evaluate whether their emotions and desires are good or bad, courageous or cowardly, useful or destructive. They form subjective judgments of the worth of their own desired states and courses of action (Taylor, 1990).

Thoughtful reflection on emotional promptings is a key part of emotional competence. This is where conscious thought plays its crucial role. Thought must be used to judge whether emotional prompting coheres with what people value as worthwhile for themselves and others. This is not just a matter of "get in touch with your feelings and follow them" but involves both evaluating the desirability of the feelings one gets in touch with and changing them when they are no longer aiding adaptation.

Therapists, thus, help people feel entitled to their need, but this entitlement should be to their need's being legitimate and not to the legitimacy of having the other person meet their need, which is an unproductive form of entitlement. Healthy entitlement is supported by clients' expressions being made through "I" statements, which help in the taking of responsibility. So, "I deserved more" is better and emphasizes agency more than "Why did you not give this to me?" which is more of a complaint. Once the person experiences "I deserve," the person is empowered, and the question "What do you need to do to get what you need?" is viable. Although the need often is interpersonal at times, it can also be from the self, so therapists can ask, "What do you need from the other or from yourself?"

Mobilizing Agency

Therapists need to work toward emotion and need activation. They see development as occurring by way of transformation of emotion rather than by learning through conditioning, skill training, or rational restructuring to change behavior. Emotion-oriented therapists also do not focus on understanding motivation; rather, they try to access emotions. Instead of analyzing clients' interactions to find patterns of behavior or explanations for actions, therapists access emotions and make sense of the motivations and action tendencies within them. Problems are seen as arising from disclaiming of emotional experience and from the perseveration of certain past emotional responses in the present as well as from lack of emotion awareness, emotion dysregulation, and faulty meaning creation.

The need and action tendency in an emotion provide direction; in adaptive emotion, they provide meaning and orientation. In maladaptive emotions, the sense of having deserved to have the unmet need met and the therapist's validation of this sense facilitate access to the adaptive emotions of assertive anger, the sadness of grief, or compassion for the self for not having had the need met. As a result, a sense of agency is mobilized in the person. Approach action tendencies (often in anger and sadness) are then able to undo the withdrawal action tendencies in the maladaptive feelings (often of shame and fear).

SESSION EXAMPLES

The following transcripts show therapists working to access the heartfelt needs within aroused emotions. Some of the examples illustrate how this work leads to new adaptive emotions.

The first excerpt is from the very beginning of therapy. The therapist is creating an alliance with Mary, a 49-year-old, depressed, White woman, of English descent, who has suffered a trauma and is scared to be assertive with her husband to express what she feels and needs. The woman has been lied to by her husband about his illegal financial dealings, and she now has to cope with the fear and humiliation of his potential incarceration. Before clients go on the path of facing their pain, it is helpful for them to have some sort of rationale as to how this may help. Telling them that getting to their need will help guide them is a good way of gaining agreement on a therapeutic goal and thereby creating a good alliance. In this excerpt, the therapist offers the rationale that by exploring together her emotions and her needs within the emotions, this exploration will help clarify what direction she wants to take, which will help her feel better. The therapist frames the therapeutic work in terms of facing her fear and identifying her need.

"I'm Game to Go Ahead"

THERAPIST: Well, I still think that, you know, it looks like something that needs to be explored, you know, that part of yourself that is most of the time contained—actually giving it a voice in the safety of this room, um, [to] actually clarify what you need to say to your husband about what that's all about (*Client: Mm-hmm.*) inside. And you know that's the first step: to unlock the feeling and unlock the emotions, and from that, we will see how it's going to come out. But typically, what happens is people get a better sense of what they are experiencing, and from that, you get a better sense of what you need (*Client: Mm-hmm.*) in the situation, um, and through that, it provides a sense of clarity (*Client: Mm-hmm.*)—well, more clarity in terms of what you need to do next (*Client: Mm-hmm.*). Yeah, so. [providing a rationale to work on emotions and need]

CLIENT: I've, um, well, that's why I'm here.

THERAPIST: What—what are you feeling, or what's your gut reaction when I say that, or . . .

CLIENT: Well, I think, um, I think that is the direction that we have to take because, um, I don't see any other, any avenues rather than a status quo, which obviously hasn't been working and, over time, is—is not getting any better. (*Therapist: Mm-hmm.*) Um, so I certainly, at the end of last session, felt more, uh, I guess you might say, game to (*Therapist: Mm-hmm.*)—to go ahead and not worry so much about (*Therapist: Mm-hmm.*) what the end result would be. I mean, it's certainly some concern. (*Therapist: Mm-hmm, sure.*) I'm not just sort of (*Therapist: Sure.*) blowing all kinds of caution to the wind (*Therapist: Mm-hmm.*), but, you know, I need to not, um (*Therapist: Mm-hmm.*), fear change. [agreeing]

THERAPIST: And, certainly, you have control in this process, too, it's (*Client: Mm-hmm, mm-hmm.*)—and you have ultimate control in what you decide to do. That's not something that I would be telling you what to do. (*Client: Mm-hmm, mm-hmm.*) It's—this process evolves from within yourself. Yeah, I sense that you are kinda feeling like, okay, um, maybe really let go a bit of this fear and just take a chance? And see what happens? Is that kinda what you are feeling? [providing safety of control]

CLIENT: Yes, I need to do this.

THERAPIST: Mm-hmm. What do you—what do you *need from him*, what would you like to tell him what you need from him? [getting at need conceptually]

CLIENT: Well, I need his trust. I think that this has eroded our, um— I needed him to let me know the bad parts as well as the good parts, even if, maybe, he doesn't think well of himself. I know he thinks I'm critical of him, and I am. There are a lot of things that definitely offend me, and he doesn't want to hear that. He thinks by hiding, um, enough of the stuff that's going on, maybe I won't notice all the things that will back up my feelings that he's not a good person.

THERAPIST: So, you are saying, "I need you to basically let me hear about parts of yourself and what's going on. I need to hear that."

CLIENT: My husband always has this great fear that, um, he would be in court or somewhere, and if I am called to testify—and

I wasn't—testify against him or let things out that work against him (*Therapist: Mm-hmm.*), and some of it comes from the fact that he knows that I can't lie very well. (*Therapist: Mm-hmm.*) And I think some of it comes from the fact that he thinks, in his own mind, "She thinks I'm wrong," and under that kind of pressure, it's going to come out that "she thinks I'm wrong." (*Therapist: Mm.*) Um, there it will be in front of everyone (*Therapist: Mm-hmm.*), um, it would be on public record, it would be (*Therapist: Mm-hmm.*) used against me by my, um, accusers (*Therapist: Mm-hmm.*), and there will be, uh, nowhere to hide (*Therapist: Mm-hmm.*), no way to save myself, and . . .

THERAPIST: What's happening to you, what's happening to you now, what are you experiencing?

CLIENT: Well, it's a very sad thing. It's a very, um, destructive thing.

THERAPIST: Very painful, isn't it, to . . .

CLIENT: Yeah, to a certain extent, I think, um (*cries*) . . . [activated emotion schematic processing]

THERAPIST: Can you stay with that, just the feeling, hold that feeling?

CLIENT: I feel so untrusted, so left out (*cries*).

THERAPIST: What do you need from him? [heartfelt need]

CLIENT: I needed him to respect me enough to trust me, to keep me in the loop. I—I didn't know what to expect. I feel myself getting more and more angry with him. (*Therapist: Mm-hmm.*) (*Client now speaks as if to her husband.*) "Why did you let things come to this stage where I had to be in here defending myself, defending you without the tools to be able to do it?" (*Therapist: Mm-hmm.*) I was just so angry.

THERAPIST: Mm-hmm. "I feel betrayed almost . . ."

CLIENT: "I felt (*Therapist: Yeah, it's not fair.*) very much betrayed, very much set up (*Therapist: Mm-hmm.*) so that I had no—no way to defend myself (*Therapist: Mm-hmm. "I was left out."*), very little knowledge about how to help you [husband]. I need you to trust me." [heartfelt need]

THERAPIST: "Just so betrayed. So, painfully sad, too."

CLIENT: "I feel so sad (*cries*) that this is what it's come to, such a loss. Married for 26 years, and you didn't trust me, and now I can't help you. In fact, I hurt you by what I've said in those interviews, and we have lost all we had. It's like our history is being shattered, and you will in some way die to me even though you will be alive. (*Sobs*) Just such a loss, and now I have to carry on without you. I needed you to trust me more, and now I'm now all alone. Just so sad . . ."

After stating her need, the client begins to access her anger and then her sadness. She works through her sense of betrayal to get to her loss and begins a grieving process.

In the next excerpt involving a different client, the therapist guides the client to regress to an earlier adolescent time to get to the emotion and the unmet need. After accessing her sad, lonely feeling, the client gets to her unmet need for contact/comfort and to be liked, which leads to a sense of deserving anger. Her fear is touched on but not worked through in this segment, but she accesses the unmet need for protection and safety—which most often is the organismic need—in the face of violence. This need, over time, would be followed and may lead to boundary-setting anger, the healthy sadness of grief, and compassion to the self.

"I Need You to Like Me"

In this excerpt, the client, Chloe, a 33-year-old, Black, Jamaican woman who is employed as a nurse, is working on her childhood abuse and neglect. She presented with difficulties in interpersonal relations and in adjusting to a new job.

THERAPIST: Let's go back and be 13 years old, and speak to your father. As a 13-year-old, tell him what you told me: "I'm really trying to . . ."

CLIENT: "I'm really trying to get your attention to get your love, to show you: Look how good I am in school. Look at all the awards I've gotten. Look at all the awards I've gotten."

THERAPIST: As a 13-year-old, what's it like? Tell them [both parents], "I'm really . . ." [focus on internal experience]

CLIENT: (*Speaks as if to her parents*) "You know, I'm really turning to my friends because there's nothing at home for me—there's nothing here. The only thing I get at home is discipline and work. And when I'm done with my homework, it's clean the house or do this or go down to the basement, you know, like go play in the cold basement. It was never, 'Let's go out together,' 'Let's do this together,' or 'How was school today?' It felt cold and lonely."

THERAPIST: What did you feel? [focus on internal experience]

CLIENT: Just unloved (*cries*). Sad, lonely, and empty. [focus on internal experience]

THERAPIST: Yes, so unloved, unwanted. Tell him what you needed, what you missed: "I needed . . ." [heartfelt need]

CLIENT: (*Speaks as if to her father*) "You know, I needed to have some type of contact, conversation with you to find out how my life is going, to find out how your life was going, you know, there was nothing there. You're just people that I feared. I didn't—going home was not a nice experience. I didn't like being at home, particularly all the fighting."

THERAPIST: Go back. Be the 13-year-old and tell them what it's like. It's hard to go back there, but you were there at one time. Do you feel any of the fear? [age regression]

CLIENT: If I was 2 minutes late, I was terrified 'cause I knew I was going to get hit.

THERAPIST: Tell them about this fear . . . as the 13-year-old. [focus on underlying fear]

CLIENT: "Yes, I'm afraid. I'm terrified. I just want you to like me. I'm really trying to be good. I'm really trying to be good so you'll like me. So, you know, you'll like me and see that I'm a good kid, and you'll want to do things with me." [fear and need]

THERAPIST: Tell them, "I need you to like me." [heartfelt need]

CLIENT: "Yeah, well, yeah, I need you to like me."

THERAPIST: What do you feel now as you say this? [focus on emerging new feeling]

CLIENT: I feel so deprived. I'm angry. I deserve to have parents who like me. Goddammit, you were my parents. I deserved to be loved. I was just a kid trying so hard. [deserving of assertive anger, which is self-affirming]

The preceding sequence demonstrates that the need is pivotal. When the client expresses her need and feels deserving, a new adaptive emotion of anger is generated. She now feels more deserving and is more of an agent who is stronger and less of a passive recipient of the mistreatment. Allowing and acceptance her initial feelings of sadness, fear, and loneliness are necessary and important yet insufficient for change. What is central is that once an unmet need is accessed, a new emotion, in this case, anger, mobilizes the person to get what she needs to promote her own survival and growth. Her newly felt adaptive anger provides a sense of direction and an action tendency to achieve this.

"I Needed a Mother"

In the next example, Walter is a 47-year-old, White man suffering from depression. In a previous session, he had just become his 6-year-old self and was experiencing his fear. He had expressed his fear by saying, "Very scared. Feel like I will be hurt by her [mother] at any time," and the therapist had responded, "Very unsafe." Here, the therapist facilitates the heartfelt need now that the client's emotion schematic fear has been activated and differentiated. This heartfelt need comes out of the sense of what he needed to make the painful feelings go away. Note how accessing the need leads to accessing newly experienced anger at not having had the need met and, ultimately, leads to beginning to grieve for what was missed.

CLIENT: Right, right.

THERAPIST: When you feel so scared, so panicked and unsafe, what do you need? [heartfelt need]

CLIENT: What do I need?

THERAPIST: Hmm. What did you need from your mother at that moment?

CLIENT: I needed a mother. . . . I needed her to make things clear. . . . Don't scare me so much. Don't threaten me like this.

THERAPIST: (*Points to the empty chair*) Tell her: "I need you . . ." [amplify the need]

CLIENT: (*Faces the empty chair and speaks as if to his mother*) "I need you . . . [to] be patient to make things clear . . . make clear what's going on and why you are so angry. . . . I don't know the consequences and impact of what I do. . . . I need you to be patient and tell me that it's wrong and why it's wrong (*cries*). I need you to be clear. . . . Then, if I understand, I won't do it again next time." [heartfelt need]

THERAPIST: So, I need you to make it clear, what's going on, not to scare me. What do you feel right now? [focus on emerging feeling]

CLIENT:	I feel angry inside now. [assertive protective anger]
THERAPIST:	Hmm. What is the anger like?
CLIENT:	I want to attack her back.
THERAPIST:	What do you want to say or do?
CLIENT:	I would like to beat her back.
THERAPIST:	Do it.
CLIENT:	He hits a pillow with his hand. [symbolically aggressive anger]
THERAPIST:	What is the anger like if it is expressed in words? If the anger can speak, what will it say? . . . You can feel your anger . . . You say you feel angry.
CLIENT:	The anger is here (*points to his stomach*). There's a fire which wants to come out from here. It wants to attack, to destroy, to say . . . [differentiating]
THERAPIST:	Hmm. Feel the fire which wants to come out. If the fire could speak, what would it say?
CLIENT:	Now I want to swear. "You're a bitch. A fucking bitch. You were cruel and mean, and you just used me. You never loved me."
THERAPIST:	Tell what you are most angry at her for? What makes you most angry? [differentiating]
CLIENT:	I feel she is unreasonable . . . totally unreasonable. She only can use violence to attack others. [differentiating]
THERAPIST:	Tell her.
CLIENT:	"I'm furious. I'm so angry."
THERAPIST:	Yes, some more, tell her. [intensification]
CLIENT:	"I'm angry at you. . . . I'm angry at you for that you seem like a mad person. I feel you're really sick."
THERAPIST:	Only in violent ways.
CLIENT:	"Just a mad person. You can only be mad. . . . You're the one who has no brain in the family. . . . Feel like you don't treat me as a family member, just like we are your enemies. I feel like you treat me as your enemy. If I do something wrong—even little

things at home—not just me, including my father, you will go crazy like a mad person."

THERAPIST: What do you need from your mother? [heartfelt need]

CLIENT: I need my mother to speak well . . . to think clearly . . . to think clearly whether I am your family or your enemy. I need my mother to have a certain attitude—to treat us as your family.

THERAPIST: Yes, tell her what it was like to not get this. Tell her what you missed. [shift to sadness]

CLIENT: I need her to have a consistent attitude. I missed the safety of knowing what was coming, of what would happen next. It was scary, and it's sad that I lived so long in fear. I missed a lot of my childhood.

At this point, the client begins to focus more on the grief of what he had missed, but he continues to oscillate between anger and sadness.

"It Wasn't My Fault": Confronting the Internal Critic

In this next example, the client, Jina, a 32-year-old, White, European woman who had been sexually abused as a child, is confronting her own internal critic, who blames her for her abuse and pushes and criticizes her. She begins in the self chair, speaking to the critic. This later evolves into a dialogue with a mother who ignored the daughter's sexual abuse. At this point in the transcript, the client is telling her critic to stop abusing her. Essentially, the critical voice is blaming her for making mistakes based on her blaming herself for the abuse when she was a child. This excerpt again illustrates that when the unmet need for love and acceptance from the self and the need for protection from the mother is accessed by going into and allowing the painful feelings of being unprotected, it leads to the emergence of more healthy adaptive emotions:

CLIENT: (*Talks to the critic*) "It's not needed" (*sniffs*).

THERAPIST: Yeah, tell her, "I don't want that abuse anymore."

CLIENT: "I don't want you to abuse me anymore. I don't want it."

THERAPIST: "Yeah, and I'm really angry."

CLIENT: "I'm angry at you for making me feel so pressured, and I act out of guilt, and I do stupid things, and then I feel worse, and it's just a vicious cycle [access emotion scheme] (*blows nose*), and then I second guess myself, and it just (*cries, sniffs*) interferes with everything."

THERAPIST: "Yeah, you interfere with my whole life."

CLIENT: "And I don't want you to interfere anymore."

THERAPIST: Yeah . . . What do you want? [heartfelt need]

CLIENT: I want her to be able to forgive me and let it go (*cries*) (*Therapist: Yeah.*)—let me make mistakes if I need to (*cries*).

THERAPIST: "Let me be human."

CLIENT: (*Cries*) That feeling I had when I was 5. [scheme activation]

THERAPIST: What is it?

CLIENT: (*Cries*) "That's when you told me it was my fault that I was sexually abused, and I hate that feeling. I feel so guilty and worthless (*Therapist: Yeah.*), and I think that's the connection I have."

THERAPIST: Yeah. Tell her—take a step.

CLIENT: "It wasn't my fault. I was just a little girl."

THERAPIST: Yeah, "I was a little girl."

CLIENT: I felt pressured. I should have said no, but I didn't, but it was because I was pressured, and any little kid would have done it.

THERAPIST: Yeah.

CLIENT: I'm not abnormal.

THERAPIST: "I was young and scared and nobody was there."

CLIENT: (*Blows nose*) Nobody was there to keep me safe.

THERAPIST: Yeah, yeah, that's right. "I was in danger, and I just did what I could, what I had to, to survive. It wasn't my fault."

CLIENT: "It wasn't my fault (*cries*) (*Therapist: Yeah.*), and it wasn't my fault. Stop telling me it's my fault. (*Therapist: Yeah, yeah.*) It wasn't my fault (*cries*)." [assertive anger]

THERAPIST: Yeah, yeah, it's really heavy to hold that.

CLIENT: "It's been like a rope around my neck just waiting to be tight enough to choke my life out, and I have a life worth living, and I don't need to die."

THERAPIST: Yeah.

CLIENT: "I can be productive."

THERAPIST: Yeah, yeah.

CLIENT: "And I can stay productive if I can just get you to work with me instead of against me [referring to her critic]."

THERAPIST: And how could she work with you? What do you need from her?

CLIENT: "I need you to forgive me, to realize that it wasn't my fault, (*Therapist: Yeah.*) to love me." Because she hates me for being so stupid to let that happen, and I could have had control, but I didn't . . .

THERAPIST: So, you want her to realize that the truth is that little children can't stop . . .

CLIENT: Abuse.

THERAPIST: And it's not their fault—yeah, so you need forgiveness and you need comfort.

CLIENT: I need love (*Therapist: Yeah.*) I need to be loved for who I am. [heartfelt need]

THERAPIST: Yeah: "Love and accept me for whatever way I am, yeah, all of me."

CLIENT: And to let that go because that destroys everything.

At this point, the dialogue shifts to the mother who ignored her abuse.

CLIENT: (*Speaks to her mother in an empty chair*) "I resent you for not loving me, even when I changed and was . . ."

THERAPIST: So, "I resent you for not seeing my pain (*Client: Yeah.*) all those years"?

CLIENT: "And I bottled it so much to the point where it was just exploding, and you didn't see any of it, you didn't recognize it. (*Therapist: Yeah*) I needed you to help me feel better about myself, for it happening, I was just so afraid of you (*blows nose*), and I was afraid that if you ever found out, you would hate me and throw me out of the house." [heartfelt need]

THERAPIST: Uh-huh, uh-huh, so you needed to feel that I could tell you to feel safe.

CLIENT: "I didn't feel that I could approach you and say this happened (*Therapist: Yeah.*), and that makes me angry. Why couldn't I tell you? (*Therapist: Yeah.*) I was just a little kid." [emerging assertive anger]

CLIENT: "I was just a little kid."

THERAPIST: "So I'm angry at you for silencing me."

CLIENT: "For not listening to me when I did talk, and . . ."

THERAPIST: Yeah, yeah, so kind of like she didn't create an environment where you felt . . .

CLIENT: Safe at all.

Again, it is not only accepting the painful feelings but also that sense of agency that is provided by access to the need that gives the whole process a sense of direction. The process can be described as a deepening downward and inward movement to arrive at the painful underlying feeling, followed by an emergence—an upward and outward leaving and moving toward new possibilities.

CONCLUSION

Getting at heartfelt needs, which are embedded in underlying painful emotions, helps people access more adaptive emotions. This chapter looked at what needs are, how they are developed, and how to activate them to promote change. In addition to activating clients' recognition of their own needs, it is important that therapists help people feel that they deserve to have their needs met, especially in situations of past deprivation. Doing so provides clients with a sense of worth and helps them move from a passive position toward a more active, assertive position in which they feel deserving of having had their needs met.

Accessing a feeling of deserving to have a previously unmet adaptive need met is a central part of the change process of undoing old feelings with new ones. It is best achieved by dealing with unfinished business from the past, so the next chapter looks at reexperiencing the past in the present.

10 REEXPERIENCING THE PAST IN THE PRESENT

As demonstrated in Chapter 9, identifying the unmet needs in a painful emotion can often involve a journey into the client's past. In this chapter, I go into greater depth to share several methods of reexperiencing past emotional events to access and transform maladaptive emotions. I discuss different memory processes—episodic, autobiographical, and semantic memory as well as declarative and procedural memory—and their implications for practice with a focus on exploration of the role of memory reconsolidation in promoting therapeutic change. I then describe various ways of accessing memories to make them accessible to change and outline, in particular, age regression interventions. In these interventions, clients are invited to go back, become the child, and speak as the child as well as talk to themselves as a child in imagination or in a chair dialogue. These evocative interventions can be disorganizing for some highly fragile, severe personality-disordered clients. Clinical judgment based on degree of client fragility and the strength of the therapeutic relationship need to be used in the decision to engage in going back into childhood memories (Bateman & Fonagy, 2004; Yeomans et al., 2015).

https://doi.org/10.1037/0000248-011
Changing Emotion With Emotion: A Practitioner's Guide, by L. S. Greenberg
Copyright © 2021 by the American Psychological Association. All rights reserved.

EPISODIC, AUTOBIOGRAPHICAL, AND SEMANTIC MEMORY

Emotion and memory are highly interrelated. Emotion schematic memories of painful experiences that need therapeutic work are most accessible by activating episodic memories. An *episodic memory* is a memory of a past personal experience that occurred at a particular time and place. It is the unique, subjective memory of a specific event so always will be different from someone else's recollection of the same experience. Episodic memories are of events that can be explicitly stated, such as one's spending the first day at a new job, attending a relative's 100th birthday party, or a bride's recalling her wedding day. These memories are not just memories of the bare facts of the event itself; rather, in these memories, people see themselves as actors in the events, and the emotional charge and the entire context surrounding the event are part of the memory. Episodic memories give the best access to emotional experience. A good way to access episodic memories is through *age regression*, a type of intervention in which clients are invited to go back and become their child. This intervention activates memories of experiences and specific events to help unfold the sequence of the actual events that took place at any given point in a person's life so that it can be reconstructed.

"Episodic memory" is sometimes confused with "autobiographical memory." The two are related, but different. *Autobiographical memory* is a memory system consisting of a number of recollected experiences from an individual's life based on a combination of episodic memories plus semantic memories (general knowledge and facts about the world). Autobiographical memory thus contains the information one has about themselves that builds across episodes. This memory process includes several domains of which self-description—the source of a large part of a person's sense of identity—is an important one and contains information, such as one's occupation, favorite color, and ice cream flavor preference.

Autobiographical memories are also important in therapy. Autobiographical memory narratives disclosed by clients are often related in the landscape of action in terms of what happened and generally are initially told in a more external than internal manner. They provide the client with the chance to engage in storytelling to create a visually rich, detailed picture describing what happened. Whereas autobiographical memory may involve episodic memory, it also relies on *semantic memory*, which has to do with the knowledge and rules governing behavior that have been acquired through a lifetime of experiences. Semantic memory is factual and typically devoid of emotion or reference to the self or to specific times and places. In semantic memory, for example, one knows the city they were born in and the date, although they do not have specific memories of being born there. Autobiographical recollection, on the other hand, involves thinking about past events in a personal way, is emotionally meaningful, and has great relevance to people's sense of self and the meaning of their lives. Although semantic knowledge conveys meanings, it is rarely the kind of personal meaning embodied in autobiographical and episodic memories. Semantic memories, therefore, are far less relevant in a therapy focused on emotion because they usually are recounted with little or no emotional arousal.

The critical distinction between semantic and especially episodic memory is not so much the type of information being processed but the depth of experience involved in each. Episodic memory is highly experiential and provides the person remembering with the lived experience of remembering. It is the most powerful memory process for accessing affect because it makes possible a type of mental time travel through subjective time—from the present to the past—thus allowing one to reexperience previous experiences. This simply does not occur when recalling factual knowledge through the semantic memory system.

Here is an example of memory processes in which the client shares both autobiographical and episodic memories:

CLIENT: The memories I have preceding age 4—they are always like in regards to pleasing people and making them feel good. . . . My mom was working during the day, but in the mornings, and she always would bring in this baby bottle for me, and I remember one morning, she brought it, and I took it, and I started sucking. . . . Ooh, God, ugh! I hate this taste, but, somehow, I knew it is important for her, you know, like part of her daily routine and also like the contact between me and her and the preparations and everything. . . . I couldn't say anything, and this is what I do all the time . . .

THERAPIST: So, it's pretty amazing at 2½, you were already so attuned that this would hurt her, that I'm going to drink this anyway and not ruin it for her, like, "I sacrifice myself."

Here, the client relates an autobiographical memory demonstrating her inability to assert her needs, and the story includes an episodic memory in which she actually almost tastes the bottle and feels the disgust. This sensory detail makes the experience accessible now to reprocess at the experiential level. If the client had relayed information about this time of her life as a more general semantic memory (e.g., "Mom worked during the day, but she always brought me a bottle to drink every morning when I was little"), she could reprocess the experience at a conceptual level of insight. Insight can be helpful for understanding that her mother cared for her, but reprocessing the experience means changing the feeling of it so she no longer feels lonely abandonment in her body.

DECLARATIVE VERSUS PROCEDURAL MEMORY

Episodic, autobiographical, and semantic memory together are known as *declarative memory*, which refers to memories that can be articulated as opposed to another type of memory, *procedural memory*, which is responsible for knowing how to do things but not knowing what it is that one knows in one's body. Procedural memory stores information on how to perform certain procedures, such as walking, talking, and riding a bike at a level below conscious awareness or, as in the preceding example, the experience of the daughter's subsuming her own needs to please the mother despite the disgust. Semantic memory, then, is a more structured recorded memory of what happened; it can be articulated in language, whereas procedural memory cannot.

Procedural memory is important because it carries *scripts*, the unconscious, automatic sequences of experience and action that constitute a lot of people's psychological lived experience. A lot of emotional schematic reactions are operating at the procedural rather than the declarative level. They are triggered by cues without deliberate intention. For example, when the boss raises their voice, it automatically activates fear and an action tendency to withdraw. Or, when a spouse frowns, the partner does not consciously know that their spouse's expression of disappointment is actually covering their anger, which, if expressed, would activate guilt, which would lead the spouse to block their expression of anger. None of this is conscious, but it is a script stored in memory at the procedural level and requires activation in therapy to transform this sequence.

Personally-relevant events appear to be stored in memory at their "emotion addresses" through the emotion schematic processing system. One memory of sadness is connected to other memories of sadness. When people feel angry, anger memories are activated. This form of mood-dependent memory means that a current disappointment links to other disappointments, a feeling of shame to other diminishments. Present emotional experiences, thus, are always multilayered, evoking with them prior instances of the same or similar emotional experiences. Therapists need to access memories in therapy to transform much of people's maladaptive emotional experience. We first have to arrive at painful emotions from the past, predominantly by activating episodic memories, and only then can we help people leave them through transformation by having new lived experience in psychotherapy sessions.

Boritz et al. (2008, 2011) directly investigated the relationship of expressed emotional arousal and autobiographical memory in the context of early, middle, and late phase sessions of the treatment for depression. They found a significant increase in autobiographical memory specificity from early to late phase therapy sessions. Treatment outcomes were predicted by a combination of high narrative specificity plus expressed arousal in late phase sessions. So, as opposed to providing generic memories like, "My father was never there," remembering a specific time when he was absent was therapeutically more productive. In addition, the combination of expressed emotional arousal and narrative specificity was associated with complete recovery at treatment termination. Recovered clients were significantly more able to emotionally express their feelings in the context of telling specific autobiographical memory narratives than clients who remained depressed at treatment termination. Interestingly, some cognitive experimental research findings (Williams et al., 2007) have consistently identified difficulty retrieving specific personal memories as a consistent marker of clinical depression. Accordingly, therapists need to shift clients to be more specific by asking the client to give a detailed concrete example or life event to exemplify a general concern or issue and by facilitating a reexperiencing of episodic memories as opposed to a global retelling of past memories and significant events.

The following excerpt drawn from a therapy session with a 47-year-old, married, Caucasian client with complex trauma demonstrates the therapist empathically supporting the narrative retelling of a trauma event involving the episodic memory embedded in an autobiographical narrative memory. The focus of the exploration, whether it was an internal experience or external description, is noted in brackets:

CLIENT: I said that to my sister yesterday, that night is so clear to me.

THERAPIST: The night she died.

CLIENT: The night she killed herself. It's so clear, I can remember everything.

THERAPIST: Can you tell me?

CLIENT: Just like it happened yesterday, and I remember, and it sort of came into clear focus for me as a kid, and I hate it, I mean, I hate it. I remember the night that my mother died, that's what it was like. [emergence of episodic memory narrative of suicide scene] I was walking home to my brother and sister, my sister was supposed to be babysitting my brother in the house, and, um, it was quiet, and I thought they were waiting to jump out and go, "Boo!" you know? Kids' stuff. [external track describing what happened] (*Therapist: Mm-hmm.*) So, I tiptoe—tiptoe up the sidewalk and open the front door very carefully and listen, still nothing, just the sound in my eardrums. [shift to internal]

THERAPIST: This deafening silence. [therapist evocative reflection of internal experience]

CLIENT: So quiet, and I'm thinking this is really berserk, really crazy, because usually by now, they've jumped out and scared the living daylights out of me, and we've all laughed (*Therapist: Mm.*) and punched each other, or whatever kids do. And I remember walking in and still nothing, and thinking this is really funny, and I took my boots off, and I went creeping down into the kitchen, and I saw my mother's foot first, and—I was in absolute shock and not knowing what to do. [shift to internal experience]

THERAPIST: And your heart almost stopped. [evocative elaboration of internal experiencing]

CLIENT: And I started shouting because I thought my sister was supposed to be there, and I started screaming for my sister, and then I noticed that on the table there was a note saying that she was over at my aunt's and uncle's at a New Year's party, and they had put my little brother to bed there [shift to external], and that was really because of all the turmoil as a child, too. I was frightened to call anybody because you know your own business stays within the four walls of your house, so (*Therapist: Sure, sure.*) it felt like 10 hours, I'm sure it was a minute, but it seemed like 10 hours.

THERAPIST: So, then you walked in and saw what had actually happened. [Therapist invites a return to the scene and shift to external.]

CLIENT: I tried waking her up. I thought she might just have, you know.

THERAPIST: Who knows as a child?

CLIENT: And I'm just shaking her and shaking her and trying to wake her up, and thinking, you know, oh, God, what do I do, who do I call, what do I do (*Therapist: Mm.*). So, the first thing I did, I called my aunt, she came over with my sister because, of course, I said,—I don't know what I said, I have no idea—and, of course, when she came in, my heart also goes out to her because I can't imagine an adult, myself now walking in on a situation like that—with your family.

In this segment, the client and therapist work together in a detailed unfolding of a trauma scene. The client presents a clear, episodic memory along with her internal experience.

In the next example with a client, the therapist probes for the disclosure of a specific autobiographical memory narrative:

THERAPIST: Uh-huh. So, see if any specific memory comes up of any—of a time when you really felt (*Client: Uh—oh, yes.*)—uh-huh. [focus on episodic memory]

CLIENT: I took—I remember the time when I called home. I called . . . I called my mother's home just to hear whoever's voice answered. I did it four or five times, and then I would just hang up (*Therapist: Hmm.*) just to hear [her family name], just to get in touch with that house that seemed so far away and gone and lost.

Here, the client responds to the therapist's request for a memory with a narrative that conveys the sense of the client's poignant longing for the family that she had to leave behind. She felt "lost" when she chose to leave home as a teenager to live with the father of her newborn baby. It is clear in the preceding two examples that the therapist is actively encouraging the clients to shift to the recollection of emotionally significant personal memories and to describe their internal experience.

Therapists need to invite clients to shift from external processing of what happened or from reflexive processing of what it meant to internal processing of what it felt like to facilitate deeper emotional experience. Lewin (2001) found that in good outcome, experiential therapies shift from external or reflexive to internal processing, comprising almost a third (30%) of all process shifts undertaken by therapists. In contrast, in poor outcome, therapists initiated significantly fewer shifts to internal processing (16.75%) than their good outcome counterparts. In essence, it appears as if the therapist's specific focus on emotional experience in the context of the client's reflections on their lives helps the client to enter more fully into a sustained elaboration of their own internal world of felt emotions.

MEMORY RECONSOLIDATION

Emotionally distressing events result in emotional reactions. The emotions of this experience fade unless they are "burned" into memory. The more highly aroused the emotion, the more the evoking situation and the emotion will be remembered (McGaugh, 2002). Then, the emotions are connected to memories of the self in the situation, and episodic and emotion schematic autobiographical memories are formed. As a result, the emotional response can be recreated again and again long after the event. For example, a memory of a betrayal or something that reminds one of it stimulates an emotional response of anger and hurt. Given that maladaptive emotion schematic memories result in such painful emotions as fear, shame, and sadness, which are at the center of many disorders, the possibility of disrupting previously acquired emotion schematic memory by adding new input has important clinical implications.

As discussed in Chapter 4, memory reconsolidation provides a way of understanding how distressing emotional memories can be both strengthened over time and also altered through the corrective experience. Consider, for example, an emotionally distressing event, such as a betrayal or abandonment. The emotional reaction is an integral component of the memory connected via the spatial and temporal context to the event and bound to the self, thus forming an autobiographical memory. The more highly arousing the emotional reaction, the more likely an episodic memory will be formed and the evoking situation will be vividly remembered later on. When a memory is recalled, the emotional response is reengaged, and the sympathetic nervous system is reactivated via the amygdala. According to reconsolidation theory, the recollected event and its newly experienced emotional response are reencoded into a new and expanded memory trace. Thus, memory for the original traumatic incident is strengthened, making it (and the now intensified emotional response) even more likely to be accessed in the future.

This theory also provides a mechanism for understanding how this same emotional memory might be revised. During therapy, patients are commonly asked to recall and reexperience a painful past event, often eliciting a strong emotional reaction. If the psychotherapy process leads to a new, more adaptive emotional response, this plus the feeling of being in the context of the safe, therapeutic, relational environment can then be incorporated into the old memory through reconsolidation. In this view, change in psychotherapy is not simply the result of a new memory trace being created or new semantic structures being developed. Instead, reconsolidation leads to the transformation of the components of the memory structure itself. It is conceivable that once this transformation has taken place, the original memory, including the associated emotional response, will no longer be retrieved in its previous form. By this view, psychotherapy is a process that not only provides new experiences but also changes our understanding and experience of past experience in fundamental ways through the transformation of memory.

It is important to reiterate that, in this process, transformation is not simply the result of a new memory trace being formed; the original event memory itself is transformed in fundamental ways. Psychotherapy, then, is a process that not only provides new experiences and different ways to evaluate new experiences but also changes emotion schematic memories of past experiences in fundamental ways through the reconsolidation of memory. Accessing a new emotion in response to the same situation is one of the best ways to change the experience of an old emotion memory. Once a previously inaccessible emotion memory is evoked, the new emotional experience is integrated into it, and when the memory reconsolidates it, the new emotion fuses with the old memory and transforms it. Thus, for example, feeling adaptive anger to overcome shame leads to changing the memory of the experience and thereby the narrative. As pointed out in Chapter 4, two things are essential in this process: The old memory needs to be activated so it is being currently experienced; then, novelty should be introduced only after at least a 10-minute delay. New experience too soon or not in conjunction with memory activation, like in a subsequent session, will not produce incorporation of new experience in the reconsolidation phase.

For example, consider the client mentioned earlier who recounted her episodic memory of her mother's suicide scene. Whenever she thought of her mother, she had horrifying memories of her mother lying in a pool of blood on the kitchen floor. Whenever this image came to mind, it left her feeling cold and clammy with awful feelings of fear and emptiness. After working through her anger, shame, and sadness, and after finally letting go and forgiving her mother, the client talked about how this awful memory had changed by remembering previous happy memories of her mother. These memories, in contrast, left her feeling all warm and cozy. These new feelings toward her mother changed the old cold, clammy feelings. They fused with the old feelings to form a more integrated picture of her mother. This client reported later at follow-up that when she thought of her mother, she no longer imagined her lying in a pool of blood but, rather, remembered her alive mother and felt warm and loving feelings. Ultimately, a full transformation of her emotion memory occurred, and she thought of her mother as the loving mother she had known before the suicide, and she had good warm, feelings remembering having felt loved by her mother.

Evoking the emotion schematic memory, reducing the intensity of previous emotions by putting words on them, processing them further in terms of the needs embedded in them and their impacts on the person's experience, and then introducing new emotions allow the memories to be reconsolidated in a new way. Thus, in relation to, say, a betrayal, if the offending other is eventually seen with more compassion than anger, and the situation is experienced with sadness at loss rather than shame of humiliation, the experience of the memory changes. With new feelings, the emotion schematic memory is changed, and now the amygdala is no longer activated by memories of the offending incident. To achieve this change, it is necessary to activate the painful memory and then to experience the memory of the betrayal without the attendant pain and fear and, instead, with some new feeling, such as anger or compassion. We need to see that what leads to change is the emotional mechanism of changing emotion with emotion rather than a process of reason triumphing over emotion.

New emotion memories, however formed, also help change autobiographical memories and ultimately personal narratives. Narrative and emotion are intricately interwoven. No important story is significant without emotion, and no emotions take place outside of the context of a story (Angus & Greenberg, 2011; Greenberg & Angus, 2004). The stories people tell to make sense of their experience and to construct their identities depend, to a significant degree, on the variety of emotion memories that are available to them. By changing their memories and by accessing different memories, people change the stories of their lives and their identities. Thus, for the client discussed earlier who thought about her mother's suicide scene, her access to positive memories of her mother and a new lived experience in the session supported a view in which she saw her mother as loving and caring rather than as recklessly abandoning, as she had previously seen her.

In discussing memory reconsolidation, it is important to distinguish it from the behavioral phenomenon of extinction. In animal studies of both reconsolidation and extinction, an element of the learning situation, the context (a conditioned stimulus), is presented without its previous consequence (the unconditioned stimulus). In most of the experiments with rats, the unconditioned stimulus is a shock administered through the grid floor. Because of this similarity, there has been some question about how to separate the two—and this has considerable importance in the present context because reconsolidation is assumed to actually change components of the reactivated memory, whereas extinction is assumed to merely create a new memory that overrides the previously trained response. Thus, an "extinguished" response is not really gone because it can spontaneously recover over time or be reinstated if the organism is exposed to a relevant cue in a new context. Recent work has shown that the cellular/molecular cascades in these two cases are different and that whether reconsolidation or extinction is initiated depends on the temporal dynamics of the test procedure and how recently the memory in question was formed or reactivated, or both (de la Fuente et al., 2011; Inda et al., 2011; Maren, 2011). At this time, it is clear that reconsolidation and extinction represent distinct reactions to reactivating a memory (Lane et al., 2015).

WOUNDED CHILD WORK

A central part of an emotion-oriented therapy involves processing unresolved painful emotional experiences from the past, predominantly from childhood. Children have less capacity than adults to adequately process their emotions, and this can result in the development of core maladaptive schemes. These past painful experiences generally lead to maladaptive ways of responding in the present to others and themselves. When children are ignored, rejected, or physically or emotionally hurt, they will tend to respond to others in similar ways to show they coped with earlier difficulties.

All too commonly, perhaps resulting from direct physical threats, shame, or a lack of available confidants, painful experiences are never discussed with anyone or processed. When a parent is the instigator of abuse, it is often a double whammy, first because of the violation or harm and, second, because the parent is not available to assist the victim in dealing with it. The lack of an available caregiver to provide comfort and support may be a critical ingredient in what makes the experience(s) overwhelming or traumatic. What this means emotionally is that the implicit emotional responses were never brought to the conscious level of discrete feeling through symbolization in language. As a result, the traumatized individual knew the circumstances of the trauma but did not know how it affected them emotionally. This lack of awareness contributes to the tendency to experience traumatic threats in circumstances in an overly generalized manner that reflects the inability to distinguish circumstances that are safe from those that are not. It is often only in therapy when the experiences are put into words that the emotional responses are formulated for the first time.

Putting these feelings into words present opportunities for work with the *wounded child*, a metaphor for a vulnerable wounded part of the self. This metaphor helps people reown their feelings by talking about and symbolizing them in language, identify where these feelings originated, and, most importantly, facilitate transforming these feelings. Ultimately, in this work, the goal is to help people regain strength and access nurturing feelings toward their own pain and hurt. The wounded child metaphor is important because it is easier for an adult to allow, and to experience, their vulnerable feelings when they imagine themselves as a child. They can more easily connect with how they feel now as an adult when they take a child position in imagination. Identifying with their younger self helps get past the adult protective coping measures developed over a lifetime. It is easier for a 50-year-old adult man, for example, to experience his fear of being alone when imagining himself as his 6-year-old self—taking the position of being afraid of being alone at night in his bedroom that is far away from the safety of his parents' bedroom—than it is to feel his fear of being alone as a 50-year-old. As an adult, he is supposed to have all kinds of adult resources, both internal and external, to slough off his lonely fears as childish and not befitting his current situation in life. All people develop these coping methods or what Winnicott (1965) called a false self that protects the more vulnerable parts of self. Usually, the more wounded a person was, the more they build these false self-protective walls.

Every adult has vulnerabilities and feelings of weakness that are well represented by the image of a vulnerable or wounded child. This, however, is not suggesting that the person is fixated at an early stage of development but, rather, is a way of describing an adult feeling: At some time, all adults feel vulnerable, afraid, alone, and insecure. These are adult feelings too often disallowed as childish. Society tends to put weakness into the hospital as though it were sick rather than accept it as a healthy adult need for comfort, nurture, and safety. I am not talking about a child self, stuck at some early stage of development, but an adult feeling of weakness. The vulnerable feelings may retain the remnants of childhood feelings that have developed from these, but they are most definitely adult feelings. So, therapists are working with an actual present, adult emotion, and the notion of it being a wounded child is symbolic, not real.

Representing adult experience as a wounded child within is an intervention method that helps people access the feeling and the full range of memories of this feeling had their origins in childhood (Bradshaw, 1988; Webster, 2019). It provides the context for reexperiencing feelings that were felt but never were adequately processed and have remained in memory and represent themselves in the present. The wounded child metaphor therefore facilitates access to feelings and provides a lead into age regression interventions. I use this term "regression" not in the way that Freud did to denote a defense mechanism leading to the temporary or long-term reversion of the ego to an earlier stage of development (Freud, 1917/1976) but as the name for an intervention to help access feelings of adult vulnerability or weakness. The aims of working with the wounded child with age regression are to help arrive at the painful emotion memories and, ultimately, to leave them by transforming them with new emotional experiences.

The aim of all emotion work is to access the dreaded core maladaptive emotions, which are so painful that people do whatever they can in life to not feel them or even to not feel any emotion at all. The therapeutic skill to help clients approach dreaded feelings is to ask the client to stay with the emotion and to talk from it. This is both a general skill of emotion-focused work and a specific skill needed to help clients approach their pain in the context of wounded child work. The therapist, thus, invites the client to stay with the feeling, make space for it, and become the wounded child to give a voice to the painful experience as the child. The therapist then helps the client differentiate the experience and validates how painful it was. The process generally ends with self-soothing by which the therapist helps the adult self respond to the woundedness in the child with compassion and support.

The Process of Wounded Child Work

Clients come to therapy because they are feeling bad, and therapy generally starts with the therapist helping client unfold their narrative and begin exploring their concerns. Generally, the clients talk in the landscape of action about "what happened." Sometimes, they move into the landscape of meaning and talk about what "what happened" meant, but they spend little time in the landscape of feeling. The therapist's task, initially, is to empathize and combine that with a gentle, consistent pressure toward the internal, toward the client's core affect. However, when clients talk about their feelings, these often are secondary feeling reactions, such as saying, "I'm frustrated or angry" when talking about situations in which their needs have not been met and they primarily feel hurt, or they may be crying in helplessness or hopelessness when they are primarily angry. Sometimes, however, right from the start, clients may present experiencing primary, painful, maladaptive feelings like feeling "lonely" or "worthless," but then they often are talking about these painful feelings in a helpless or protesting manner rather than experiencing them in a productive manner. The therapeutic task is to help clients process these core feelings productively.

After the first few sessions focused on listening to the narrative and developing an alliance, the therapist works to coconstructively develop a focus on the client's core painful, maladaptive emotions. In our research (Greenberg & Goldman, 2019), we have found that the core painful feelings that most often appear are fear, sadness, or shame. These emotions are identified by the therapist, who, in addition to listening to the content of the narrative, is emotionally attuned to what is most painful in the client's narratives. The origins of these painful emotions are explored and related to the client's attachment and identity histories. By exploring their histories, clients access disowned emotions—emotions that are too dangerous or frightening to feel, so they block them, treat them as "not me," and disclaim the feelings and action tendencies. When their needs for security and validation are not met and their painful feelings are not soothed, people protect themselves by cutting off their feelings and needs. They, however, now also anticipate and come to expect negative treatment from others, and they react to minor cues of abandonment or criticism using their survival strategies. These strategies that were designed to protect them have now become an important part of the problem. Driven by the desire to survive, they disclaim their painful feelings and needs in an attempt to best cope with the situation. It is important in working with emotion to always see people as doing the best they can, in their context, in their efforts to thrive and survive.

After agreeing on goals and tasks, and establishing a safe, trusting bond, the focus shifts collaboratively to working with the client's memories, emotional reactions, and survival behaviors from their past. A key way of working is to have the client reexperience childhood situations and feelings by means of age regression to childhood. The client is invited to enter episodic memories as a way of accessing the dreaded painful feelings to rework them in the present. Here, they deal with past traumas, experiences of abandonment, invalidation, neglect, and unprocessed hurt and grief. A helpful approach is to imagine going back progressively or, more appropriately, regressively, in imaginary small steps to help the client get into the experience of being a younger self. The therapist can use a metaphor of going down in an elevator or being on a journey by saying, "Now you are moving down from 30 years old to 20, to 15, to 12, and now you have arrived. You are 8 or 6 years old." Alternately, before immediately becoming the 6-year-old, the therapist might also ask the client to imagine their 6-year-olds sitting in front of them in a chair, or on their knee, and have the adult client describe how they see their child self. This helps evoke memories of being the child. Ultimately, therapists want to help people identify with and speak as the wounded child self.

The most usual process in wounded child work is that in which the therapist guides the client to move from a discussion of current feelings or events to memories related to the feeling or event. For example, in discussing unresolved feelings toward parents, the therapist might say, "So, you have this feeling of never being seen by them. Let's go back to when you remember feeling this as a child." Or, the person may be talking about how much of a bully the father was to her and to her mother, so the therapist invites her to go back by saying, "So, if you are willing, let's go back when you were 8 years old and get at what it felt like for you as a child growing up in that environment." Sometimes, clients of their own accord might reenter and reexperience a childhood scene—not as a flashback, but they may suddenly feel themselves, when they are talking about an adult experience, reexperiencing a childhood scene. They spontaneously go back to an experience and reexperience it in the present. A client, for example, may talk about having been humiliated by a coworker and suddenly go back to having been shamed in class at school by a teacher and remember the other kids making fun of her. Clients need to feel sufficiently safe within themselves and with their therapists to do this reexperiencing.

Compassion and Self-Soothing

The expression of anguish or emotional suffering has been identified (Greenberg, 2015) as a marker for self-soothing work in which a more adult part of the self soothes the wounded child. Typically, the anguish occurs in the face of powerful interpersonal needs (e.g., for love or validation) that were not met by others. Intervention involves some soothing agent that provides soothing where none was available before. This can be done in a chair dialogue: Clients are asked if they, as an adult, could soothe their wounded child. The goal is to evoke compassion for the self. Therapists can use chair work to try to evoke compassion, but one does not have to use chair work because accessing and soothing the wounded child can be done as part of a more dialogical intervention.

In this type of imaginary transformation, the therapist might say,

> Try closing your eyes and remember your experience in this situation. Get a concrete image if you can. Go into it. Be your child in this scene. Please tell me what is happening. What do you see, smell, hear in the situation? What do you feel in your body, and what is going through your mind?

After a while, the therapist can ask the client to shift perspective by saying,

> Now, I would like you to view the scene as an adult. What do you see, feel, and think? Do you see the look on the child's face? What do you want to do? Can you do it? How can you intervene? Can you try it now in your imagination?

Changing perspectives again, the therapist can ask the client to become the child and ask the following questions:

> What do you as the child feel and think? What do you need from the adult? Can you ask for what you need or wish? What does the adult do? What else do you need? Ask for it. Is there someone else you would like to come in to help? Can you receive the care and protection offered?

This intervention concludes with the therapist asking,

> Check how you feel inside right now. What does all this mean to you, about you, and about what you needed? Can you come back to the present, to yourself as an adult now here with me? How do you feel? Can you say goodbye to the child for now?

A helpful intervention to help evoke compassion is to ask clients to give examples of times when they have been empathic to another person or to an animal. It is the client's capacity to be empathic and caring of another in need or pain that therapists try to build on to help the client become more aware of their compassion so that they can access it in the service of soothing themselves.

However, when the self-soothing dialogue is introduced to clients who are not sufficiently differentiated from the hostile negative caretaker and they are asked to start with their own child, the contempt or destructive reaction of the other may be evoked. It is precisely this type of negative reaction that needs to be transformed over the course of treatment. In such cases, it can be initially difficult for the client to feel compassionate about their own wounded child state; instead, they invalidate their own vulnerability. At these times, it is better not to ask the person to see themselves as a child in the other chair or to imagine the part of the self that needs soothing, which may evoke negative feelings or condemnation of the child or the vulnerable self. It may be more helpful to symbolize the anguish as being that of a universal child or a close friend who has experienced the same things that the client has experienced and that are the source of their anguish. Even though people understand the implication of what they are being asked to do by being compassionate to a universal child in similar circumstances, they may be able to soothe a universal child more easily than their own child, who automatically evokes self-contempt. Once compassion has occurred in relation to a child in need, it is easier to transfer this feeling to the self.

Strength to Protect the Self

Sometimes the adult self may feel overwhelmed by seeing a hurt, damaged child because they do not yet have a sense that they can protect themselves effectively, or they may fear that they will disintegrate and drown in their pain. At these times, therapists can become surrogate protectors. For example, when a client is overwhelmed or frightened by the pain they see in themselves as a young child, the therapist and the child can work together to confront the abusive or neglectful other. The client can feel safer in their therapist's presence, drawing strength from the therapist. The client can be encouraged to imagine the therapist right behind them or even in front, telling the abusive other to stop. In empty-chair dialogues, the therapist can help the client put their need into words.

At times, the client may be unable to offer solace and comfort to the distressed self for a number of reasons. A client's feelings of vulnerability and fear may not have been validated sufficiently, or the feelings are still too entangled and confusing, and the client has not yet begun to differentiate out from an unresponsive parent. Or the client may still be distraught about their own behavior and feel too ashamed, or, for whatever reason, cannot access their resilience. Sometimes clients may feel angry and betrayed by significant others who did not provide for them, and this can also hinder their desire to assume any responsibility for self-care. However, slowly, as therapy progresses, and with a continued and repeated discussion of the importance of self-compassion, clients, over time, are helped to accept that if they are to heal and thrive, they need to be compassionate to themselves for their own protection and well-being.

What follows is an example from a session with a 28-year-old woman from mainland China who is working in therapy, speaking in English. The session addresses the client's core wounded feelings of fear and shame from childhood maltreatment by both her mother and father. The cross-cultural applicability of this type of work with core emotion is important because there is the misapprehension that it may be more difficult to work with emotion in Asian and more collectivist cultures in which concern for the other supersedes concern for the self in individualist culture. The situation of this client is that, as an adult, she has difficulty in intimate relationship and relates this to her treatment by her parents. In this ninth session, she is dealing with a memory related to being slapped by her father and how this relates to her current marriage.

Clinical Example: Hatred Toward Father

CLIENT: Ya. It's just that . . . my father would never hit me or my mother. There was, however, an instance when he picked up a chopper [an ax] and attempted to hurt my mom. I was shocked. And when my husband put his fist up to my face . . . it reminds me of my father waving the chopper at my mom.

THERAPIST: I can only imagine how it affected you. How did you feel as a child?

CLIENT: I have some hatred towards my father.

THERAPIST: Hatred. This seems like the root.

CLIENT: Same—same pattern with my partner.

THERAPIST: It haunts you. It will be good to address it? Let's try and go back to that time in your life to that experience feeling scared and of hating. [age regression]

CLIENT: Okay, what do you mean?

THERAPIST: Imagine you are going back to when you were young. Go back. You're now 20, 15, 12, you're 7 years old. Be your 7-year-old and speak as her. What was it like for you?

CLIENT: (*Nods*) When I was much younger, he used to buy things for me. I have some gratitude towards him, but as I was growing up and until he passed on, I have a lot of hatred towards him.

Especially the way he treated my mom . . . the way he remarried and cheated on my mom.

THERAPIST: He's someone you feel gratitude towards but also a lot of hatred. Be the 7-year-old and tell me what you feel. [Speak as the child.]

CLIENT: He doesn't give me an allowance—he always takes from my mom. Since I was young, he doted on me. He had never hit me. I just recall one thing that one moment. . . . In the beginning, I loved him as a daughter should. I make sure he took care of his health and take his medications.

THERAPIST: There's love and hate.

CLIENT: Hate—there was this once because of my mother and how he treated her, and . . . regarding my stepmother, and he slapped me across my face!

THERAPIST: Slapped you . . .

CLIENT: Yes, at the dining room table. Slapped me.

THERAPIST: Such a shock? Go back to that. How old were you? What do you feel? Speak as the little girl.

CLIENT: I was 10 years old. I remember, at that moment, when he slapped, I felt pain . . . I have felt it. In my whole life, he had never beaten me . . .

THERAPIST: He hit you. What's it like for you, you feel so much pain? Describe what it was like, the pain. [episodic memory]

CLIENT: The pain is like . . . a lot of stones crashing down on me—my heart is broken. The fatherly love was all spilled on the floor. I wanted to gradually forgive him, but I couldn't . . .

THERAPIST: After that moment, it was impossible to forgive as your heart has broken. That slap caused the pain in your heart.

CLIENT: (*Nods*) Since that moment, my brother also realized that he has changed. He has totally changed. I felt that since that moment, he changed. No longer my dad. He changed to become . . . became a stranger. Someone I don't know him anymore.

THERAPIST: As a child what would you want to say to him if he were here? Tell him how you feel about his treatment towards you, your mother . . .

CLIENT: I'm 10 years old that year—I'm in Primary 3; my parents are divorced already for 1½ years, I help out with household chores—cook, clean. As a 10-year-old, it's too much. I want to play like my friends.

THERAPIST: A lot of responsibility. So burdened and alone.

CLIENT: Yeah, I feel so alone and afraid. I need a father who takes care of me. Protect me, not scare me. It's not supposed to be my problem or responsibility to look after everyone and everything. I have no parents. I need my parents. [emotion schematic memories and needs]

Coconstruction of What an Experience Was Like

Therapists, as shown in the preceding case, need to repeatedly guide toward the focus, toward the core painful maladaptive emotion—in that excerpt, to the feeling of being alone and afraid. The work needs to always move toward the focus but without losing the more nondirective following aspect. The therapist is not imposing their view of what it felt like but, rather, is helping coconstruct how it was for the client. Coconstruction is an art that involves being able to empathize and validate as well as simultaneously refocus on core issues, deepen experience, and evoke emotion.

For example, a 29-year-old client who comes into the 12th session expressing sadness and anger about her bad relationship with her parents says she is sad that they have not reached out to her despite her telling them that she does not want to talk to them. She says, "It's so painful that even my distancing from them feels like nothing to them." She is distressed about what is happening now with her parents. However, it is important in these situations of current interpersonal difficulties for the therapist to guide toward the unfinished business of her childhood because of a history of neglect and abandonment as well as core feelings of sad loneliness and insecurity rather than for the therapist to stay on the current interpersonal conflict. The client's current distress with what is going on with the parents needs to be treated as a doorway into her past relationship with her parents that was filled with neglect and invalidation. It left her with a big hole inside from her feelings of emptiness and unsureness. The client wants to vent about how bad her parents are, but the therapist, after validating the client's present anger by affirming—"It's so infuriating to get no response, not even a nod in your direction"—guides toward her core emotional pain by saying, "So much hurt, so much anger. All your life, you've felt you've never been considered, never been seen. Let's go back to those early days that have left you feeling so invalidated."

GUIDELINES FOR AGE REGRESSION WORK

This section discusses a set of steps that act as a therapist's guide to age regression work (but Webster, 2019). First, when an experience of concern related to childhood abandonment, neglect, or trauma emerges, this is a marker for age regression and possible work on imaginal transformation. For example, a client may say, "My parents just always left me to myself. They were too involved in their own stuff to even know what I was doing, never mind feeling almost like I didn't exist for them." The therapist empathizes and guides the client to pay attention to what is being felt in the body in the present: "Just left so alone, feeling I'm not important? Just stay with that feeling. What do you feel in your body right now?" The therapist then guides the client to go back to an earlier time when they felt this before:

> If it's okay with you, let's go back to an earlier age. Do you remember a specific age or time when you were aware of feeling that? Take your time. . . . Let's go back: You are 30, you're 20, 15, 10, now you are 6 years old. Okay, so you are 6 years old. What's happening and what are you feeling?

At this point, the therapist follows five steps to focus the client on the feelings in the event as a child:

1. Guide the client to be the child and talk as the child in the present. Say, "As your 6-year-old, what are you feeling in your body? There you are; your mother is talking to her friend. What's it like for you? What do you feel? Be the 6-year-old and tell your mother." Guide the client to reexperience the feelings in the present. Help the client stay with and accept the painful feeling: "Just stay with those feelings and welcome them." Validate the child experience: "Yeah, it was so painful and must have been so lonely."

2. Once the feeling is felt deeply and is validated, focus on the unmet need. Ask, "What did you need?"

3. Validate the need and promote a feeling of having deserved to have the need met: "Of course you needed attention and support. You deserve it. Tell them again: 'I deserved some of your attention.'" Transformation now occurs by accessing a new feeling that arises in response to the need having not been met (usually, assertive anger or grief at the loss or compassion). "What comes up in you now as you say that?" is a good question to assess new feelings. Sometimes a new feeling comes without an explicit statement of the need but asking for the need often helps access a new feeling.

4. Once the pain and the need have been felt, one of the new feelings that may emerge is compassion. The therapist encourages the experience and expression of compassion by asking the client to be the adult self

and speak to wounded child self: "If you, as your adult, looks at your wounded child here feeling so alone and unimportant, feeling all this, what would you want to say to them or do?"

5. The therapist generally finishes the session by bringing the client back to the present and debriefing the client's experience of the work: "How are you feeling now? What do make of this? Are you ready to go back into the world? Anything you need right now?"

When the therapist invites the client to be compassionate to the wounded child, it is ideal to have the client enact this compassion. The therapist can ask the client to see the child sitting in a chair in front of them or in their imagination and then talk to the imagined child and express care, support, compassion, and love. Enacting compassion embodies the experience more deeply than just having the therapist and client talk about it.

Using Imaginal Reentry and Imaginal Transformation

Another variant of regression work is imaginal reentry into a past scene in which the child felt unprotected or abandoned. Here, the therapist asks the client to go back to the scene but to bring in a person to protect or nurture the child self. The aim is not self-soothing but imaginal transformation.

The therapist says, "Imagine yourself as a child in a scene related to the painful memory. Imagine yourself now as an adult or a protective other entering the scene and intervening to assist." The therapist guides the client to imagine a protective other to support and protect the vulnerable wounded self. The other may be a police officer who protects against an abusive father; or perhaps it is the therapist, who set limits or educates; or it might be a mythical figure to take the child to a safer place. The therapist asks the protective other, "Is there anything that you want to say to the child or to anyone on the child's behalf?" and makes sure that the child feels safe and protected by the support of the adult. The therapist initially and along the way, at appropriate moments, asks the child questions related to the child's sensations, emotions, thoughts, and behaviors. So, in guiding the client to enter the scene and during the process, the therapist might ask, "What do you see, hear, smell, sense in your body? What do you feel? What is going through your mind? What do you want to do? What is happening?"

Speaking as the Child or to the Child

In age regression, the client can take two major positions: speaking as the child or speaking to the child. When clients are being the child, it is good for them to speak as much as possible in the present tense, such as saying,

"I feel afraid" as opposed to "I felt afraid." When speaking from the adult position, the client could be both an observer and an actor who does things like support and express love and caring to the wounded child self. Different self–other combinations can be used. The most classical form as previously described involves saying, "Imagine yourself being the wounded child and speak from that position" and then asking the client to speak from the adult position. The adult then can be asked what the child needed or what the adult could say to the child that would help the child—or even if the adult could take the child away and protect them.

However, in some self-annihilating clients, being the wounded child or speaking to the wounded child brings up too many feelings of contempt for the child. In such cases, a different form is best. For example, when invited to speak to her wounded child, one middle-aged woman who had been sexually abused by her neighbor immediately chastised her 8-year-old for knowingly going to the neighbor's house because he had a big TV. But when asked to imagine another child, in this case, her daughter, in the same situation, the client was able to access feelings of care and protectiveness rather than blame. She was then able to feel more compassion toward her own child self. To sidestep the negative feelings clients might have about themselves as a child, the therapist can ask what they would feel and want to say to a universal child who has suffered the same things as the client had as a child: "Imagine a child who was abandoned this way by their parents. What do you feel or want to say to this wounded child?"

A variant intervention, as mentioned earlier, involves asking the client to imagine a very close friend: "So similar that they have had the same experiences as you and are feeling the exact same way as you. What do you want or wish for them? What would help them? What can you give them to help this?" The therapist asks the client to imagine an ideal parent or significant other in the other chair—not as they were but as the client needed them to be—and then has the client ask that other for what they need. Next, the therapist has the parent speak to the wounded child as a good parent.

Developing Capacity to Care for the Self

In the resolution process, clients typically move from anguish, through the main steps of accessing painful primary maladaptive emotions, and toward a statement of unmet needs and the sadness of grief at not having had those needs met (Goldman & Fox-Zurawic, 2012; Ito et al., 2010). At times, however, there is fear and interruption of emotion, and also protest about having to soothe oneself rather than having received soothing from others. These difficulties have to be worked through before the client can access the primary painful emotions. It appears that it is not simply enacting compassion for the self that leads to resolution but also access to the unmet need and grieving its loss that are important in accessing compassion for the pain of the loss and the provision of the missing compassion that is so healing. As clients go through this process with a supportive and empathic therapist, they develop feelings of compassion for themselves and for what was lost. Over time, doing this in conjunction with receiving empathic soothing and acceptance from therapists, who are emotionally attuned, clients eventually develop the capacity to soothe themselves and transform their painful emotions.

It is important to reiterate that therapists are not assuming that there is a child within. It is just that an earlier self-state of vulnerability or woundedness experienced as a child is evoked in the session, which, in turn, activates the emotions they experienced at the time of the injury. It can be highly poignant to clients to have the hurt they experienced as a child soothed and comforted by their adult self to provide the affective attunement that was never received.

The timing of this intervention, particularly for the questions regarding how the client feels toward the younger self who was wounded, is important. It must not occur too soon in therapy because that can lead the client to feel invalidated or overburdened once again. When clients have been overburdened and responsible for caring for themselves, they need a period during which they can lay down the burden and relax. They want someone else to provide the care and support that was missing before they, once again, assume the mantle of self-care. Of course, when they take it up again, it is in a different way—one that acknowledges their feelings and needs as well as supports them to find better ways to meet their needs in the present.

Clinical Example: Viewing the Child Self Through Grandmother's Eyes

The following example shows a process of a client entering her wounded child position and transforming her core emotion schematic memories of worthlessness. The client is a 30-year-old Korean woman who has suffered from depression most of her life. She struggled as an adolescent with her very strict parents; as a teenager, she had self-harmed. The excerpt begins with the therapist guiding toward memories and helping the client stay with and focus on her core feeling of worthlessness until she accesses resilience and her need for validation of what she does have to offer. She then accesses compassion for herself through her grandmother's eyes:

THERAPIST: So, partly it's about things you have observed in your family, sort of, right? With the people around you, right? With your brother, in particular. Expectations. But there's also memories, I mean emotional memories, not just scenes but also experiences of being shut out, receiving hurtful remarks, in different ways being told that you don't fit in or something like that, you're not allowed to join in.

CLIENT: Yes, I repeatedly felt I didn't fit in, I was failing.

THERAPIST: You say they linger in you. So, that means they're there now, right? (*Client: Mm.*). So, that means they are with you; they do something to you now.

CLIENT: Unfortunately, they do.

THERAPIST: So, let's stay with that feeling Yes, so, that's an important— important thing. There is a threat there, like, "I have to meet their expectations."

CLIENT: (*Sobs*) Yes, yes.

THERAPIST: So, what do you feel now? Just hold on to it, it's important.

CLIENT: I don't want to give these people the power.

THERAPIST: I understand that very well. It's like there's some injustice in . . . not only have they done this, but in addition, it affects you even now.

CLIENT: Yes, many years later.

THERAPIST: I understand that . . . there's an inner protest inside of you against it. But if you look up inside of it, it's like you carry with you many different forms of experiences of, "If I don't . . . If I'm not performing or don't master it all, then the truth is that I'm nothing. Then I'm worthless." (*Client: Yes, mm.*) And these memories, these different events, are triggered almost daily. (*Client: Yes.*) It's not that you necessarily remember what happened . . . (*Client: No.*). But the threat that you are not good enough is triggered almost daily.

CLIENT: It does, and I'm very anxious that people don't actually like me—that they are just nice towards me (*laughs*).

THERAPIST: Like it's a secret that is kept from you or something like that. (*Client: Yes, yes.*) That, in reality, they dislike you or think you're no good.

CLIENT: Yes, I'm afraid of that because during my entire education, apart from the 2 years spent at university, there have been people letting me know that they don't think I'm any good. And I don't understand why because I can't remember ever doing anything towards anyone. On the contrary, I've been taking care of people, and I've tried to make sure nobody felt left out. So if anyone in class or at handball—there was one girl in particular that was a lot by herself and was bothered, so me and a friend of mine took care of her. I can't understand what I have done that makes people annoyed with me, and it's not the same person. There were some people at elementary and middle school, not so much at high school, there wasn't, so, there I was actually doing all right.

THERAPIST: It's like you're under constant . . . I mean your inside has been under constant threat of being told that you're not . . . (*Client: Yes.*) don't like you, sort of, right? (*Client: Yes.*) But deep inside, there's a truth that threatens you, right? That you're not likeable . . . (*Client: Yes.*) or that people can turn against you at any time. (*Client: Yes.*) If I may direct you a little bit inwards, sort of, right? So, to listen to this feeling . . . it's actually a quite deep . . . If we peel off all the attempts of trying to cope with it, sort of. There's actually a deep feeling of not being good enough. Not being adequate. Not being enough, right? What is it that this part would have needed to hear? [preliminary attempt at need]

CLIENT: I don't know because I don't know whether I'll be able to say that.

THERAPIST: No, it's hard to say it. Right. So, if we just keep focusing on that, when we sort of direct the flashlight in there (*points toward their own stomach*). (*Client: Mm.*) It's just like something arises: "I don't even want to say it because it's so . . . hurtful?" . . . or . . . ? (*Client: It is . . .*) Yes, so, if we go there anyway . . . (*Client: Yes, um . . .*). It's vulnerable, right? (*Client: Yes.*) Just like opening something that no one is supposed to see or no one is supposed to know about. [validate the fear and guide toward the core emotion]

CLIENT: (*Cries*) It's so hard.

THERAPIST: I understand. I can see it hurts, right? But it's almost like it's also . . .

CLIENT: Yes, I think so. I need to give myself a chance. Rome wasn't built in 1 day.

THERAPIST: So, if we try even more (*points toward stomach*), I understand this happens because it's vulnerable, it's a little bit like you need to give yourself the time or something like that, but it sounds like deep inside, there's an experience of being worthless, sort of, right?

CLIENT: (*cries*) Yes. Worthless. [The client has hit rock bottom and feels anguish core maladaptive pain.]

THERAPIST: Mm, and it feels that way when I say it. Just like that part sort of . . . boils down to the feeling of not having anything to offer anyone or something like that, right? (*Client: Yes.*) So, just stay with it, it's really important. (*Client: Mm.*) This is what gives us the chance to make a change, to go there. (*Client: Yes.*) Yes. What is it deep inside this wounded part of you . . . that feeling worthless part of you would have needed to hear? [heartfelt need]

CLIENT: It's . . . You also have a lot to give. That . . . there's someone that needs you, too. [With the help of the therapist focusing on her organismic need, the client begins to mobilize and bounce back.]

THERAPIST: So, that you are significant, is that it? (*Client: Yes.*) You need to hear that you're significant. (*Client: Yes.*) Can you feel it when you say it? Yes . . . Right, just like, I don't know . . . you have said something about your grandmother, a picture of her eyes. (*Client cries.*) Yes . . . Yeah . . . Mm . . . So, just welcome it. It's just like this is what that part needs deep inside. Those eyes. That warmth. The deep acceptance, sort of. (*Client: Yes.*) Yes, mm. [Therapist evokes a soothing other.]

CLIENT: (*Drops her tissue*) Oops. Um, she was very unique (*mumbles*). She could make anyone feel . . .

THERAPIST: So, what would she have told this part of you? (*Client: Um . . .*). What is it that her eyes and her warmth communicated? And what does she see?

CLIENT: She sees her grandchild . . .

THERAPIST: What does she see when she sees you? What does she see in you? Her eyes. If you keep her eyes lifted up, the warmth, the voice . . .

CLIENT: Um . . . That I primarily . . . I think for her, it was most important that I'm kind and good, caring, and take good care of the people around me.

THERAPIST: So, that's the actions, but deep inside, what she tells you. It's sort of the things she likes about you, so that's really important, so it's like you can imagine something even more fundamental, sort of, when she sees you, she tells you . . . ?

CLIENT: That . . . she loved me no matter what and is proud of me . . . and . . . thought I had a lot going for me.

THERAPIST: What does that do to . . . (*points toward stomach*) If we sort of bring back that part of you that feels useless, sort of . . .

CLIENT: Mm . . . (*laughs*) . . . Yes, I—it makes me feel good to see myself from her . . . or with her eyes. Things like that. Thinking that she did see me.

THERAPIST: So, it means that it feels a little bit like what? A little bit alleviating?

CLIENT: Yes, that I can. . . . My chest tightens when I think about me being useless, and it's' almost like I can breathe a little easier when I think about her.

THERAPIST: (*Gesticulates with own hands*) It's just like there's two very different . . . things, right? One is what was stored in you, right? The bullies, the different people signaling that "We don't want you" or "We don't like you," or something like that. (*Client: Yes, mm.*) The hurtful, really bad feeling of not being anything, not being valuable, right? (*Client: Mm.*). And then it's just like the picture of those warm, loving eyes, and the love, sort of, which came through words and action, and in every possible way. (*Client: Mm, yes.*) It's just like there's something important in letting the one catch up with the other. To bring the first into the latter. [changing emotion with emotion by synthesizing two feelings]

CLIENT: I never tried to prove anything to my grandmother (*Therapist: Yes.*) We were . . . good enough the way we were.

THERAPIST: So, the safety in that . . . the safety in that no matter what happens, no matter what shows up, that love will remain. It's absolute, sort of, it's not conditioned by anything, or . . .

CLIENT: (*Cries*) No, mm, that's right.

THERAPIST: What do you feel now?

CLIENT: (*Exhales*) That I . . . right now, I feel like I miss my grand-mother (*cries*).

THERAPIST: Yes, right. There was so much . . . like we talked about. You got so much from her, sort of, right? Yeah. (*Client: Yes.*) It's just like allowing her warm eyes and love affect you . . . and especially let it affect that inner, deep, hurtful feeling, sort of, right?

CLIENT: (*Eyes tear*) Yes. It feels warm and comforting. She accepted me, and it makes me feel worthwhile.

BRIDGES TO THE PAST

As stressed, the first phase of emotion-focused work involves arriving at emotions by attending to and becoming aware of them mainly through the therapist's empathic attunement to affect and attention to bodily sensations and feelings. Initially, the client might be expressing secondary feelings of anger in reaction to some primary feeling to a situation that evokes fear of abandonment. By empathizing with these feelings but then putting the focus on the more primary feeling of, say, the abandonment anxiety under-lying the anger, the client can be helped to track back to the deeper feelings of fear of abandonment.

This work begins by paying attention to what is occurring in the present, what feelings the client is expressing, or what is occurring in the client's body while they are talking. The therapist can then guide the client to go back in time by means of questions such as; "Have you felt this feeling before in your life?" or "When did you first have this feeling?" If, for example, a client is saying they are feeling so frightened at work or so lonely and that even though they are married, they feel this loneliness, the therapist might ask, "When did you first have these feelings?" or "Have you felt this feeling of loneliness before in your life?" The current feeling state of aloneness is used as a launching pad to explore its origins.

Similarly, therapists can build a bridge to the past by moving from present body sensations and experience to the origins of these experiences. They do this by asking clients to stay with a body experience and to arouse memo-ries: "Just stay with those sensations in your chest. Do they remind you of anything?" or "Just follow that body experience back to where it started." For example, if people, as they are talking, feel shaky or queasy, therapists can ask them to stay with their body experience by saying, "Just stay with those sensations in your stomach. Can you let words come from the sensations?" followed shortly thereafter by, "Do these sensations and feelings remind you of anything from an earlier time?" or "Just follow your body experience back to where it takes you." In addition, if clients present with symptoms, the therapist can focus on the bodily experience associated with the symptoms. For example, if a client talks about obsessive rituals like checking under the bed repeatedly before sleeping, the therapist might explore what bodily sensations are occurring in the sequence leading up to these behaviors. Once the client becomes aware of some bodily experience triggering the symptom, the therapist can help the client track backward to earlier times when those sensations played a role in the client's life.

After a feeling or body experience has been identified and located in the body, the therapist guides the client to put into words and speak from it, a method that can help access the wounded child. For example, in a session, a man says that even though he is an accomplished professional, he still feels anxiety making presentations. As he talks about this, the therapist asks what he is feeling in his body, and he says he has butterflies in his stomach. The therapist asks him to pay attention to the sensation in his stomach and just follow it. The client slows down, focuses on his bodily felt sense, and connects it to his experience of his father giving him tasks as a child but with an attitude of "I know you will mess this up," and how this left him with this great performance anxiety to not screw it up. The aim, of course, is not insight but to go back into the experience, access the unmet need, validate the deservingness of the need, and transform it with new experience.

In general, it is helpful to ask clients when they felt certain sensations before and to then guide them to go back to the earlier experiences and the memories associated with the sensations. This going back should be done by traveling on the wave of the feeling, not by logical deduction. The therapist does not ask, "When have you felt this before?" which is a request for information and more likely to get a cognitive response, but, rather, "Follow that feeling back to when you have had it before. What was it like?"

Clinical Example: "Like the Walking Dead"

The following example involves another client from mainland China. She is a single 27-year-old suffering from childhood trauma and social anxiety.

I mention the client's nationality as in the previous example as a way of demonstrating the cross-cultural application of emotion-focused work. In my experience in Asian cultures, metaphors are often used to express emotions. Moreover, descriptions of body sensations are more common because word labels for emotion are not as familiar or common, but emotions are definitely available and can be worked with. The discussion following illustrates how important emotion work is.

The client in this session talks about when her girlfriend ignores her and how that evokes the feeling of being ignored by her mother. The session moves to wounded child work. Note the client's reference early on to body sensations and the use of the metaphor "like the walking dead" in response to an exploratory question from the therapist about what she felt. Also note how following her sensations acts as a bridge to past memories:

THERAPIST: Wow, yeah, that sounds really sad, really feels like . . . Does it feel like that feeling is being triggered again? "When I was little, with my mother . . ."

CLIENT: I guess what I was feeling was that I hadn't been connected to my girlfriend lately, a feeling I'm having right now.

THERAPIST: It's like feeling . . . ?

CLIENT: Right. I just feel like if she doesn't talk to me (*Therapist: Yes.*), my hands and feet are gonna be cold and I'm gonna panic. It's like this walking dead feeling I have. [body sensation]

THERAPIST: Wah, cold hands and feet, and panicking inside your heart. That feeling is so deep in memory, and also terrible, because I am not like a normal person, almost like a walking dead. Mm-hmm. Do you feel it that way now? Does it remind you of how Mom made you feel when you were a kid? [bridging to past]

CLIENT: Yes. I feel it now like I used to feel.

THERAPIST: Can you remember how old were you the first time you felt this way?

CLIENT: (*Furrows eyebrows*) I can't remember, but, in my memory, when I was a baby, I wasn't connected to my mother. I felt like I was there alone. It was hard. I felt like I was the only one in the world. (*Therapist: Yes.*) I couldn't do anything, and I felt like if Mom didn't show up, I would be screwed.

THERAPIST: "Yes, I was so young, I needed someone to take care of me, but if my mother didn't come, my hands and feet would be cold, and I would be disconnected with the world."

CLIENT: Also, once I was in the factory with my mom, and she went to the bathroom and left me outside, and then an uncle told me, "Your mom doesn't want you anymore."

THERAPIST: Wow. Oh, my God. What would you like to tell Mom? Be the child: "What I felt is . . ." [childhood regression]

CLIENT: Because Mom likes boys more than girls, I'm afraid of being abandoned because I'm a girl.

THERAPIST: Uh-huh. "Mom doesn't want me, she doesn't want me, and then she can give birth to another boy."

CLIENT: Actually, those feelings resemble my feelings now.

THERAPIST: Yeah, so it's rooted in Mom.

CLIENT: I mean, it's like Mom doesn't want me anymore. It's over. (*Therapist: Hmm.*) And then I . . . I couldn't live alone.

THERAPIST: Yeah, helpless. Yeah.

CLIENT: I'm an orphan. (*Therapist: Well, yes, yes.*) I can't live any longer.

THERAPIST: "Yes, I'm going to die."

CLIENT: And then, trapped in a terrible panic.

THERAPIST: Yes, let's slow down now. Can you stay in the feeling of panic? If you can, look at the panic, put the panic in here, as if it were between me and Mother, with me by your side. Look at the panic, now . . . feel it here. You're afraid, but I'm here with you now. Can you be that frightened child, maybe 5 or 6 years old, and talk from that fear? "I'm afraid I'll be alone." [age regression]

CLIENT: Yes, I'm afraid I'll be abandoned alone and how will I survive. I'm really afraid who will look after me. It's like, please don't get rid of me. [core emotions scheme of fear of abandonment]

Having entered the child state, they then work on the client's fear of abandonment as a child and on providing a feeling of safety to help transform the fear. She ends up both asserting her right to have a parent who loved her or at least took care of her, and validating her worth as a girl and a daughter who did not deserve to be so neglected because she was a girl.

Clinical Example: "I Am So Scared"

In this example, the therapist guides a 32-year-old, single, male client suffering from depression and interpersonal difficulties back in an age regression to be his 5- or 6-year-old. The client did not feel safe in his relationship with his parents that included a mother who was very harsh and a father who could not protect him. When he was young, his mother always scolded him, which made him feel that his mother did not love him:

CLIENT: When I was a child, I was so eager for a good mother. When she showed in front of me that she was burdened, I was willing to take care of her and tried to understand her feelings . . . because I believed that she loved me or liked me (*eyes tear*). (*Therapist: Hmm. Hmm.*) . . . And I also loved you, liked you (*moves into direct contact with the mother, imaging her in front of him*). But when I gradually feel maybe you cheated me, you used me, I am very angry, very sad (*cries*).

THERAPIST: Hmm. Really heartbroken.

CLIENT: Right (*wipes tears with a tissue*).

THERAPIST: Yeah, so what are your tears saying?

CLIENT: Tears say, "I have endured so much pain to take care of your feelings, but this is meaningless. It was all being used by you."

THERAPIST: Thinking of that, you must feel such heartache.

CLIENT: Right. I feel heartache for myself.

THERAPIST: Are you thinking of yourself when you were a child?

CLIENT: Right.

THERAPIST: How little?

CLIENT: Heartache for my whole childhood. Heartache because I was a good child when I was little and took too much care of your [mother's] feelings.

THERAPIST: When did this feeling begin? How old were you? When you started to feel this heartache.

CLIENT: How old? Five to 6, or 6 to 7. At that time, I thought my mother was very fierce and not tender.

THERAPIST: Hmm. When you think of your time in 5 or 6 just now? Do you have any picture coming up in your mind? [evoking image of child self]

CLIENT: It's just like that I did something wrong. I recall when I was young, one day at home, I played with the meat that my mother bought and made it bad. Then when she came back, she became furious and punished me fiercely.

THERAPIST: You are the 5- or 6-year-old you. You hear your mother say that she is so furious, scolding and humiliating you, and then beat you. What do you feel? [age regression]

CLIENT: I am so scared.

THERAPIST: Hmm. Very scared.

CLIENT: I am scared, I am scared, I am stunned. I look at her and listen to her. All I have in my heart is scared feeling. [core fear]

THERAPIST: As you sit there and now you talk about this fear, do you get the sense of that scared feeling? Right now in your body?

CLIENT: Yes.

THERAPIST: What is your scared feeling like?

CLIENT: Scared that she will hurt me. I just feel she will really hurt me.

THERAPIST: Feels like you'll be hurt. So scared, so afraid and unprotected, just wanting to run away or be protected.

CLIENT: Right, right. Feels like she is going to do something to me at any time. [fear of danger]

THERAPIST: Hmm. So scared. When you come here, you are like this (*portrays the client's gesture of curling up*).

CLIENT: Right.

THERAPIST: It looks like you want to shrink. Disappear. Yes, good.

CLIENT: The whole me wants to shrink, very scared.

THERAPIST: Just hold this position. Feel the scared feeling. [action tendency]

CLIENT: Hmm (*continues to do the action of curling up*).

THERAPIST: You can say more about that scared feeling.

CLIENT: Tell her?

THERAPIST: Yes, tell her.

CLIENT: "I feel that I don't know what happened . . . just all of a sudden . . . why all of a sudden . . . suddenly so furious and suddenly feels like you want to beat me. Right. What happened? This meat . . . this meat . . . is this meat so important? To knock over the meat . . . to make it bad . . . is it such a serious thing? . . ."

THERAPIST: Feel what you feel there (*points to the part of body curling up*).

CLIENT: Feel it's horrible. Really want to hide myself.

THERAPIST: Hmm. Really want to hide. So scared.

CLIENT: Hmm. Very scared. . . . Feel like I will be hurt by her at any time.

THERAPIST: Very unsafe. What do you need?

CLIENT: I need to feel safe. I need some protection, someone—something to hide behind.

In this excerpt, the client arrives at his core fear of danger, and this makes it accessible to new input by accessing new feeling. He takes the first step of leaving the painful maladaptive state by accessing his need, which, with his therapist's help, validates that he will begin to feel deserving of having a mother who did not terrify him or having protection against her rage. Once his brain appraises that his need for safety was not met, it will automatically feel both angry at having been robbed of and sad at having missed a safe childhood.

CONCLUSION

A central part of an emotion-oriented therapy involves processing unresolved painful emotional experiences from the past, predominantly from child-hood. In this chapter, I discussed different methods of reexperiencing past emotional events in the present and highlighted the importance of episodic and autobiographical memories. Memory reconsolidation was offered as a key change process. In addition, the chapter presented guidelines for age regression work and demonstrated wounded child work and bridging to the past through body sensations.

For some clients, a potential difficulty on this path is when intensely painful emotions become too overwhelming. Therefore, Chapter 11 looks at emotion dysregulation and methods to enhance regulation. In that chapter, I also examine ways of soothing core anguish to transform it through self-compassion.

11 EMOTION REGULATION

The inability to regulate emotion is rapidly being seen as a core form of psychological dysfunction (Barnow, 2012; Bradley et al., 2011). That inability can result in being overwhelmed by strong, painful emotions (increased sympathetic nervous system arousal) or, alternatively, becoming numb and distant from emotions (increased parasympathetic arousal). Good emotion regulation, on the other hand, is having the desired emotions at adaptive levels, at the right time, and in the right way. Clients who come to therapy frequently are experiencing conditions related to underregulation of emotion, such as depression, anxiety, substance abuse, and eating disorders. In addition, emotional dysregulation is the problem that leads to dysfunctional behaviors in disorders involving self-harm, trauma, and borderline functioning (Warwar et al., 2008). These are often dysfunctional attempts by clients to regulate underlying painful emotions (Linehan, 1993). Emotion regulation, therefore, is a topic of central interest in psychotherapy and is becoming a transtheoretical factor in understanding a variety of symptoms and maladaptive behaviors. It is being proposed as a possible unifying transdiagnostic emotional change process.

https://doi.org/10.1037/0000248-012
Changing Emotion With Emotion: A Practitioner's Guide, by L. S. Greenberg
Copyright © 2021 by the American Psychological Association. All rights reserved.

Whether in everyday life or in a therapy session, when emotions are over-activated, can no longer be connected to cognition, and are outside the client's zone of tolerance, some form of regulation of emotion is helpful. However, there is some ambiguity about what process is being referred to talking about "emotion regulation." The term *emotion regulation* has predominantly come to be used to mean a second-level, deliberate management or control of emotion (Gross, 1999). This type of regulation occurs after the emotion has been activated or to prevent its activation, and it involves reducing and reining in emotion. It is used in this way chiefly in cognitive behavior, modification-oriented therapies and involves the teaching of skills, such as a change in the situation, distraction, cognitive reappraisal, or calming.

On the other hand, another term, *affect regulation*, is used mainly by more affect-focused, intrapsychically oriented therapies to mean the implicit modulation of emotion or the relational coregulation of affect. This clinically and neuroscientifically based view focuses on automatic processes involved in the generation of emotion as an aspect of regulation. In addition to deliberate emotion regulation skills, automatic regulation processes are involved in managing negative affect. An affective neuroscience perspective supports a one-factor view of emotion regulation in which regulation is seen as being automatically integrated with emotion generation (Campos et al., 2004; Cozolino, 2002). This view differs from a two-factor, conscious control view of deliberate emotion regulation in which emotion is first generated and then managed. Emotion regulation in which the client can deliberately regulate emotion is necessary, but a second-level, deliberate process acts after the emotion is generated and needs to be combined with the development of automatic affect generation capacities.

Automatic regulation of emotion is achieved implicitly at the point of generation. This automatic regulation is developed by internalizing the empathic soothing of the other so that the self feels more secure and is less intensely activated, or by transforming emotion at its point of generation so that when it arises, it is already regulated. Therefore, affect regulation occurs much more implicitly by coregulating affect or by changing emotion with emotion such that the emotion that needed regulation is no longer being activated. With affect regulation comes an automatic soothing or transforming of emotion so that the experienced emotion is already regulated or is modulated (Jurist, 2019).

Deliberate emotion regulation involves some form of conscious strategy that helps reduce arousal (e.g., breathing and soothing techniques) to enable calm and meaning-creation in sessions, and skills to be used outside the session to help people cope. In general, the dysregulated emotion is either a secondary, symptomatic emotion, such as anxiety, anger, helplessness, or hopelessness, or a maladaptive primary emotion, such as traumatic fear of danger, overwhelming sadness of lonely abandonment, or the debilitating shame of self-loathing. Clients enter therapy to rid themselves of these painful emotions so they can cope better in their lives.

BUILDING CAPACITY FOR SELF-SOOTHING

Automatic affect regulation occurs more implicitly by coregulating affect via internalization of safety and the therapist's empathic soothing. Experiencing an aroused emotion being soothed by the therapist, often nonverbally, is a right hemispheric process and is one of the best ways to build the implicit capacity for self-soothing. Being able to self-soothe develops initially by internalizing the soothing functions of the protective other (Stern, 1985). For example, I have had clients who say they hear my voice in their head during the week. Having a constant reminder of empathy from someone else is helpful; empathy from the other is internalized as empathy for the self (Bohart & Greenberg, 1997).

Other affect regulation processes involve the transformation of emotion intrapersonally at the level of generation. For example, transformational soothing is focused on internally bringing soothing and compassion to painful emotions from the past by the adult self or by evoking a soothing figure from the past to help resolve the past threat, as demonstrated in Chapter 10. This strengthens the self by changing emotion with emotion and developing automatic soothing so that the emotion that is experienced is already regulated when it emerges.

Deliberate Coping Regulation

Deliberate emotion regulation skills have been studied as a general factor in coping. A large body of research has implicated difficulties in emotion regulation as central to the development and maintenance of psychopathology. Recently, a systematic review identified 67 studies that measured changes in both emotion regulation and symptoms of psychopathology following a treatment for anxiety, depression, substance use, eating pathology, or borderline personality disorder (BPD; Sloan et al., 2017). Results showed that regardless of the intervention or disorder, use of both a maladaptive emotion regulation strategy and overall emotional dysregulation was found to significantly decrease following treatment. Symptoms of anxiety, depression, substance use, eating pathology, and BPD were also reduced. The findings of this review provide evidence supporting the notion that emotion regulation is a transdiagnostic construct and is for treatments that target emotion regulation for individuals presenting with multiple disorders.

A number of meta-analyses have shown mixed results about which deliberate strategies appear to be the most effective. Aldao et al. (2010) examined the relationships between four symptoms—anxiety, depression, eating, and substance-related disorders—and the following six emotion regulation strategies:

- reappraisal—reinterpreting the meaning of an event to change its emotional impact
- acceptance—remaining in contact with feelings, thoughts, and sensations
- problem solving—making a conscious attempt to change a situation or its consequences
- avoidance—behaviorally avoiding situations to have an emotional impact as well as experientially avoiding internal experiences
- rumination—focusing passively and repetitively on distress or negative mood
- suppression—pushing away thoughts, emotional expression, or both

They found a large effect size for the maladaptive effects of rumination, medium-to-large maladaptive effects for avoidance as well as medium-to-large adaptive effects for problem-solving and suppression, and small-to-medium adaptive effects for reappraisal and acceptance. These results are surprising given the prominence of reappraisal and acceptance in cognitive behavior and acceptance-based treatment models. The authors also found that internalizing disorders were more consistently associated with regulatory strategies than externalizing disorders.

Another meta-analysis by Webb et al. (2012) revealed that attentional deployment had no effect on emotional outcomes, whereas response modulation had a small effect, and cognitive change had a small-to-medium effect. Although attentional deployment and concentration were not effective, distraction was found to be an effective way to regulate emotions. Suppressing the expression of emotion also proved effective, but suppressing the experience of emotion or suppressing thoughts of the emotion-eliciting event did not. Reappraising the emotional response proved less effective than reappraising the emotional stimulus or using perspective taking.

Daros and Williams (2019), in another meta-analysis and review, ascertained the relative endorsement of six of the most commonly studied emotion regulation strategies. They compared strategies in individuals with elevated symptoms of BPD to strategies used by individuals with low symptoms of

BPD and healthy controls as well as to individuals with other mental disorders. Results indicated that symptoms of BPD were associated with less frequent use of cognitive reappraisal, problem-solving, and acceptance, and more frequent use of maladaptive strategies of suppression, rumination, and avoidance. When compared with individuals with other mental disorders, people with BPD endorsed higher rates of rumination and avoidance and lower rates of problem solving and acceptance.

These aforementioned studies show that deliberate regulation skills help with symptom alleviation; however, which skills to use when and by whom remains to be understood. The studies produced mixed results of what was most effective, but of interest is that cognitive reappraisal and acceptance— the most strongly advocated cognitive behavior therapy strategies—may not be as effective as either distraction or suppression of expression in helping people regulate. It was found, though, that BPD clients used less cognitive reappraisal, problem-solving, and acceptance than non-BPD clients, thus lending some support to these strategies as correlates of healthier functioning.

Self-Soothing: Learned Through Direct Instruction

In the emotion-focused approach I present here, I recommend that explicit regulation strategies be taught as a first step—as coping strategies to deal with down-regulating emotion in people whose emotions are so dysregulated as to impair their coping. This work, in general, needs to precede working on processing of underlying emotions, but it may, at times, be done in conjunction with it. However, when there is sufficient capacity to regulate emotion, I recommend focusing on accessing and transforming the emotion schematic processes that underlie the presenting dysregulation.

A two-stage treatment framework, thus, is potentially useful for highly dysregulated clients. It begins with the teaching of deliberate down-regulation skills followed by work on automatic regulation by targeting underlying primary emotion generation processes. The notion of stages here, though, is not meant to suggest a hard-and-fast sequence rule. Rather, it is applied in a marker-guided fashion to fit the current state of the client in the session and in how they are coping with life outside the session. If a client at a particular juncture is so overwhelmed by emotion in the session or in life, then down-regulation and use of skills are needed to help cope. When the emotion is sufficiently regulated and the client can bring cognition to bear on emotion to make sense of it, the therapeutic process can profitably shift to access the underlying generating processes that, in the first place, led to the emotion that needs to be down-regulated.

Thus, if a client is panicking in an out-of-control fashion or is so filled with despair to want to harm self or others, then skills of distraction, calming, and distancing from emotion are needed. If, however, they are able to talk about these emotions and their triggers in a more modulated fashion—and not be swamped by them—then it is time to explore the underlying emotions to which these dysregulated emotions are a reaction: for example, the underlying attachment insecurity, shame, or sadness that leads to the panic or self-hatred. In these situations, down-regulation is a second-level process in which emotions that have been generated are acted on to control and manage them to help people cope. Thus, when a person gets to unmanageable levels of anxiety, coping self soothing is helpful to manage the intensity of the feelings.

Transformational Self-Soothing: Learned Through Experience and Internalization

A different type of self-soothing is more transformational in nature. As discussed in Chapter 10, it involves ways of being with the self to moderate and transform core pain. It is rooted in a client's ability—based on inner resources, probably derived from the internalization of compassion received from others—to soothe their own core painful, primary maladaptive emotions. This enables them to achieve lasting change by transforming their pain. The brain functioning involved in affect is inherently complex; the primary level of emotion regulation is best understood as involving a rapid cascade of effects moving up and down different subcortical and cortical areas. People do not have deliberate cognitive control of this type of primary regulation of affect. Rather, lots of implicit processes involve massive feedback loops and syntheses of different levels of processing in which different parts of the brain interact with each other, leading to synchronization, which results in the self-organization of the entire brain.

The development of automatic transformational self-soothing, then, is different from the development of deliberate coping self-soothing. Transformational self-soothing involves the activation of unresolved emotional suffering to enhance its regulation at its point of generation rather than to control it once it has been generated. Thus, it is the painful emotions that never received the needed soothing in the past or the present experienced threat of abandonment or disintegration that can be changed by feeling compassion toward the self, grieving the loss, and soothing the anguish of the self. Once a painful emotion schematic memory has been evoked, soothing can be provided both by the individual themselves or by the therapist. Coping self-soothing is a deliberate skill used to address symptomatic dysregulation that one needs to overcome, whereas transformational self-soothing focuses on bringing soothing to unresolved painful emotions from the past. This helps transform past threat and strengthen the self by the development of automatic soothing so that emotion now is experienced in a regulated way.

Deliberate forms of regulation by cognitive and behavioral means are more of a left hemispheric process and are useful for people as coping skills when they feel out of control. However, emotional dysregulation problems that occur in more fragile personalities and arise more from deficits in the more implicit forms of regulation possibly are more right hemispheric and, therefore, cannot be modified by direct procedures. It is the building of implicit or automatic emotion regulation capacities over time that is important for these highly fragile personality disordered clients. Implicit forms of regulation often cannot be trained or learned as a volitional skill.

ADDRESSING EMOTIONAL DYSREGULATION

The term *emotional dysregulation* refers to the inability to regulate unwanted emotional states. As mentioned earlier, emotional dysregulation is an aspect and possible cause of many psychological disorders, such as personality disorders, bipolar disorders, anxiety disorders, depression, addictions, and posttraumatic stress disorder. Emotional dysregulation is the person's inability to control or regulate their emotional responses to evocative situations. It can also be thought of as having high emotional reactivity: The person often reacts in an emotionally exaggerated manner to such things as criticism, perceived abandonment, or relational conflict. Environmental and interpersonal challenges such as these lead to overreacting, crying, blaming, having angry outbursts, engaging in passive–aggressive behaviors, or causing conflict. Emotional dysregulation often involves avoiding abandonment and rejection or having difficulty maintaining stable relationships. Emotional dysregulation is frequently relational and is triggered in intimate relationships or in relationships with people who have power or control over one.

Dysregulation can be arranged on a continuum ranging from an overregulated style to an underregulated, overactivated, hyperaroused regulatory style. An important characteristic of dysregulation and disorganized affective responses is unpredictability involving oscillating between excessive or diminished affective responsiveness A central characteristic is difficulty with both soothing oneself and returning to a baseline of emotional experience. There may also be difficulties being stimulated and feeling a sense of liveliness. Either style, under- or overregulation, can lead individuals to engage in external regulation in the form of self-harm, eating disorders, substance abuse, sex addiction, or some form of excessive risk-taking. These behaviors often are central in personality disorders and posttraumatic stress disorder.

Emotional dysregulation probably develops from an interaction between the temperament of the child and the early experiences of abandonment, deprivation, or frustration of the child's attachment and identity needs. Emotional dysregulation may derive from early interpersonal traumas in childhood or latter traumas in life. Early traumatic events create a hyperactive central nervous system that is sensitized to cues related to early stressful events. Traumatic events and emotional neglect lead to the development of maladaptive emotion schemes.

When to Regulate and When to Activate

An important issue in any treatment is to consider when emotions should be regulated and when they should be activated. In addition, one needs to consider what types of emotion are to be regulated and how this is to be done. Emotions that require down-regulation generally are either secondary emotions, such as anxiety, anger, despair, and hopelessness, or primary maladaptive emotions, such as the anxiety of basic insecurity, fear of danger, and the shame of being worthless as well as any emotions that currently are not able to be connected to adaptive cognition because they are so overwhelming. Maladaptive emotions of shaky vulnerability, overwhelming sadness, or feelings of core shame all benefit from down-regulation to create a working distance from these feelings rather than become overwhelmed by them. Suppressing feelings, however, can lead to a rebound effect, also known as a bottle-up, blow-up effect. Total distancing from emotion in many situations, then, is not helpful. In some cases, however, people can effectively distance themselves from their emotions, and this disengagement can facilitate learning and memory. Likewise, too much emotion at too high an intensity can, at times, be countertherapeutic. A crucial clinical judgment is when to down-regulate, distract, and modulate and when to facilitate approach and intensification.

There are a variety of indications for when to down-regulate emotions. First, it is important to promote regulation when the therapeutic relationship cannot yet provide the safety needed for emotion activation or deeper work. A clear indicator for emotion regulation is when a client feels overwhelmed by emotion or when emotion does not inform or promote adaptive action. When a person is in a crisis, then down-regulation and crisis management are needed. A previous history of violence or uncontrolled anger, or, alternately, prior experiences of disintegrating and being unable to cope are strong indicators for promoting either anger regulation or anxiety management. If clients engage in destructive coping, using substances to self-medicate, if they binge eat, or if they engage in self-harm to deal with distress, then coping skills are needed (Linehan, 1993). If the problem is a skills deficit, then training in the development of emotion regulation or problem-solving skills is called for.

Which Emotions to Target and How

The therapist needs to make a judgment about which emotions need regulation and which type of regulation is necessary. They need to distinguish among primary, secondary, and instrumental emotions, and between adaptive and maladaptive primary emotions—and help clients to do the same. It is generally secondary emotions of global distress that need down-regulation, except for trauma related experiences for which it is primary maladaptive emotions that need down-regulation. Let's look at anger regulation as a case example.

Therapists should distinguish among primary adaptive anger, which needs to be supported; secondary anger, which masks hurt; or primary maladaptive anger, which is an immediate and overly general response to perceived threat, and frequently is associated with posttraumatic stress reactions. For instance, a rape survivor might, for years after the assault, react consistently with rage at being touched by a person of the same gender as their rapist. This anger probably needs both deliberate skills to initially help cope but also, in the long run, deeper work to transform the underlying fear memories. Secondary reactive anger, however, is often defensive anger that masks more vulnerable core emotion, such as sadness, fear, or shame. Here, it is better to work on the underlying vulnerable feelings than on skills to regulate the anger. Instrumental anger is anger one uses consciously or unconsciously to manipulate or control others; one's use of it is not a candidate for regulation, but the person needs work on personality problems and to learn to express that anger in more direct ways. Each of these distinct anger problems requires different intervention strategies. Skills are then needed for improved coping related to maladaptive and secondary anger, but adaptive anger at unfairness needs facilitation rather than regulation.

Also, the same individual can experience and express a variety of types of anger, so each situation needs to be treated differently. For example, therapy for a client who was abused by his father and sexually molested by a male relative involved several ways of addressing his anger:

- His secondary defensive anger covering shame when he felt slighted by his wife needed to be bypassed rather than regulated to get to his underlying shame.

- Blowing up at perceived signs of disrespect from his children, however, needed deliberate regulation skills. His use of instrumental anger and aggression to control others needed learning of new, more direct ways of expressing himself.

- The difficulty he had acknowledging feelings of healthy anger about his father's abuse because he feared doing so would jeopardize the current relationship he had with him needed discussion and problem-solving. Resolution of the past trauma needed acknowledgment of his appropriate anger at the abuse but for him to let go of it and not react to things with his father in the present in terms of the past.

Therapists themselves, thus, need to distinguish and help clients distinguish among different types of emotions so they know when to regulate and when to express, when to modulate, or when to bypass their anger and attend to a more core vulnerable experience.

There are a variety of forms of treatment for emotional dysregulation. Medication, when appropriate, combined with effective psychotherapy can improve sleep and stress management. Plus, psychoeducation sometimes can significantly improve the quality of life of people with emotional dysregulation. Teaching clients skills to regulate has been proved useful as have relational processes of validation; development of a secure attachment relationship with the therapist; and development of *mentalization*, the ability to reflect on the contents of one's own and others' mental processes. What is clear is that emotion needs to be the target of treatment, so methods of working on changing how emotions are both generated and managed once generated are central. Next, I discuss deliberate skills, which are useful coping skills for people who are highly dysregulated—but are not a full treatment. Then, I discuss an emotion-focused approach to changing the emotions underlying dysregulation.

DEVELOPING EMOTION REGULATION SKILLS

Distraction and distress tolerance skills are useful for regulating emotions (Linehan, 1993). They involve identifying triggers, learning to avoid triggers, establishing a working distance from emotion, allowing and tolerating emotions, increasing positive emotions, engaging in self-soothing, doing diaphragmatic breathing, and relaxing. Tolerating distress includes mindful breathing and awareness of emotion. Regulating breathing and observing one's own emotions—letting them come and go—are crucial processes that help regulate emotional distress. It is the development of these skills that is the focus of this section.

At first glance, many activities may seem like they help people keep their emotional balance, but on further consideration, they reveal themselves to be unhealthy: They help in the moment, but, in the long run, they actually hurt. These include such things as abusing alcohol or other substances, engaging in compulsive sex, inflicting self-injury, avoiding or withdrawing from difficult situations, engaging in physical or verbal aggression, or excessively using social media. These activities tend to help people feel good in the moment, but they usually function to delay the inevitable: that people have to face the emotion.

Overt dysregulation of emotion like yelling or overwhelming weeping plus acting out behaviors can benefit from learning skills to manage emotions more effectively. The first step in the practice of self-regulation skills is for people to recognize that they have the choice in how to react to situations and to deliberately choose to use the skill. Using the power of choice is a primary self-regulation skill that empowers people to work with the disruptions and challenges that they face. People also have to accept that they never have complete control over how they feel.

Choice, but Not Control

Developing the motivation to choose is an important aspect of therapy. A quote attributed to Viktor Frankl (1959) states that "between stimulus and response there is a space. In that space lies our freedom to choose our response." The ability to stop and take a breath is a crucial skill because it allows one to take an observer's perspective in relation to internal experience to observe one's sensations, feelings, and thoughts; where one's focus of attention is; and to what one is reacting. This skill helps develop a working distance from emotions rather than being overwhelmed by them. Learning how to pause in between an intense emotional reaction and ensuing actions is one of the most valuable skills a person can have.

Having chosen to regulate and having managed to take an observer's perspective, one of the most powerful tools in emotion regulation is simply to identify and name the emotion one is feeling. Here, it is good to know about the difference between primary and secondary emotions, and how to address each in the most helpful way. Therapists can provide this information as part of their psychoeducation for clients and their orientation to what therapy will be like or in an ongoing fashion as part of the process. In addition, receiving support and understanding is helpful in regulating emotions, and therapists should certainly discuss with clients how they will provide support and understanding during sessions. If appropriate, they can also discuss available family and community supports.

Caring for body, mind, and spirit aids being emotionally regulated and is an important responsibility. Engaging in physical activity, eating well, and getting lots of sleep are critical to having resilience and balanced emotion regulation. A healthy body is also an important step on a path to a healthy mind. Eliminating physical issues, such as feeling, tired, hungry, or sick, will make it easier to maintain emotional balance. Negative emotions should not be ignored, but leaving room for the positive as well and increasing positive emotions is almost always good. Focusing on the positive helps put worries and insecurities aside.

A mind-set of living life in the present instead of being stuck in the past or the future, first advocated in Western psychotherapy by Gestalt therapy, has now been adopted by a variety of approaches, as have specific mindfulness practices. Facilitating a present-living mindset often means helping people become more aware of emotions, thoughts, and body sensations. Mindfulness practices can help increase the ability to regulate emotions and decrease stress, anxiety, and depression. It also can help to focus attention as well as to observe thoughts and feelings without judgment. The more integrated the practice of mindful awareness becomes in life, the more emotions become regulated.

Acceptance

Allowing oneself to be vulnerable takes strength and courage. Acceptance of suffering—no longer running away from difficult emotions but facing them instead—is an attitude more than a skill but is of great help in regulating emotions. Accepting vulnerability is crucial to explore emotions and ask questions to get in touch with how one is feeling in a given moment. Learning to let go of emotion and move on can be difficult but is perhaps one of the most important emotion regulation skills. People often become stuck when attempting to process negative emotions. Negative emotions seem to stick in the brain. Instead of simply letting them go and moving forward, people often hold on, obsessing over every little bit of emotional experience and bemoaning, "Why did this happen to me?" It seems paradoxical, but accepting that one is feeling emotions that one would rather not feel can be the key to letting go of those emotions. When people accept that they are suffering, they stop running from the difficult emotions and turn to face them, and when they find they do survive feeling them, they experience that it was more manageable than the beast they had imagined.

Allowing and accepting an emotion involves observing it, welcoming it, acknowledging that it exists, and accepting it. Then, one needs to stand back from it and experience it as a wave—let it wash over them and then move past and away. It is helpful to concentrate on some part of the emotion, like how one's body is feeling or some image about it. The person needs to observe the emotion coursing through their body to symbolize the experience of it in words (Lieberman et al., 2007). For example, they can create a safe distance from an overwhelming emotion by adopting an observer's stance so they then are able to describe the fear as, say, a black ball located in one's stomach.

It is helpful to recognize that a person is not their emotion and that emotion is a part, but not all, of the person. People are more than what they feel; they do not necessarily have to act on the emotion, but they may just need to sit with the emotion. Often, acting can intensify and prolong the emotion. Paradoxically, becoming aware of an emotion is one of the most effective ways of helping to contain an emotion. Accepting an emotion helps clients become aware of it, express it, and decide what to do about it as soon as it arises. Suppressing emotions and not doing anything tend to generate more unwanted emotions and thoughts, making them more unmanageable and more distressing. When people become aware of what they feel, they are able to reconnect to their needs and are motivated to meet them.

People need to practice welcoming, accepting, and validating emotions. This can be a difficult concept. They need to learn to accept their emotions just the way they can learn to accept things about themselves or their experience that they cannot change: their age, height, allergies, and so on. Accepting what one cannot change and approving or liking it are two different things. One does not have to like their allergies or acne, but those things are there and can be managed. They are not easy to change; however, if a person just accepts or, in some instances, comes to appreciate them, they feel a lot better than if they keep fighting the idea that those things are there.

A Safe Place

Therapists also can help by explicitly guiding their clients to self-soothe in the moment. Promoting clients' abilities to regulate and achieve a working distance from their emerging painful emotional experience is an important skill that helps them tolerate their emotions and self-soothe. A central strategy to promote self-soothing is to suggest to clients when they are in high distress and before they become overwhelmed that they imagine a place where they feel safe and to access that place in their imagination. Once they have an image of that safe place, they are asked to feel what they experience there (Elliott et al., 2004; Watson, 2002). Therapists can say, for example, "Imagine taking yourself somewhere safe, where you feel secure and comforted. Where do you take yourself? Can you describe what it's like? What do you feel there?" In this exercise, clients go to a safe place in their imagination where they can list their concerns and set them out in front of them or imagine placing each concern in a separate container. In this way, clients are encouraged to relieve the tension of their concerns and anxiety in the moment. It gives them a sense that they can create some distance from their anxiety to feel more relaxed and calmer. Alternatively, therapists can encourage their clients to "clear a space" (Elliott et al., 2004), that is, ask clients to create a space in their mind by acknowledging their troubling concerns one at a time but then push them to the side of their mind to create an internal space of calm emptiness.

These imagery exercises help clients soothe high secondary distress in the session and are also given as homework to cope with high distress experiences outside the sessions. Therapists use these exercises to teach clients that they are capable of imagining and providing a safe place for themselves. Having the ability to access a safe place when they are in a distressed state helps clients to shift into a more soothing stance and achieve a calm state—a deliberate skill that helps clients handle immediate feelings of anxiety in specific situations and cope better by building the capacity to calm and reassure themselves.

Other ways of teaching clients self-soothing to down-regulate intense feelings is to direct their attention to experiences that feel comforting. When clients do not find it easy to call up a safe place, therapists need to provide compassion and help clients identify their need for safety or comfort. Once that has been done, therapists can then ask clients to identify experiences they do find comforting—perhaps having a cup of tea or coffee, taking a warm bath, curling up with a good book, listening to certain pieces of music, or watching TV. When clients feel overwhelmed or emotionally flooded in the session, therapists guide them to engage in self-soothing strategies to regulate their emotions. Attending to their breathing is central. Therapists need to guide clients to breathe more regularly, put their feet on the ground and become aware of what is happening around them, name what they see around them, feel themselves sitting in their chair, or look at their therapist and describe what they see. Relaxation exercises and relaxation audio recordings can be useful to teach clients relaxation skills. It also is important to explore with clients ways that they personally find comforting and soothing. Some clients have difficulty knowing what is comforting because they have never been able to comfort themselves. It is important to encourage these clients to pay attention to times in their day-to-day lives that provide them comfort. Doing so helps them to begin to build up strategies and ways of caring for themselves when feeling distressed and alone.

Emotion Awareness Exercises

Two emotion awareness exercises can be used to help people identify their emotions as the first step in emotion labeling. The first is a training sheet (see Exhibit 11.1), which therapists can provide to clients as a handout for them to fill in either during therapy or in between sessions. It is helpful to go through each step during therapy first, possibly over multiple sessions, to allow time for defining key terms (e.g., "action tendency") and to do the deeper work, such as matching needs to emotions. The second exercise is a therapist-guided imagery sequence to help clients identify how they respond to their own emotions (see Exhibit 11.2).

REGULATING EMOTION AT THE LEVEL OF AUTOMATIC GENERATION

The ability to regulate emotions comes, in part, from early attachment experiences with parents and caregivers (Schore, 1994; Sroufe, 1996). If our parents were good "emotion coaches," they would recognize our emotions as opportunities for intimacy, validate and empathize with our emotions, and help guide us toward socially appropriate expression and action. The optimal method of emotion work to help clients become emotionally regulated is approaching and accessing previously avoided emotions and being able to tolerate, accept, validate, and understand them.

Providing a Corrective Relationship and Environment

Emotional dysregulation has been attributed to failures in dyadic regulation of affect early in the life cycle (Schore, 2003; Stern, 1985). Early attachment trauma and affect dysregulation result from early misattunements between mother and infant (Schore, 2003; Sroufe, 1996; Stern, 1985), and any approach to therapeutic treatment of these clients must involve repair of these early and implicit relational experiences. Repeated experience of emotional stress reduction through affective soothing in therapy is vital for developing regulation. The relationship with the therapist can provide a powerful buffer or psychobiological coregulation for a client.

EXHIBIT 11.1. Emotion Episodes Awareness Training Sheet

Step 1:	Step 2:	Step 3:	Step 4:	Step 5:
What is your emotion or action tendency? Is it best described by an emotion or feeling word, or by an action tendency?	What is the situation to which you are reacting? • An event? • An internal experience? • Another person?	What are the thoughts accompanying the emotion?	What is the need/goal/concern being met/not being met: • In the emotion? • In the situation?	Establish your primary emotion. Is your emotion in Step 1 primary? If not, is it secondary or instrumental? Your primary emotion is the one that fits with your unmet need. For example, if your need is to be close, then sad would be primary, not angry. If your need is for nonviolation, then anger would be primary, not sad. If your need is for security, then fear is your primary emotion, not anger.

Adapted from *Emotion-Focused Therapy: Coaching Clients to Work Through Their Feelings, Second Edition* (p. 363), by L. S. Greenberg, 2015, American Psychological Association (https://doi.org/10.1037/14692-000). Copyright 2015 by the American Psychological Association.

EXHIBIT 11.2. Guided Imagery Sequence

1. Invite the client to close their eyes and remember a time when they struggled with a difficult emotion, a feeling of being criticized, or an argument with a partner. Ask them to picture the situation and enter into it to relive it now. Ask: "Where are you? Who is there with you?"

2. Encourage the client to identify the strongest emotion they feel in this situation, feel what it's like in their body, and label it (e.g., legs shaking, heart speeding up, a huge foam ball in the throat).

3. Help the client identify how they responded to their emotion. Ask: "What do you feel like doing now?" It is important to make clear that it's how they react now—not how they reacted at the time.

The first step in helping clients develop automatic emotion regulation is the provision of a safe, validating, empathic environment. How the therapist joins with clients and connects emotionally with them is the first experience in therapy that influences emotion regulation. Therapists' empathic attunement to affect, acceptance, and validation is, as discussed in Chapter 5, emotionally soothing. Being able to soothe the self develops initially by internalization of the soothing of the protective other (Sroufe, 1996; Stern, 1985). This internalization helps clients develop implicit self-soothing and the ability to regulate their own feelings automatically.

Internal security and comfort develop by having the feeling that one exists in the mind and heart of the other. Most clients feel safe when their therapist offers a soothing, affect-attuned bond and an accepting emotional climate. The climate has to do with the total attitude of the therapist communicated by means of verbal expressions as well as body posture and facial expression. Facial expression is an important part of relational attunement. People read facial affect automatically at very high speed, especially those affects that are crucial to survival, such as fear and anger. Vocal tone is also important; rhythm, cadence, and energy need to be appropriate to the emotion being worked with. A soothing, slower tone and manner are crucial in accessing core vulnerable emotions. A more energetic, enthusiastic tone may be helpful in supporting the more boundary-setting emotions of anger and disgust.

Treatment of emotional dysregulation needs to recognize the importance of the therapeutic relationship in providing a corrective emotional experience. The good therapeutic relationship provides a corrective emotional experience by being responsive to the client's feeling and validation of their needs in contrast to the abusive or punitive relationship that the client experienced during their childhood. The therapy situation becomes a safe place in which the client can affirm and express their feelings and needs and desires. This corrective relationship is experienced in most sessions as the therapist explores and empathizes with the client's present difficulties. After exploring present life difficulties, the discussion often goes back to childhood and adolescence. During these explorations, the goal is to help the client access their core painful emotions of the past and to experience empathic soothing of the therapist, who helps the client reown disowned needs from their childhood so that they can recognize and satisfy their current needs. This is an experiential, not a conceptual, process that helps access emotion schemes and activate emotional structures of the brain, such as the amygdala, as well as parts where emotional memories are stored. The therapist helps the client activate painful memories to access the painful emotions and helps them transform by revitalizing the previous unacknowledged needs. Emotional memories are then rewritten and changed by the memory reconsolidation process (Nader, 2003). This is all based on developing a secure attachment between therapist and client.

Using Empathic Clarification

A particular form of empathic responding is helpful in dealing with the emotional dysregulation that often occurs with clients with complex personality problems. One of the difficult processes with these fragile clients is when there appear to be discrepancies between what clients say and what they do or feel. For example, they may deny any responsibility for their actions and attribute blame to others in situations in which they were blatantly at fault. Many therapists often deal with this aspect of dysfunctional coping by using a form of confrontation. However, given that the internalization of the therapist's soothing presence is an important aspect of developing affect regulation, confrontation is contraindicated.

As an alternative way of responding to situations of dysregulation in client interpersonal patterns, I recommend balancing emotional validation of dysfunctional coping modes with a push for change. When a client adopts dysfunctional patterns of coping based on their maladaptive emotion schemes and self-organizations during a session, their therapist needs to show empathic understanding that validates the coping effort but highlights how the dysfunctional pattern fails to get the client's needs met.

Therapists do not focus on skill training or point out clients' contributions to problematic interpersonal patterns, denial of underlying motivations, or avoidance behaviors, as might occur in confrontations. Confrontations of this sort usually raise clients' anxiety and defensiveness, which is contrary to forming a safe, secure relationship. However, something more than the safety of the relationship is needed for dealing with these difficult patterns— something that is an alternative to confronting discrepancy or skill training. What is needed is for the therapist to convey understanding of the client's behaviors in terms of the client's protective coping efforts, underlying emotions, and unmet needs. Therapist responses that I have found work best when their components occur in a particular sequence.

An emotion-focused response for clients who are depressed or anxious but not emotionally dysregulated is sequenced more or less like this:

1. Begin with an empathic reflection of the client's secondary emotion.
2. Focus empathically on the client's primary painful maladaptive emotion.
3. Identify the unmet need in the primary emotion.

As an example of the preceding sequence, the therapist would say, "Yeah, you are feeling so angry at the way you were treated. It left you feeling so unimportant, and you really need to feel seen and respected." The first step is to *reflect* a secondary feeling that the client has explicitly expressed, and the next steps are to *conjecture* about the primary underlying vulnerable and painful emotion, and the need.

But, in situations in which the client's reactions are highly dysfunctional and their emotions are dysregulated, it is better to change the sequencing in the response. The therapist needs to:

1. Reframe, through reflection or conjecture, the client's difficulty in terms of underlying needs.
2. State an understanding of the client's core painful disowned emotion that is under the more surface secondary/instrumental emotion or behavior.
3. Restate that the secondary reaction makes sense as an attempt to satisfy the unmet need.
4. Refocus on core pain and unmet need at the end.

This sequence is shown in the following response to a client's statements about his present girlfriend and past ones, who he says left him "because he loves them too much." The present girlfriend's view was that she left him because he was too needy. He broke her finger in an altercation. He says this is not true and that the girlfriend is being unfairly influenced by couple therapists the pair had seen. The emotion-focused therapist, rather than saying something like, "Could it be that the girlfriends left you because of your anger?" responds by saying,

> So, as I understand it, you so need and want closeness. All your life, you have yearned for closeness. When you didn't get it with your girlfriend, it left you feeling so painfully lonely and abandoned. So then you got to feeling hopeless and angry, and began to fight for what you are missing. But what you really need is closeness, and it's so painful when you don't get it.

The client's attention is guided by this response to the need and pain underlying the dysfunctional behavior. The therapist does not have to contradict or invalidate the client's experience.

It is helpful to think of three Rs to guide this intervention: reframe, restate, refocus. As shown in the preceding example, the secondary reaction is *reframed* as a reaction to a primary underlying vulnerable and painful feeling and need. The understanding is validating and conveys "it makes sense" that you react this way when you have this painful feeling and unmet need, and the client feels understood and accepted. Then the focus is shifted to the exploration of the painful feeling without any confrontation or raising of the client's protective defenses. The therapist then repeatedly *restates* the understanding in terms of the painful unmet need and feeling that, at a deeper level, drive the problematic behavior. It's important to *refocus repeatedly* on the painful feelings that need to be processed, as in: "But what we really have to focus on is to help you deal with this feeling of loneliness and inadequacy because this is what drives the anger."

Do not focus on insight into unconscious motivation or modifying behavior, or on problem solving and skill training. Rather, follow the sequence:

$$\text{Need} \rightarrow \text{Core pain} \rightarrow \text{Secondary emotion or behavior}$$
$$\text{that fails to get the need met}$$

Throughout the process, the therapist maintains therapeutic presence, empathic attunement to affect, acceptance, respect, and genuineness.

In another example, a client says,

> There is no way for me to find a girlfriend, and I'm really desperate. It's a social problem. It is much easier for women to find a partner. That is so unfair! I tried everything, but it didn't help. I was on Tinder for 1 year, and I only got one match from somebody I know. Laura is my only chance. She has to come together with me. She really owes this to me, and she needs to understand this. If it doesn't work with her, I'll kill myself, and she'll know that she was the reason.

The therapist responds,

> Yeah, all of this is very painful. You want desperately to be together, and when she is hesitant, this leaves you feeling so afraid of losing her and so powerless, and this understandably makes you angry. But, somehow, this anger doesn't really help you to get what you want, and what seems most painful is this feeling—sort of a fear, a fear of being rejected, abandoned, and being all alone without her. Can we talk a bit about what that's like?

This form of responding ties the client's dysregulated emotions and actions to core needs and emotional pain (and to historical origins, if possible), and takes a subjective view, not an objective view. Rather than blaming clients, which is essentially what confrontation implies, therapists are empathic, have positive regard (the client tried the best possible solution at this moment), view blocks as self-protection, and are compassionate to clients' suffering. Rather than making explicit a client's dysfunctional pattern, the underlying motivation driving the pattern, and the cost, therapists focus on understanding the painful emotion and validating the need.

Empathic clarification as discussed here involves a repeated switching among emotions, behaviors, and needs: The therapist validates the client's means of coping as an understandable outcome of the situation and the client's life history, and as driven by the unmet need. At the same time, the client's attention is brought, without blame, to the negative consequences of the behaviors.

Developing a Case Formulation

The first strategy in using experiential methods for treating the deeper layers of emotional dysregulation is to develop a case formulation that helps guide intervention toward the core painful emotion. The therapist's initial step is to collaboratively identify and come to agreement with the client on what the client's core painful emotion and self-organization are that govern their way of functioning. Case formulation provides both participants with an understanding of what the client's core painful emotion schemes are as well as the client's associated needs. From this understanding, the therapy develops a focus on the client's core concerns and operating self-organizations, such as, being sensitive to abandonment, feeling deprived, feeling unworthy, and feeling wronged. It is these self-organizations that generate the dysregulated emotions and that are worked with at an experiential level with the aim of their transformation, not their regulation. Their transformation leads to the client's no longer being emotionally dysregulated. What often is in need of regulation is the dysregulated secondary emotions that are reactions to the more primary, painful emotions in these organizations. Thus, the dreaded fear of abandonment leads to dysregulated rage or panic and the shame of feeling unworthy leads to overwhelming self-loathing and to self-harm, whereas suppression of underlying anger or shame leads to substance abuse.

Case formulation helps clarify what to focus on in treatment and to move beyond the many secondary reactive states characterized by exaggerated emotions of sadness, anguish, anger, and shame. In addition to dysregulated secondary emotions, core maladaptive states from childhood maltreatment can leave people dysregulated and experiencing overwhelming feelings of sadness, feeling emotionally empty, feeling lonely and socially unacceptable, and feeling not worthy of being loved. Clients suffer from feeling sad, scared, alone, unworthy, and unlovable, and feel the enormous pain and fear of abandonment caused by their abusive histories. These histories, however, express themselves through secondary depressive, fearful, and desperate feelings as well as feelings of inferiority.

Other forms of dysregulation involve excessive anger, frustration, and impatience because needs have never been considered or satisfied. Some clients react with uncontrolled aggression and can hurt people or damage objects. Others use a "wall of anger" to protect themselves from others whom they perceive as threatening. Other clients manage emotions with impulsive discharge, reacting immediately in an attempt to meet their needs or desires. They are unable to postpone their gratification or to predict the consequences of their actions. Some attempt to regulate by eating, watching TV, abusing drugs, or having promiscuous sex. Others are organized to withdraw or suppress their feelings and depersonalize. All these different types of dysregulation emanate from underlying core painful emotions and the client's patterned self-organizations, and it is the underlying schemes and self-organizations that need to be the target of treatment. If change takes place at this deeper level, dysregulated emotions will disappear. If people feel worthy, grieve their losses, let go of or forgive past hurts, let go of anger and resentment, and feel better, they no longer have a need for the secondary emotions.

Building New Meanings and Behaviors to Get Needs Met

Most of the methods covered in this book, such as focusing, attuning, reexperiencing the past in the present, overcoming blocks, and changing emotion with emotion, can be applied to the activation of the specific emotion schemes and self-organizations involved in emotional dysregulation. These methods give the client the possibility to experience adaptive anger and sadness and compassion, to build new narrative meanings and behaviors related to getting needs met, or both. Imagery work and chair dialogues (Greenberg, 2017), which are helpful in treating and transforming emotion schemes and self-organizations, are the two main methods for treating dysregulation. These methods, described in previous chapters, are briefly discussed next in terms of their use for emotional dysregulation.

Imaginal Transformation

Imagery can be used in a number of different ways to evoke clients' core painful emotions and to transform their anguish by accessing the transformative emotion of compassion. The visual system and emotion are highly related, so imagination is a good way to evoke unresolved painful emotions. Imagination can be used to enact dialogues between self and other or even between parts of self, or to experience new emotions. It can be helpful for clients to evoke compassion toward the self or imagine adding comforting people or resources to situations or scenes so they can experience different scenes in new ways. In imaginal transformation, schemes and self-organizations related to traumatic memories are activated with their associated painful emotions. In working with a client's present distress of, say, feeling rejected or ashamed, the therapist can ask the client to find, in their imagination, a situation in which they experienced an emotion similar to the present negative emotion. Here, an emotional bridge is being formed between present and past. In this way, traumatic experiences, often from childhood, can be changed and can acquire new meaning through support experienced in the imagery of reliving the past with new outcomes. The therapist or another adult protective person chosen by the client is asked to enter the old scene to help the client meet the child's needs. Alternately, the client's soothing capacity can be activated by imagining the self as one's current adult reentering the evoked scene and providing a reparative response.

Thus, the therapist can ask the client to reenter, in their imagination, a scene in which they were being bullied or neglected and to access their core emotions. These painful feelings can be transformed by the client's expressing what was needed or by imagining having a safety-providing protector who helps them get what they needed. Clients can imagine a police officer, or even the therapist, who offers the protection that was missing. Alternatively, other aids to empower or protect the client can be imagined; for example, having clients being able to hide from the perpetrator, handcuffing them, or locking them outside the room. Imaginary experiences like these can help generate new emotions of assertive anger and compassion toward the self that help change the old maladaptive emotions of fear, shame, and sadness.

In this type of imaginary transformation, the therapist might say,

> Try closing your eyes and remember your experience in this situation. Get a concrete image if you can. Go into it. Be your child in this scene. Please tell me what is happening. What do you see, smell, hear in the situation? What do you feel in your body, and what is going through your mind?

After a while, the therapist can ask the client to shift perspective. The therapists says,

> Now, I would like you to view the scene as an adult. What do you see, feel, and think? Do you see the look on the child's face? What do you want to do? Can you do it? How can you intervene? Can you try it now in your imagination?

Changing perspectives again, the therapist asks the client to become the child and also asks,

> What do you as the child feel and think? What do you need from the adult? Can you ask for what you need or wish? What does the adult do? What else do you need? Ask for it. Is there someone else you would like to come in to help? Can you receive the care and protection offered?

This intervention concludes with the therapist asking,

> Check how you feel inside right now. What does all this mean to you, about you, and about what you needed? Can you come back to the present—to yourself as an adult now here with me? How do you feel? Can you say goodbye to the child for now?

During imaginal transformation, emotions of fear, shame, and sadness are changed both by the therapist's presence in the room or by another's entering the scene in imagination and meeting the child's need. This process helps clients realize that they deserve to be recognized and protected. In addition, the client has a different experience of the traumatic situation: a possibility to experience similar situations in the future in a safe way. With the continuation of treatment, the relationship with the therapist and the schematic transformation that is created during the imagery create a healthy organization in the client, who is now able to get needs met in a constructive fashion.

Chair Dialogues

When clients experience dysregulated emotional states, chair work can help to fight the critic or develop a sense of deserving to have unmet needs met by others. The effect of the use of chair dialogues is a transformation of the painful emotions; the ensuing down-regulation of the symptomatic dysregulated emotion; and the experiencing of an up-regulation of positive, self-soothing emotions.

A primary source of emotional dysregulation often is self-attacking and self-blaming, which create an unbearable negative affect. Frequently, this dysregulation originates from the internalized voice of critical, demanding, and punitive attachment figures. This internalization of negative voices makes clients afraid that they did something wrong, see themselves as bad and worthless, and believe that their feelings and desires are unacceptable. They feel under tremendous pressure and set excessively high standards and goals. Then, they become angry at themselves, hate themselves, and punish themselves in some way.

Different types of chair work involve dialogues between different parts. For example, in self-critical splits, one aspect of the self is critical or coercive. In this work, the punitive voice attacks the self, which reacts. Thoughts, feelings, and needs within each part of the self are explored and communicated in a dialogue to achieve working through the painful feelings—often of shame—and accessing a sense of deserving to have had needs met until there is a softening of the critical voice. Resolution involves integration between sides. Two-chair enactment at self-interruptive splits, as discussed in Chapter 8, are worked with by making the interrupting part of the self explicit. Clients become aware of how they interrupt their emotions and are guided to enact the ways they do it, and then to react to and challenge the interruptive part of the self. Resolution involves expression of the previously blocked experience. Empty-chair dialogue is used to work on unfinished business with a significant other. Here, the client's internal view of a significant other is activated, and the client experiences and expresses their emotional reactions to the other to access the unmet needs. Resolution involves shifts in views of both the other and self and either holding the other accountable or understanding or forgiving the other.

Self-soothing dialogues, as discussed in Chapter 10, are helpful when clients experience anguish about past trauma, neglect, abandonment, or humiliation. Self-soothing is facilitated in a chair dialogue in which clients are asked if they, as adults or some other compassionate figure, could soothe their vulnerable or wounded self. The goal is to evoke compassion for the self (see, e.g., Gilbert, 2010). This intervention is a more active way, over and above the relationship with the therapist, to directly facilitate self-soothing by assisting the client to offer compassion to the suffering self, which can be done by activating compassion and comforting self-talk in chair dialogues.

Therapists introduce this task when clients are in anguish and have difficulty being self-compassionate and accepting of themselves. To facilitate the evocation of self-compassion and caring for the self, therapists, as in age regression work, can suggest to their clients that they engage in a dialogue with an imagined vulnerable self or themselves as a wounded child and soothe and care for that self. Clients are encouraged to be responsive, caring, and comforting to themselves. Compassion toward the self transforms negative emotion with the more positive emotion of compassion, which undoes the negative feelings (Greenberg, 2011; Tugade & Fredrickson, 2004).

When clients become dysregulated, there is a possibility that they may enter dissociated states. Modified chair work can enhance the client's metacognitive ability and prevent dissociation. Rather than activating the painful emotions, the chairs are used to recognize different parts of the self and understand how they affect each other (Pos & Greenberg, 2012; Pos & Paolone, 2019). Chair work interventions normally are used to intensify experience to activate adaptive alternate emotional resources and self-organizations. For the client with problems of dysregulation, though, these interventions may be too emotionally dysregulating and disorganizing. They may be unwise because, instead of contact between the parts and ultimate integration, these clients can experience increased emotional disorganization. Chair work has the potential for intensively activating clients' object relations (Kernberg, 1967), including the self's primitive defenses (McWilliams, 1994), such as black-and-white thinking, polarization, or primitive freezing in response to the overwhelming activated affect (Pine, 1986; Porges, 2004). Getting a working distance and externalizing the emotion, then, are more helpful than increasing arousal. Maintaining contact in the relationship is important because chair work can leave clients feeling somewhat "abandoned." Dysregulated clients often display limited reflective functioning or mentalization capacity. Emotional activation could lock clients more deeply into whatever self-organizations were online and lead to behavior coming fully from the presently active state with little capacity to meta-observe it from a reflective position or experientially remember a previously more organized state.

Chair work, however, can provide structure to the dysregulated client's experience of self, stimulate metacognitive awareness, attenuate emotional activation, and increase the experience of self-coherence. Chair dialogues that are conducted in this more reflective, cognitive manner to create awareness of how different aspects of self function can help regulate emotion. Strategies can be used to work with the maladaptive relationships between self states in conflict and can help the client take a more reflective and metacognitive stance toward their warring parts and what binds them in conflict. Once adjusted, chair dialogues, rather than disorganize and dysregulate clients, can provide a particular kind of "scaffolding" for these clients' self-reflective processes or mentalization (Fonagy et al., 2002), and this scaffolding has the potential to contribute to their sense of integration. An example of therapy with a more fragile client follows.

ENTERING THE REGULATION PHASE OF TREATMENT: A CASE DESCRIPTION

The client, Lily, a 27-year-old Caucasian of Russian descent, entered therapy with problems of self-harm and emotional outbursts. The initial phase of treatment emphasized identifying emotions and needs and developing an understanding of how emotions were a result of Lily's childhood unmet needs that had, at the time, been an adaptive response to attachment needs that had not been satisfied in childhood, adolescence, and at present. To facilitate this process, the therapist asked open-ended questions of what it was like for Lily growing up in her family and questions about her childhood and adolescence. The therapist maintained as much eye contact as possible to show sincere interest in Lily's life story and to validate her emotional experiences, except when she was self-punitive. Self punitive self-blaming states were dealt with according to the sequence laid out earlier in this chapter of seeing the anger at self as secondary and going underneath to the unmet need and core pain.

The second phase in therapy involved developing automatic regulation. This had been occurring all along by internalization of the safe, soothing, and empathically attuned relationship with the therapist. For example, when Lily began therapy, she was detached. The therapist empathized with and validated her feelings of detachment, and then bypassed them and went to the underlying feelings of lonely abandonment, neglect, or abuse. The therapist used imaginal transformation and chair work to access the core painful maladaptive emotions. Once contact with underlying emotion had been made, new, healthy, adaptive emotions were accessed to change the old emotions. In preparation for going in to Lily's most painful feelings and to enhance her tolerance to her dreaded emotions, a safe place was installed. The therapist did this by having Lily close her eyes and visualize her safe space, going into it, and experiencing the emotions of comfort and the feelings of safety. Then, at times when Lily was in a more calm and relaxed mood, the therapist invited her to visualize the past situation that had led to those strong emotions. Once visualized by Lily, the therapist focused on what Lily was feeling, allowing her to feel both what she needed and her related emotions. Present emotions are used to bridge to childhood situations in which Lily had felt a similar emotion.

The therapist then asks Lily questions. Ideally, this questioning is done using the present tense as though it is happening now—maintaining the "as if" condition. So, the therapist asks Lily, "Where are you? How old are you? What is happening?" The therapist asks if Lily can see the child, what she looks like as the child, and how the child feels. The client now begins to slowly take on the facial expression of a scared child. Her voice changes to a more childlike voice—softer—and she whispers what she sees and the vulnerable feelings have been reached. The therapist empathizes with and validates the emotions, and invites in a knight in shining armor to stop any aggression so that Lily can know what being protected feels like. If anywhere in this process Lily becomes, or approaches, feeling overwhelmed and unable to tolerate the pain, the therapist asks her to go to her safe place. By doing this, the activation of dissociative processes is staved off.

Once Lily's need for a sense of safety, genuine interest, and value is met, the therapist takes her back to the current scene. Now that she has felt protection and care for her vulnerable self, Lily does not feel as frightened or invalid any longer; instead, she feels deserving of needs and acts to satisfy them in a functional way. In this way, the client interiorizes a new, healthy model of self in relationship.

Lily is now able to recognize her emotions. She connects them to her childhood experiences, expresses and satisfies her needs in the present, and automatically feels emotionally regulated. During therapy, she sometimes would rapidly shift states, which were triggered when a critical or hostile voice emerged that made her feel she was bad or unlovable. In those situations, the therapist used chair work to help Lily notice how the self-critic was activated and triggered her painful feelings. Such work enhances a client's awareness of different parts of themselves and their interactions, and by enacting what they do to themselves, they enhance their metacognitive abilities.

Another central part of therapy was dealing with Lily's punitive self-critical voice of always putting herself down and blaming herself, saying, "You are stupid, wrong, will never be normal or liked." The process of resolution involves going through the collapsing into hopelessness and getting to the underlying shame and fear until the client accesses their needs for comfort and safety, and they begin to assert themselves against the critical voice. This process was modeled and validated in two chair dialogues many years ago (Greenberg, 1984), and it has been developed and tested in a variety of studies (Greenberg, 2017). By asserting the self and a softening or the weakening of the punishing part, an integration occurs between the punitive critic and the vulnerable experiencing self. The client is able to recognize and diminish the punishing part when it arises, letting the healthy part that recognizes their emotions and needs have a voice. This constant coactivation of Lily's vulnerable part and her healthy part enhanced her emotion regulation capability.

By the end of therapy, Lily stated that she felt much more connected to her vulnerable feelings and needs, and that she listens to them and no longer feels overwhelmed by emotions, nor is she a victim to them. The therapy allowed Lily to experience possibly her first responsive and caring relationship—and the first time she trusted anyone and showed her vulnerable side—and to share her vulnerability and work with it using the imaginary chair work. Sessions lasted for a little over a year: biweekly for the first 5 months and once a week thereafter.

CONCLUSION

Emotion regulation can be deliberate, as in coping self-soothing, or automatic, as in transformational self-soothing. Each has its place and needs to be applied at the right time. When people are so highly dysregulated that they are acting destructively and are unable to cope with daily living and maintaining relationships, they need direct instruction in coping skills. When this is not the case, deeper work is needed to access underlying painful emotions to work on and to transform the processes of emotion generation. This perspective also suggests thinking of a two-stage process in which the first stage for highly dysregulated people is skill-based treatment to be followed by a transformation of underlying self-organizations and emotion schemes. Ultimately, the goal is to eventually access new, adaptive feelings. Once this happens, therapists can focus on helping their clients construct new narratives. In Chapter 12, I discuss the construction of new narratives to consolidate change.

12 NARRATIVE AND EMOTION

Being human involves creating meaning and using language to shape personal experiences into narratives. We are born to create meaning and we are born into meaning systems (Frankl, 1959). We cannot, not create meaning. As we have seen, people have both an emotion system and a meaning-creating system, and although emotional experience provides information and action tendency, it does not carry fully formed meaning within it. Emotions give people direct feedback on a moment-to-moment basis about what is important and meaningful for them in a specific situational context, and that information organizes them for adaptive action in the world. Emotion has an aim and moves us in a direction, but we need to guide the tendency by making sense of what it is telling us, and we need to decide how to achieve its aim. We need to bring cognition to emotion to make sense of it, create meaning, and decide on actions. Human beings' primary way of making meaning is through the stories we construct (Angus & Greenberg, 2011; Bruner, 1986, 1990). Accordingly, in this chapter, I discuss the role of narrative in working with emotion (Angus & Greenberg, 2011; Greenberg & Angus, 2004).

https://doi.org/10.1037/0000248-013

In making sense of what people feel, we not only label what we feel by symbolizing bodily felt emotion in words, but, most importantly, we organize our emotional experience into narratives. We organize our experience into stories, which allow us to reflect on what has happened to us and to create new meaning. Clients externalize emotionally meaningful experiences in stories such that their "lived stories" become "told stories" that they can then share with others and reflect on for further meaning-making. The narrative organization of emotional experiences supplies a sequential time frame so that experience is organized in stories with beginnings, middles, and ends. Causal connections can then be made between actions and emotions and meanings, which helps to organize experience that may have been confusing or disorganized. In addition, meaning—and the language it is expressed in—is not simply the private property of any particular individual but, rather, belongs to the larger social context of shared forms of language-based understanding. People, thus, learn to make sense of life events in forms that fit their culture, and the meanings they make are sustained in their most important interpersonal relationships (Angus & Greenberg, 2011; Bruner, 1986, 1990; Greenberg & Angus, 2004; Sarbin, 1986).

Therapy, then, is a process of clients' coming to consciously articulate and possibly change their stories. The act of storying experience in psychotherapy is an essential self-organizing process that provides a platform for subsequent reflection and further personal meaning-making (Angus & Greenberg, 2011). Therapists need to listen carefully to their clients' most important stories because the stories give them access to how people are attempting to make sense of their emotions, themselves, and their worlds. In psychotherapy, clients' narratives are the essential starting point for meaning-making (Angus & McLeod, 2004). In the process of articulating and reflecting on life experiences in psychotherapy, personal narratives become deeper—fused with emotional meaning and significance—taking more information into account and becoming more integrated. There is more than one way to tell a life story, so therapy helps people tell new stories (Angus & Greenberg, 2011).

Personally significant narratives are often indicated by the experience and expression of emotion; therefore, it is important for therapists to listen for stories that are emotionally charged and experientially alive. Narrative organizes and gives meaning to emotions by identifying what was felt, about whom, and in relation to what need or issue. Storying disconnected emotional experiences helps self-understanding and meaning-making. So, what powers the mechanism of story change in psychotherapy? Moving from primary maladaptive to adaptive emotion.

UNDERSTANDING THE NARRATIVE EMOTION RELATIONSHIP

From a neuroscience perspective, Damasio (1999) suggested that the first, essential impetus to story an experience is the awareness of an inner bodily felt feeling, thus indicating the intimate relationship between emotion and narrative. People's first narrative is a nonverbal imagistic narrative of our feeling of what happened. It is through the storying of affect that we come to know what has happened to our body. Knowing, which is the most fundamental level of consciousness, springs to life when changes in the status of the body-self—such as emotional responses—are connected to environmental impacts (Damasio, 1999). The first stories were constructed by prelinguistic primitive human beings who coded experience into something like, "You throw a stone at me, and when it hits my body, it hurts." Thus, meaning was created long before language. Prelinguistic narratives, such as the preceding one, organize the experience into ones that have beginnings, middles, and ends as well as agents, actions, and intentions.

Narrative meanings can be formed without words, and they are formed about people's most personal experience: what happened to their emotional bodies. In essence, knowing springs to life in the unfolding story of changes to the body's state. People, thus, live in a world that is experienced and organized as an unfolding story in time. Knowledge, from nonverbal imagining to verbal literacy, depends on the ability to map what happens over time, inside and around our organism, and to and with our organism. Both narrative and emotion processes also operate at tacit levels of consciousness, and both are fundamental in the generation of conscious meaning.

The self then emerges from the dialectical interaction between ongoing, moment-by-moment experience and higher level meaning-making processes that attempt to interpret, order, and explain elementary experiential processes (Greenberg, 2015; Greenberg & Pascual-Leone, 1995). Affectively toned, preverbal, preconscious processing is a major source of self-experience that is articulated, organized, and ordered into a coherent narrative (Greenberg, 2011; Greenberg & Angus, 2004; Greenberg & Pascual-Leone, 1995). Individuals constantly create the self they are about to become by synthesizing biologically based information and culturally acquired learning. And although biology and culture may sometimes conflict, they are not inherently in opposition to one another. Rather, they are both necessary and important streams of a dialectical synthesis that, together, form meaning. People live most viably by managing to integrate biological and social, emotion and reason, and head and heart.

To better understand themselves, people continually work at making sense of their experience, and they do so by symbolizing, storying, and explaining their lived experiences to themselves. They, thereby, construct an ongoing narrative that organizes their emotions into personal stories that enhance a sense of continuity over time. It is in this manner that a stable sense of personal identity emerges. Within this framework, it is the narrative framing of emotional processes, at both tacit and conscious levels, that leads to the development of new views of self, other, and world that are key to change experiences in psychotherapy.

MAKING SUBJECTIVE EXPERIENCE AVAILABLE FOR EXPLORATION AND CHANGE

Narrative framing of emotional processes is important in promoting personal change experiences in psychotherapy. Roger Schank (2000) went so far as to suggest that people need to tell someone else a story that describes our experiences because the process of creating the story creates the memory structure that contains the gist of the story. For Schank, telling a story is not a rehearsal; rather, it is an act of creation that, in turn, becomes a memory. Narrative and memory are intimately intertwined.

In my view, all significant stories are based on a core emotion, and all core emotions are embedded within a significant story (Greenberg & Angus, 2004). Narrative organization of emotional experience in which intentions, purposes, expectations, hopes, and desires are articulated allows us to understand what an experience means to us. The meaning of an emotion is only truly understood when its occurrence is organized into a coherent story within a sequential framework that identifies what is felt, about whom, and in relation to what need (Angus & Greenberg, 2011). There are stories of loss, of pride, of love, of ecstasy, of jealousy, of anger and of despair. Each story is characterized by an emotional theme, and emotional experience is a key indicator of the personal significance of the narrative.

Angus and colleagues (Angus et al., 1999, 2017) developed a measure, the Narrative-Emotion Process Coding System, that codes client process in session into three possible categories: (a) *external narrative mode*: talking about what happened; (b) *reflexive narrative mode*: talking about what it means; and (c) *internal narrative mode*: talking about what it feels like. Client narratives, therefore, can be coded as working within the landscape of action, meaning, or feeling. In working with emotion, the therapist needs to guide clients who generally present by talking about what happened to talk about what it meant and, ultimately, what it feels like.

One of the important insights generated by the narrative processes research program (Angus et al., 1999; Boritz et al., 2011, 2014, 2017; Lewin, 2001) at York University has been the discovery that good outcome cases can be distinguished from poor outcome cases by a particular pattern of narrative processing. In good outcome emotion-focused cases, therapists focused clients inward when the clients were themselves engaged in reflexive processing. The clients, once they focused internally and having been guided by their therapist's internally focused response then, of their own accord, reflected on their emotional experiences to create new meaning. Therapist shifted clients' focus from meaning to feeling, and then clients shifted from internal emotional differentiation back to meaning-making.

The program also found that therapist movement from external—what happened?—directly to internal—what it feels like—was not as effective. Thus, if a client says, "I saw my ex-boyfriend yesterday and immediately walked away," it is not good for the therapist to focus on what the client feels or to ask, "What did you feel?" Instead, it is better to first follow the client into what it means before going to what it feels like. If the client says something like, "This breakup was so sudden. He must have been planning it without telling me," it is now better to go to what it feels like. This finding should act as a reminder that this key focus on what it feels like and the attendant question "What do you feel?" that is frequently used in working with emotion can be highly overused—and asked at the wrong times. Therapists working with emotion should not automatically use this as a catchall phrase. Going into the landscape of feeling is best to deepen meaning or put words to feeling when clients are already implicitly aroused in the body and are trying to make sense of their experience, not when a person is in a nonaroused, external mode of processing and simply is describing what happened.

When introducing a topic, clients often start off by talking about what happened—what my colleague and I termed the "same old story" (Angus & Greenberg, 2011), which provides a generalized description of experiences and relationships. Therapists then help clients to access specific personal memories that make what is being talked about more concrete and specific. In doing so, the client's subjective emotional experience becomes more available and begins to be explored. A process of sense-making takes place, which helps to develop a perspective on the "problem," and what is felt is clarified. If, however, there is a lot of unstoried affect, the client will feel disorganized, which will lead to emotional dysregulation. Emotion regulation then is enhanced by organizing these experiences into a coherent narrative.

WORKING WITH NARRATIVE CONSTRUCTION

The construction of a narrative based on emotion can be thought of as involving four steps. The initial step is similar to that described in focusing and awareness in Chapters 3 and 6. This first step involves the rapid *synthesis* of tacit affective responses from sensations and emotion memories to generate an inner bodily felt sense. In the second step, the person *symbolizes what is felt* by attending to the bodily felt sense to differentiate and name the feeling to create meaning. Next comes *the conscious articulation of new meaning by means of narrative construction*. At this stage, a conscious narrative account is constructed that provides a causal explanation of emotional experience. The fourth step entails *the consolidation of an identity narrative* by integrating different aspects of experience into the narrative. This new narrative is an explicit indicator of significant client change events in psychotherapy (Angus & McLeod, 2004).

Attending

The first key processing strategy involves paying attention at a sensory motor level to the bodily felt sense like a sinking in the stomach and the action tendency of withdrawal associated with feeling humiliated by, for example, being unable to answer a question at a business meeting. This complex felt sense needs to be attended to before it can be symbolized. As Gendlin (1996) described, the felt sense incorporates the whole situation; it is not just the word for an emotion. A complex bodily felt sense of, for example, the aforementioned shame-based experience includes the emotion of shame about failure but also contains narrative elements, such as the sequence of events, the desire to appear knowledgeable to colleagues, the experience of feeling the judgment of others, and the tendency to "want to hide and disappear." This fundamental experience is coded first as a wordless narrative in imagistic sensory and kinesthetic form, and it is to this that clients must attend to turn their lived story into a told story.

The therapist works with clients to attend to and become aware of their emotionally salient lived experiences so they can tolerate, accept, and eventually explicate and story their vulnerable emotions. Consider how this process occurs when a client is telling the following story about a surprise encounter at a movie theater that happened the night before. He states that, while standing in line for a movie, he turned around to look at some movie posters and suddenly realized that standing behind him was someone whom he either wished desperately to avoid or whom he was amorously longing to meet. Depending on which set of emotions, desires, and feelings prevailed in the moment, he would be able to narrate two entirely different senses of internal complexity that were generated in the context of the unfolding story of the chance meeting at the theater. In relation to each story, he could talk about how he felt in and about the unfolding narrative scene, and explicate complex felt meanings, such as the intentions, beliefs, purposes, and goals of self and other.

Many of these tacit meanings—and the "story" of the event—were not processed consciously in the moment before opening his mouth to greet the other person at the movie theater. What was actually said would either be coolly dismissing or charmingly disarming, depending on, in part, the past history of the relationship of the client and the other person as well as current goals, intentions, expectations, and appraisals. If no clear experience had emerged at the moment of the surprise encounter at the theater, this person's performance might have appeared to be awkward in response to feeling overwhelmed by a complex tangle of mixed emotions and feelings. Thus, beyond the specific performance generated—what is actually said or done—there lies at the periphery of awareness a host of tacitly synthesized, bodily felt meanings that, with attentional allocation, can be brought to focal awareness, symbolized, and their meaning articulated (James, 1890; Perls et al., 1951).

It is from this experiential ground that personal meanings are differentiated and symbolized, articulated in the context of an unfolding narrative scene, and meaningfully understood. It is the quest for knowing and naming what is felt, and for knowing what it means or says about me in the context of a specific situation or relationship, that heralds the shift to the next level of experiential processing: symbolizing.

Symbolizing

Symbolizing and differentiating embodied feeling states, now in awareness, compose the first step to new meaning-making (Angus & Greenberg, 2011). Clients need to symbolize their emotion, such as feeling sad, usually in words, and embed the words within a broader narrative context, such as: "I feel sad that my mother never asks me about myself, not even about my children." Undifferentiated states of high emotional arousal, or what we (Angus & Greenberg, 2011) have called *unstoried emotions*, are almost always experienced as painfully disorganizing and are very distressing for clients. Therapists, then, need to help clients symbolize—in words—what they experienced in a particular situation. This type of differentiation of emotional experience leads to the creation of new meaning.

A crucial part of the making-meaning process is the making of linguistic distinctions that help capture an implicit bodily felt sense of meaning. For instance, one might symbolize a given internal sense as feeling sad or disappointed or rejected in the context of when a partner forgets one's birthday. All of these synthesized meanings of internal felt senses—sad, disappointed, rejected—convey different aspects of the same experienced situation in a way that, for example, "dismayed" or "afraid" would not. The words "sad," "disappointed," and "rejected" are all adequate but capture different aspects of the whole experience.

Conscious experience does not sit fully formed "in" us. Rather, it emerges from a dialectical synthesis that involves the integration of (a) attention to an internal bodily felt sense (a tension in the chest) and (b) a naming of that felt sense ("I feel disappointed") in the context of having my birthday forgotten ("I was looking forward to being recognized"). Engaging in this dialectical synthesis helps clients to find words to capture and express the inner felt sense of a lived story, which now, as a told story, provides a launching pad for the further differentiation of new personal meanings. How people articulate their feelings—in language embedded within a narrative—is crucial for the creation of new conscious experientially based understanding.

In experiential processing, the bodily felt sense acts as a constraint on the possible conscious conceptual constructions that can satisfy it, eliminating many other possible meanings (Greenberg & Pascual-Leone, 1995, 2001). As such, preconceptual, tacitly felt meanings carry implications that act to constrain, but not fully determine, the construction of personal meanings. Rather, felt meanings are synthesized with conceptual, explicit meanings to form narrative descriptions of personal events. It is the reflexive ability to decenter from the direct experience of the emotional responses that facilitates the articulation of what was felt in relation to whom and about what issue.

It is not only the activation of bodily felt experiences and emotional responses that is crucial for therapeutic change in therapy. Emotional responses also need to be accompanied by client *reflexivity*, an elaboration and transformation of the personal meaning surrounding an emotionally charged event. It is difficult for a therapist to shift a client toward emotional differentiation and meaning-making when the client is not actively engaged in a self-reflexive processing stance. In poor outcome cases, the client plays a more passive role when exploring feelings, often providing more of a description of discrete bodily sensations rather than experienced and symbolized feelings or emotions.

Articulating Narratives

Following the description of what happened and the symbolization of what was felt in context comes the conscious articulation of narratives. Organizing symbolized feelings, needs, thoughts, and aims into a coherent story enables experience to be understood and accepted as part of a life story. Now, complex experiences of conflict, of puzzling reactions of painful memories, are organized into understandable, new stories. For instance, understanding how a condemning internal voice leads to feelings of worthlessness helps clients to recognize that they are the agents of their experience of depression. Situations that activated painful emotions now are understood in a less negative light, and new narratives, such as, "It was not me who was unlovable; it was that you were incapable of love" are formed.

The reflexive system, a conscious, more controlled level of emotional processing, generates "cooler" emotional representations (i.e., emotional representations with lower arousal levels) and provides higher level conceptualizations of who did what to whom. It creates storied understanding of what happened, what was felt, and what it means. Promoting reflection on emotional experience as well as helping people make sense of their experience encourages its assimilation into their ongoing self-narratives.

Facilitating Identity

Now, it is possible for clients to change their most important personal stories. This final step results in the emergence of new self/other identity narratives (Whelton & Greenberg, 2000). A narrative identity involves the integration of accumulated experience over time and of various self-representations across situations into some sort of coherent narrative of who one is. At core, the self is embodied, but a body needs a story to act meaningfully; to relate past and future; to situate dreams, goals, regrets, plans, lost opportunities, hopes, and all the stuff of a truly human life (Angus & Greenberg, 2011; Whelton & Greenberg, 2000). All this contributes to achieving a sense of self-understanding and identity formation in which the questions "Who am I?" and "What do I stand for?" are addressed.

Facilitating the Unfolding of Narratives

The strategic use of open-ended questions can be an invaluable tool when engaging clients in productive storytelling and meaning-making. For instance, the question "Could you provide me a specific example of that happening in your life?" helps clients shift to the disclosure and narration of specific, image-based personal memories that are more likely to activate experienced emotions and entry into the client's landscape of consciousness. Alternatively, a question like, "So, when he slammed the door and walked out on you, what was happening inside you? It felt as if . . . ?" promotes symbolizing internal experience. Questions to promote meaning-making help clients reflect on the personal significance of new emotional understandings. A question like "What does that story say about you?" helps clients to reflect on, symbolize, and acknowledge important values and aims that define who they are.

Although it is important to focus on client stories of emotional pain for narrative change, it is equally important to help clients identify and story personal experiences of positive stories of hope, resilience, and positive outcomes when they arise. Positive outcome stories challenge negative views of self and enhance a sense of client agency and desire for personal change. Focusing on painful or so-called negative emotion facilitates deepening and disclosing of implicit feelings and meaning, whereas positive emotions broaden and build (Fredrickson, 1998).

Clinical Example of an Emotion-Based Narrative Change

When a client shifts from maladaptive emotions, such as fear and shame or sadness, to adaptive emotions, such as healthy anger and sadness, meaningful story change happens, and new stories emerge (Greenberg, 2002; Paivio & Pascual-Leone, 2010). A shift to a new emotional response activates new action tendencies, and this plus the new feelings result in stories with new outcomes. Emotional change, by definition, results in narrative change. In addition, as clients shift from expressing secondary feelings, such as reactive anger and blaming, to experiencing primary adaptive emotions, such as sadness and loneliness, new and more adaptive action tendencies are evoked, and, again, this leads to narrative change.

For example, in an emotion-focused therapy session, a middle-aged man disclosed how he felt incredibly angry at his wife for choosing to go away without him for a weekend with her friends. However, with further empathic exploration of key stories of loss and fears of abandonment in his childhood, he was able to acknowledge some of his previously unacknowledged primary adaptive emotions of sadness that accompanied his early experiences of loss. The shift from secondary maladaptive anger to access to primary adaptive sadness provided the client with a new experiential awareness of how a long-held, maladaptive fear of abandonment, and the deep sadness that it evoked, was triggering feelings of anger and abandonment in his marriage. Importantly, this new emotional awareness also equipped him with a new understanding of the source of his painful feelings of abandonment. He was now able to express his sadness at loss and his need for deeper connections with his wife without blame or resentment. His wife's understanding and concern enhanced his feelings of safety and security in the marriage. Significantly, he also reported feeling less vulnerable when spending time on his own and, as a result, feeling far less resentful of his wife when she chose to be with her friends.

IDENTIFYING EMOTION NARRATIVE MARKERS

Early on, a trauma narrative marker was identified as an opportunity for trauma narrative retelling (Elliott et al., 2004). When a client first reveals a trauma, it is best to have them unfold the story in whatever way they can, retelling the incident and possibly engaging in the recounting of an episodic memory. The therapist's role is to listen empathically and provide empathic understanding responses rather than more exploratory or conjectural responses. The therapeutic goal is to provide understanding and support to help the person begin to organize a more coherent story but not to heighten or stimulate deeper experiencing or more arousal.

Subsequently, Angus and colleagues (Angus & Greenberg, 2011; Boritz et al., 2014) defined a number of different types of in-session markers of different types of narratives that help illuminate the narrative landscape. These markers help therapists identify where clients are in their narrative construction process. Although all of the different types of narrative are ideally responded to with empathic understanding, each type of narrative benefits from empathy with a particular focus—one suited to that narrative process. The markers are broken into two types: problem-based stories and change stories. The problem stories are same old story, empty story, unstoried emotions, and superficial story, whereas the change stories are competing plotlines story, inchoate story, unexpected outcome story, and discovery story.

Problem Stories: The Arriving Phase

Problem stories arise as part of the arriving at emotions stage of treatment. *Same old story* occurs when the client expresses a dominant, often overly general view of self and relationships. This story is marked by lack of agency, and the client is stuck in the story. It is often expressed in a complaining tone with fused anger and sadness. The same litany of complaints is repeated with a sense of resignation and hopelessness because people feel stuck. They are stuck in secondary emotions. The best way to respond is to empathize with the story, acknowledge the sense of "stuckness," and then conjecture about underlying primary feelings.

In an *empty story*, the client describes an event with a focus on external details and behavior and repetition of overly general, autobiographical memories (ABM) like, "My father was always absent"; these empty stories are marked by a lack of internal referents or emotional arousal. Intervention involves focusing on the missing emotions with a view to ending with a new story based on new emotions. There is a shifting from overly general ABMs to specific ABMs like, "I remember my fifth birthday. He was supposed to come and take me out, and he never came, and I was left crying on the doorstep." Therapists ask for specific examples, conjecture about what was felt, and empathize with the episodic memories and emotional experience as they emerge.

Unstoried emotions involve a process in which clients experience under- or overregulated emotional arousal without coherent narration of the experience. Intervention involves identifying cues that triggered the emotion and symbolizing emotions in words. The end state involves helping clients assimilate emotion into narrative organized into emotion episodes with beginnings, middles, and ends. In these situations, clients lack a context for understanding what the emotion belongs to, so therapists help clients engage in a safe reentry into the experience and move from the landscape of feeling to reconnect with the landscape of action by narrating what happened. They then move to the landscape of meaning to understand what they felt. This marker often occurs in the context of first disclosures of trauma. Therapists' empathic attunement in combination with reassurance and empathic validation helps the client safely reenter the lived story of a specific trauma experience to access specific ABM narratives and differentiate their subjective experience of the frightening experience. Trauma experiences are now located in a specific time; emotions are causally connected with action and intentions, and are organized within a narrative framework with a beginning, middle, and end.

In *superficial stories*, clients talk about events, hypotheticals, self, others, or unclear referents in a vague, abstract manner with limited internal focus. The therapist's aim here is to deepen the narrative mainly through empathic conjecture into underlying feelings as well as to evoke episodic memories to get at more concrete experience. *Untold stories* are also of interest. These occur when the client is not saying something that is emotionally important often out of fear or shame. This requires empathic exploration to help the client move from a lived story into a told story. The therapist helps the client to disclose implicit emotions and helps the client shift from overly general memories to episodic memories.

Change Stories: The Leaving Phase

In terms of change stories, the client now enters the leaving phase. Having arrived at emotions and storied them in awareness, it is now time to leave them and create new stories. *Competing plotlines stories* are identified when clients experience challenges to their same old stories wherein states of emotional incoherence, confusion, and puzzlement begin to emerge in therapy sessions. Here, therapists focus on developing the subdominant story to develop its voice. *Inchoate stories* are identified when clients are turning their attention inward to sort through, piece together, articulate, and make sense of an emerging bodily felt experience. These stories are facilitated by empathy and the use of client-focusing strategies (Gendlin, 1996). *Unexpected outcome stories* emerge when clients express surprise, excitement, contentment, or inner peace in response to experiencing new emotional responses, taking positive action, or both. Intervention involves elaborating and consolidating the unexpected outcome, and exploring and validating the positive outcome and narrative reconstruction. The therapist engages in reflexive inquiry of the unique outcome stories to identify client agency and enhance story salience. *Discovery stories* involve the articulation of understandings or views of self and other that result in narrative reconstruction and consolidation of client experiences of novelty and change. Therapists validate and help elaborate the newly discovered views.

CONCLUSION

In therapy, stories emerge from the body if there is a facilitative listener there to receive them and are brought into the world through the help of language. Effective therapists actively facilitate clients to shift from external narratives to the processing of emotion schematic experiences and to creating fuller reflexive narratives in a bid to help them make conscious sense of their own emotional experiences. Working at the purely conceptual or linguistic level to make narrative change does not produce enduring emotional change. Instead, therapeutic interventions are more likely to succeed if they first target the emotion schematic processes that automatically generate the emotional experience underlying clients' felt senses of themselves.

Next, the emotional experience needs to be consciously reflected on, and the tacit representation of the unfolding "wordless" narrative scene needs to be made explicit. This type of narrative construction organizes emotions and integrates them with action sequences and meanings. This integration of emotion and narrative enables the construction of a storied explanation of "what happened," "what it meant," and, most important, "what it felt like," which can then be told to others and reflected on for further understanding and meaning construction. Therapy, then, is a process of coming to know emotions—storying them—and, in so doing, changing them.

LOOKING AHEAD

A Unified Approach to Psychotherapy

Emotion is a universal phenomenon. Given its central role in human functioning, it makes sense to view the proposed principle of changing emotion with emotion as a universal change process. Likewise, we can view this and other emotional change principles as transdiagnostic, transtheoretical, and transcultural (transcultural includes gender, class, race, and religion). In this book, I suggest that maladaptive emotion and dysfunctional emotional processing is a core area of dysfunction underlying different disorders and mental health problems.

In this concluding chapter, I suggest for the field of clinical psychology and psychotherapy the beginning of an integrative, unified view of emotional change based on principles of changing emotion with emotion, empathic attunement to affect, emotion awareness, bodily focus, blocking and unblocking, focus on needs, memory reconsolidation, emotion regulation, and narrative symbolization of emotion. These are the major processes covered in this book. My hope is that this book will stimulate the examination of and perhaps, ultimately, the adoption of a view that puts emotional change as a fundamental aspect of therapeutic change and offers it as a transdiagnostic, transtheoretical alternative to the ever-increasing proliferation of disease-specific treatments

https://doi.org/10.1037/0000248-014

and therapeutic systems. Currently, there is still a vast array of psychotherapy interventions—at least more than 200 in an informal count on Wikipedia—with different approaches that rest on different philosophical and theoretical assumptions, and that emphasize different domains of human functioning and adaptation.

At a minimum, the field needs an addition of emotion to the current cognitive behavioral perspective that has dominated for the past decades. What is possibly achievable at the moment is a unified emotion-focused, cognitive behavior therapy (CBT) approach based on foundational emotional, cognitive, and behavioral change principles. Over time, even more extensive integration that incorporates more principles of change will be achieved. In the long run, the field will need to have a metatheory that allows researchers and practitioners to view the big picture and to navigate the variety of different approaches in a way that allows them to coordinate diverse treatment options.

A transdiagnostic approach suggests a more unified approach to the treatment of psychological disorders than the current differential treatment perspective commonly held over the past 40 years. It has become evidently clear that the diagnostic classifications and their corresponding disorder-specific treatments suffer from serious limitations of reliability and validity, and that there is clearly heterogeneity within diagnostic groups. For example, depression is not a consistent syndrome (Fried & Nesse, 2015), and different diagnostic groups do not represent distinct emotional disorders. Hence, there are high rates of not otherwise specified diagnoses (T. A. Brown, Di Nardo, et al., 2001; Clark et al., 2017; Le Grange et al., 2012). Some attempt has been made to rectify these problems in the fifth edition of the *Diagnostic and Statistical Manual of Mental Disorders* (*DSM*-5; American Psychiatric Association, 2013) and to recognize cultural context and common factors behind diagnoses. The issue of different treatments for different diagnostic groups, however, remains, and the field would benefit from specifying underlying principles of working with human psychological processes, specifically with emotional processes that span diagnostic groups. Establishing universal emotional change principles would be most helpful for client treatment, trainers, and clinicians alike.

Rather than adopting a medical model and thinking of mental health diagnoses as representing separate disease entities, there is increasing awareness that common processes or mechanisms operate across disorders (Brewin et al., 2010; Harvey et al., 2004; Hayes & Hofmann, 2018). Transdiagnostic treatments that target core processes—those factors that maintain disorders—are needed. The proliferation of different treatments for different disorders results in setting up a significant barrier to comprehensive treatment, dissemination, and training. Most disorders have maladaptive emotions at their base, and most treatments now include methods to work on emotion. Emotion strategies, such as awareness, acceptance, ability to change emotion with emotion, ability to overcome blocking or avoid emotion, exposure, memory reconsolidation, emotion regulation, and narrative construction, are already in wide use. A single, unified treatment that targets the essential emotional processes that cause and maintain problems in my view would benefit more clients. It would deepen therapy and promote longer lasting change by treating the underlying disease at its emotional roots rather than its symptomatic manifestations.

Originally, before the dominance of the differential treatment paradigm, which was spurred by the research question "What treatment by whom for whom?" (Paul, 1967), many approaches offered a unified treatment and were transdiagnostic. A return to this path—but now with a focus on case formulation rather than diagnosis—would help therapists apply principles of change to each client in a more individualized fashion.

Although it is important in a unified approach to realize that there are cultural and individual differences in the way emotions are viewed and expressed (examples are reviewed in Chapter 4), at the core, all human beings, clients, therapists, and people from different cultures, different families, and different diagnostic groups have emotions, and they all need to pay attention to them because they help us to survive and thrive. Despite cultural differences in emotional expression, a core set of factors is involved in treating emotional suffering regardless of the disorder and the culture. Mental health treatment would be greatly improved by the development of transtheoretical principles, which would enhance efforts at psychotherapy integration, stop the ever-increasing proliferation of therapeutic systems, and put an end to school wars.

Single-school approaches dominated the practice of psychotherapy in the 1960s and 1970s. The majority of therapists identified with a particular school of thought (e.g., psychoanalytic, behavioral, humanistic), tended to see their model as representing truth, and engaged in vigorous—and sometimes vitriolic—debates with practitioners from other approaches. The 1980s saw the rise of *eclecticism*, the unsystematic blending of ideas and techniques from the various schools of thought. Eclecticism is noteworthy because it reflected an attitudinal shift from single-school approaches to more openness to looking at complementary aspects of treatment from different angles. In the 1990s and 2000s, psychotherapy integration became a genuine movement. The Society for the Exploration of Psychotherapy Integration formed in the mid-1980s and began swelling in size and influence.

The early 1990s witnessed the publication of two handbooks in integrative psychotherapy (Norcross & Goldfried, 1992; Stricker & Gold, 1993), which detailed a multitude of important developments toward a more integrative approach to the field.

Still, fundamental differences exist in the field in epistemology and views of functioning, and a common language is lacking. The lack of agreement results in difficulties in developing an effective, integrative training program. Students often are taught one predominant approach or another, and CBT approaches dominate North American graduate programs. Training, therefore, is limiting, and practitioners cannot apply treatments that best fit different clients and problems. Instead, they can only administer the single method they were trained in. Some universities teach various schools of thought separately and then give students the option to practice from one or another, or students are left to their own devices to generate their own blend or integration. A few training programs attempt to teach integrative approaches, but even these lack a comprehensive focus and still do not give emotion a prominent role.

As the psychotherapy integration movement has grown over the years, different approaches to integration have emerged, and now, four routes to integration are generally recognized, although there certainly are other possible approaches (see Ingram, 2006). The most general approach has been the common-factors approach. Identified strongly with Jerome Frank's (1973) classic work *Persuasion and Healing*, the *common-factors approach* is conceptually grounded in a sophisticated folk psychology that emphasizes the general processes of healing that cut across all of the approaches, such as establishing a productive healing relationship, The evidence-based treatment movement begun in the 1990s has failed to overcome school wars. Rather, it has just created a presumptive CBT victory in the school wars, even though there is growing evidence from unbiased studies and reviews showing that all approaches are roughly equivalent. The claim of CBT superiority, while creating territorial dominance, has also generated much underground resistance and has not stopped the proliferation of new approaches, such as third-wave CBT approaches, schema-focused therapy, emotion-focused therapy, accelerated experiential dynamic therapy, eye-movement desensitization and reprocessing, and attachment-focused therapy.

Ultimately, I envisage and hope for a shift in how the field of psychotherapy is conceptualized. Magnavita (2008), for example, called for the construction of a unified clinical science that consists of the intersection and amalgamation of personality theory, developmental psychopathology, and psychotherapy in a way that allows for the identification of the structures, processes, and mechanisms that are involved in the major domains of human functioning. I foresee a time when students are provided with a transtheoretical, transdiagnostic, transcultural overview that allows them to understand how to work in a unified way with different systems. It would be based on an understanding of basic principles and methods of change to work with emotion, motivation, cognition, behavior, interaction, systems, culture and biology, and the relationship between these systems. This would have enormous implications for training, research, and practice.

A unified theory (Anchin & Magnavita, 2008; Magnavita & Anchin, 2014) would provide a way to assimilate and integrate key insights from the major therapeutic perspectives into a coherent whole and provide a holistic picture that would allow clinicians and researchers a map of the various ways in which to intervene. I hope to have shown in this book how working with emotion as a fundamental process and using emotion to change emotion will help develop a unified transdiagnostic, transtheoretical approach to treatment that will improve training and treatment efficacy.

References

Abbass, A. (2002). Intensive short-term dynamic psychotherapy in a private psychiatric office: Clinical and cost effectiveness. *The American Journal of Psychotherapy, 56*(2), 225–232. https://doi.org/10.1176/appi.psychotherapy.2002.56.2.225

Abbass, A. (2015). *Reaching through resistance: Advanced psychotherapy techniques.* Seven Leaves Press.

Adams, K. E. (2010). *Therapist influence on depressed clients' therapeutic experiencing and outcome* [Unpublished doctoral dissertation]. York University.

Adams, K. E., & Greenberg, L. S. (1996, June). *Therapists' influence on depressed clients' therapeutic experiencing and outcome* [Paper presentation]. Forty-Third Annual Convention for the Society for Psychotherapy Research, St. Amelia Island, FL, United States.

Adler, G., & Myerson, P. G. (1973). *Confrontation in psychotherapy.* Jason Aronson.

Adolphs, R., & Anderson, D. J. (2018). *The neuroscience of emotion: A new synthesis.* Princeton University Press.

Aldao, A., Nolen-Hoeksema, S., & Schweizer, S. (2010). Emotion-regulation strategies across psychopathology: A meta-analytic review. *Clinical Psychology Review, 30*(2), 217–237. https://doi.org/10.1016/j.cpr.2009.11.004

Alexander, F., & French, T. M. (1946). *Psychoanalytic therapy: Principles and application.* Ronald Press.

American Psychiatric Association. (2013). *Diagnostic and statistical manual of mental disorders* (5th ed.). https://doi.org/10.1176/appi.books.9780890425596

Anchin, J. C., & Magnavita, J. J. (2008). Toward the unification of psychotherapy: An introduction to the journal symposium. *Journal of Psychotherapy Integration, 18*(3), 259–263. https://doi.org/10.1037/a0013556

Anderson, E. (2015). "The White space." *Sociology of Race and Ethnicity, 1*(1), 10–21. https://doi.org/10.1177/2332649214561306

Angus, L. E., Boritz, T., Bryntwick, E., Carpenter, N., Macaulay, C., & Khattra, J. (2017). The Narrative-Emotion Process Coding System 2.0: A multi-methodological approach to identifying and assessing narrative-emotion process markers in psychotherapy. *Psychotherapy Research, 27*(3), 253–269. https://doi.org/10.1080/10503307.2016.1238525

Angus, L. E., & Greenberg, L. S. (2011). *Working with narrative in emotion-focused therapy: Changing stories, healing lives.* American Psychological Association. https://doi.org/10.1037/12325-000

Angus, L. E., Levitt, H., & Hardtke, K. (1999). The narrative processes coding system: Research applications and implications for psychotherapy practice. *Journal of Clinical Psychology, 55*(10), 1255–1270. https://doi.org/10.1002/(SICI)1097-4679(199910)55:10<1255::AID-JCLP7>3.0.CO;2-F

Angus, L. E., & McLeod, J. (Eds.). (2004). *The handbook of narrative and psychotherapy.* SAGE Publishing. https://doi.org/10.4135/9781412973496

Auszra, L., Greenberg, L. S., & Herrmann, I. (2013). Client emotional productivity—Optimal client in-session emotional processing in experiential therapy. *Psychotherapy Research, 23*(6), 732–746. https://doi.org/10.1080/10503307.2013.816882

Bagby, R. M., Parker, J. D. A., & Taylor, G. J. (1994). The twenty-item Toronto Alexithymia Scale—I. Item selection and cross-validation of the factor structure. *Journal of Psychosomatic Research, 38*(1), 23–32. https://doi.org/10.1016/0022-3999(94)90005-1

Barlow, D. H., Allen, L. B., & Choate, M. L. (2004). Toward a unified treatment for emotional disorders. *Behavior Therapy, 35*(2), 205–230. https://doi.org/10.1016/S0005-7894(04)80036-4

Barnow, S. (2012). Emotionsregulation und psychopathologie: Ein überblick [Emotion regulation and psychopathology. An overview]. *Psychologische Rundschau, 63*(2), 111–124. https://doi.org/10.1026/0033-3042/a000119

Barrett, L. F. (2017). *How emotions are made: The secret life of the brain.* Houghton Mifflin Harcourt.

Barrett-Lennard, G. T. (1993). The phases and focus of empathy. *The British Journal of Medical Psychology, 66*(1), 3–14. https://doi.org/10.1111/j.2044-8341.1993.tb01722.x

Barrett-Lennard, G. T. (1997). The recovery of empathy—Toward others and self. In A. C. Bohart & L. S. Greenberg (Eds.), *Empathy reconsidered: New directions in psychotherapy* (pp. 103–121). American Psychological Association. https://doi.org/10.1037/10226-004

Bateman, A., & Fonagy, P. (2004). *Psychotherapy for borderline personality disorder: Mentalization-based treatment.* Oxford University Press. https://doi.org/10.1093/med:psych/9780198527664.001.0001

Berkowitz, L. (2000). *Causes and consequences of feelings.* Cambridge University Press.

Bion, W. R. (1967). Notes on memory and desire. *The Psychoanalytic Forum, 2*, 271–280.

Blume-Marcovici, A. C., Stolberg, R. A., & Khademi, M. (2013). Do therapists cry in therapy? The role of experience and other factors in therapists' tears. *Psychotherapy, 50*(2), 224–234. https://doi.org/10.1037/a0031384

Bohart, A. C., Elliott, R., Greenberg, L. S., & Watson, J. C. (2002). Empathy. In J. Norcross (Ed.), *Psychotherapy relationships that work* (pp. 89–108). Oxford University Press.

Bohart, A. C., & Greenberg, L. S. (Eds.). (1997). *Empathy reconsidered: New directions in theory research & practice*. American Psychological Association.

Bohart, A. C., & Greenberg, L. S. (2002). EMDR and experiential psychotherapy. In F. Shapiro (Ed.), *EMDR as an integrative psychotherapy approach: Experts of diverse orientations explore the paradigm prism* (pp. 239–261). American Psychological Association.

Bolger, E. A. (1999). Grounded theory analysis of emotional pain. *Psychotherapy Research, 9*(3), 342–362. https://doi.org/10.1080/10503309912331332801

Boritz, T., Barnhart, R., Angus, L., & Constantino, M. J. (2017). Narrative flexibility in brief psychotherapy for depression. *Psychotherapy Research, 27*(6), 666–676. https://doi.org/10.1080/10503307.2016.1152410

Boritz, T. Z., Angus, L., Monette, G., & Hollis-Walker, L. (2008). An empirical analysis of autobiographical memory specificity subtypes in brief emotion-focused and client-centered treatments of depression. *Psychotherapy Research, 18*(5), 584–593. https://doi.org/10.1080/10503300802123245

Boritz, T. Z., Angus, L., Monette, G., Hollis-Walker, L., & Warwar, S. (2011). Narrative and emotion integration in psychotherapy: Investigating the relationship between autobiographical memory specificity and expressed emotional arousal in brief emotion-focused and client-centred treatments of depression. *Psychotherapy Research, 21*(1), 16–26. https://doi.org/10.1080/10503307.2010.504240

Boritz, T. Z., Bryntwick, E., Angus, L., Greenberg, L. S., & Constantino, M. J. (2014). Narrative and emotion process in psychotherapy: An empirical test of the Narrative-Emotion Process Coding System (NEPCS). *Psychotherapy Research, 24*(5), 594–607. https://doi.org/10.1080/10503307.2013.851426

Borkovec, T. D., & Sides, J. K. (1979). The contribution of relaxation and expectancy to fear reduction via graded, imaginal exposure to feared stimuli. *Behaviour Research and Therapy, 17*(6), 529–540. https://doi.org/10.1016/0005-7967(79)90096-2

Bowlby, J. (1988). *A secure base: Parent–child attachment and healthy human development*. Basic Books.

Bowlby, J. (1998). *Attachment and loss*. Pimlico.

Bradley, B., DeFife, J. A., Guarnaccia, C., Phifer, J., Fani, N., Ressler, K. J., & Westen, D. (2011). Emotion dysregulation and negative affect: Association with psychiatric symptoms. *The Journal of Clinical Psychiatry, 72*(5), 685–691. https://doi.org/10.4088/JCP.10m06409blu

Bradshaw, J. (1988). *Healing the shame that binds you*. Health Communications.

Brewin, C. R., Gregory, J. D., Lipton, M., & Burgess, N. (2010). Intrusive images in psychological disorders: Characteristics, neural mechanisms, and treatment implications. *Psychological Review, 117*(1), 210–232. https://doi.org/10.1037/a0018113

Brody, L. R., & Hall, J. A. (2008). Gender and emotion in context. In M. Lewis, J. M. Haviland-Jones, & L. F. Barrett (Eds.), *Handbook of emotions* (3rd ed., pp. 395–408). Guilford Press.

Brown, B. (2012). *Daring greatly: How the courage to be vulnerable transforms the way we live, love, parent, and lead.* Gotham Books.

Brown, T. A., Campbell, L. A., Lehman, C. L., Grisham, J. R., & Mancill, R. B. (2001). Current and lifetime comorbidity of the *DSM-IV* anxiety and mood disorders in a large clinical sample. *Journal of Abnormal Psychology, 110*(4), 585–599. https://doi.org/10.1037/0021-843X.110.4.585

Brown, T. A., Di Nardo, P. A., Lehman, C. L., & Campbell, L. A. (2001). Reliability of *DSM-IV* anxiety and mood disorders: Implications for the classification of emotional disorders. *Journal of Abnormal Psychology, 110*(1), 49–58. https://doi.org/10.1037//0021-843X.110.1.49

Bruner, J. S. (1986). *Actual minds, possible worlds.* Harvard University Press.

Bruner, J. S. (1990). *Acts of meaning.* Harvard University Press.

Buck, R. (2014). *Emotion: A biosocial synthesis.* Cambridge University Press. https://doi.org/10.1017/CBO9781139049825

Bushman, B. J. (2002). Does venting anger feed or extinguish the flame? Catharsis, rumination, distraction, anger, and aggressive responding. *Personality and Social Psychology Bulletin, 28*(6), 724–731. https://doi.org/10.1177/0146167202289002

Campos, J. J., Frankel, C. B., & Camras, L. (2004). On the nature of emotion regulation. *Child Development, 75*(2), 377–394. https://doi.org/10.1111/j.1467-8624.2004.00681.x

Capps, K. L., Fiori, K., Mullin, A. S., & Hilsenroth, M. J. (2015). Patient crying in psychotherapy: Who cries and why? *Clinical Psychology & Psychotherapy, 22*(3), 208–220. https://doi.org/10.1002/cpp.1879

Carryer, J. R., & Greenberg, L. S. (2010). Optimal levels of emotional arousal in experiential therapy of depression. *Journal of Consulting and Clinical Psychology, 78*(2), 190–199. https://doi.org/10.1037/a0018401

Castonguay, L. G., Goldfried, M. R., Wiser, S., Raue, P. J., & Hayes, A. M. (1996). Predicting the effect of cognitive therapy for depression: A study of unique and common factors. *Journal of Consulting and Clinical Psychology, 64*(3), 497–504. https://doi.org/10.1037/0022-006X.64.3.497

Choi, E., Chentsova-Dutton, Y., & Parrott, W. G. (2016). The effectiveness of somatization in communicating distress in Korean and American cultural contexts. *Frontiers in Psychology, 7*, Article 383. https://doi.org/10.3389/fpsyg.2016.00383

Chou, T., Asnaani, A., & Hofmann, S. G. (2012). Perception of racial discrimination and psychopathology across three U.S. ethnic minority groups. *Cultural

Diversity & Ethnic Minority Psychology, *18*(1), 74–81. https://doi.org/10.1037%2Fa0025432

Clark, L. A., Cuthbert, B., Lewis-Fernández, R., Narrow, W. E., & Reed, G. M. (2017). Three Approaches to Understanding and Classifying Mental Disorder: *ICD-11*, *DSM-5*, and the National Institute of Mental Health's Research Domain Criteria (RDoC). *Psychological Science in the Public Interest*, *18*(2), 72–145. https://doi.org/10.1177/1529100617727266

Comas-Díaz, L., Hall, G. N., & Neville, H. A. (2019). Racial trauma: Theory, research, and healing: Introduction to the special issue. *American Psychologist*, *74*(1), 1–5. https://doi.org/10.1037/amp0000442

Coombs, M., Coleman, D., & Jones, E. E. (2002). Working with feelings: The importance of emotion in both cognitive–behavioral and interpersonal therapy in the NIMH Treatment of Depression Collaborative Research Program. *Psychotherapy*, *39*(3), 233–244. https://doi.org/10.1037/0033-3204.39.3.233

Cousins, S. D. (1989). Culture and self-perception in Japan and the United States. *Journal of Personality and Social Psychology*, *56*(1), 124–131. https://doi.org/10.1037/0022-3514.56.1.124

Cozolino, L. J. (2002). *The neuroscience of psychotherapy: Building and rebuilding the human brain*. Norton.

Craske, M. G., Treanor, M., Conway, C. C., Zbozinek, T., & Vervliet, B. (2014). Maximizing exposure therapy: An inhibitory learning approach. *Behaviour Research and Therapy*, *58*, 10–23. https://doi.org/10.1016/j.brat.2014.04.006

Daldrup, R. J., Beutler, L. E., Engle, D., & Greenberg, L. S. (1988). *Focused expressive psychotherapy: Freeing the over-controlled patient*. Guilford Press.

Damasio, A. R. (1994). *Descartes' error: Emotion, reason, and the human brain*. G. P. Putnam.

Damasio, A. R. (1999). *The feeling of what happens: Body and emotion in the making of consciousness*. Harcourt Brace.

Daros, A. R., & Williams, G. E. (2019). A meta-analysis and systematic review of emotion-regulation strategies in borderline personality disorder. *Harvard Review of Psychiatry*, *27*(4), 217–232. https://doi.org/10.1097/HRP.0000000000000212

Darwin, C. (1897). *The expression of emotions in man and animals*. Philosophical Library.

Davidson, R. J., & Harrington, A. (Eds.). (2002). *Visions of compassion: Western scientists and Tibetan Buddhists examine human nature*. Oxford University Press.

de la Fuente, V., Freudenthal, R., & Romano, A. (2011). Reconsolidation or extinction: Transcription factor switch in the determination of memory course after retrieval. *The Journal of Neuroscience*, *31*(15), 5562–5573. https://doi.org/10.1523/JNEUROSCI.6066-10.2011

Dere, J., Falk, C. F., & Ryder, A. G. (2012). Unpacking cultural differences in alexithymia: The role of cultural values among Euro-Canadian and Chinese-Canadian students. *Journal of Cross-Cultural Psychology*, *43*(8), 1297–1312. https://doi.org/10.1177/0022022111430254

Diamond, G., & Liddle, H. A. (1996). Resolving a therapeutic impasse between parents and adolescents in multidimensional family therapy. *Journal of Consulting and Clinical Psychology, 64*(3), 481–488. https://doi.org/10.1037/0022-006X.64.3.481

Diener, M. J., Hilsenroth, M. J., & Weinberger, J. (2007). Therapist affect focus and patient outcomes in psychodynamic psychotherapy: A meta-analysis. *The American Journal of Psychiatry, 164*(6), 936–941. https://doi.org/10.1176/ajp.2007.164.6.936

Dzokoto, V. A., Opare-Henaku, A., & Kpobi, L. A. (2013). Somatic referencing and psychologisation in emotion narratives: A USA–Ghana comparison. *Psychology and Developing Societies, 25*(2), 311–331. https://doi.org/10.1177/0971333613500875

Ekman, P., & Davidson, R. J. (Eds.). (1994). *The nature of emotion: Fundamental questions*. Oxford University Press.

Elliott, R. (2013). Person-centered/experiential psychotherapy for anxiety difficulties: Theory, research and practice. *Person-Centered & Experiential Psychotherapies, 12*(1), 16–32. https://doi.org/10.1080/14779757.2013.767750

Elliott, R., Bohart, A. C., Watson, J. C., & Greenberg, L. S. (2011). Empathy. *Psychotherapy, 48*(1), 43–49. https://doi.org/10.1037/a0022187

Elliott, R., Greenberg, L. S., Watson, J. C., Timulak, L., & Freire, E. (2013). Research on humanistic–experiential psychotherapies. In M. J. Lambert (Ed.), *Bergin & Garfield's handbook of psychotherapy and behavior change* (6th ed.; pp. 495–538). John Wiley & Sons.

Elliott, R., Rodgers, B., & Stephen, S. (2014, June). *The outcomes of person-centred and emotion-focused therapy for social anxiety: An update* [Paper presentation]. Conference of the Society for Psychotherapy Research, Copenhagen, Denmark.

Elliott, R., & Shahar, B. (2017). Emotion-focused therapy for social anxiety (EFT-SA). *Person-Centered and Experiential Psychotherapies, 16*(2), 140–158. https://doi.org/10.1080/14779757.2017.1330701

Elliott, R., Watson, J. C., Goldman, R. N., & Greenberg, L. S. (2004). *Learning emotion-focused therapy: The process-experiential approach to change*. American Psychological Association. https://doi.org/10.1037/10725-000

Elliott, R., Watson, J. C., Timulak, L., & Sharbanee, J. (in press). Research on humanistic-experiential psychotherapies: Updated review. In M. Barkham, W. Lutz, & L. G. Castonguay (Eds.), *Bergin & Garfield's handbook of psychotherapy and behavior change* (7th ed.). John Wiley & Sons.

Field, T. M. (1998). Massage therapy effects. *American Psychologist, 53*(12), 1270–1281. https://doi.org/10.1037/0003-066X.53.12.1270

Fischer, A. H., & Manstead, A. S. R. (2000). The relation between gender and emotions in different cultures. In A. H. Fischer (Ed.), *Gender and emotion: Social psychological perspectives* (pp. 71–94). Cambridge University Press.

Flack, W. F., Jr., Laird, J. D., & Cavallaro, L. A. (1999). Emotional expression and feeling in schizophrenia: Effects of specific expressive behaviors on emotional experiences. *Journal of Clinical Psychology, 55*(1), 1–20. https://doi.org/10.1002/(SICI)1097-4679(199901)55:1<1::AID-JCLP1>3.0.CO;2-K

Foa, E. B., & Jaycox, L. H. (1999). Cognitive-behavioral theory and treatment of posttraumatic stress disorder. In D. Spiegel (Ed.), *Efficacy and cost-effectiveness of psychotherapy* (pp. 23–61). American Psychiatric Publishing.

Foa, E. B., & Kozak, M. J. (1986). Emotional processing of fear: Exposure to corrective information. *Psychological Bulletin, 99*(1), 20–35. https://doi.org/10.1037/0033-2909.99.1.20

Foa, E. B., & Kozak, M. J. (1998). Clinical applications of bioinformational theory: Understanding anxiety and its treatment. *Behavior Therapy, 29*(4), 675–690. https://doi.org/10.1016/S0005-7894(98)80025-7

Foa, E. B., Riggs, D. S., Massie, E. D., & Yarczower, M. (1995). The impact of fear activation and anger on the efficacy of exposure treatment for PTSD. *Behavior Therapy, 26*(3), 487–499. https://doi.org/10.1016/S0005-7894(05)80096-6

Foa, E. B., Rothbaum, B. O., & Furr, J. M. (2003). Augmenting exposure therapy with other CBT procedures. *Psychiatric Annals, 33*(1), 47–53. https://doi.org/10.3928/0048-5713-20030101-08

Fonagy, P., Gergely, G., Jurist, E. L., & Target, M. (2002). *Affect regulation, mentalization, and the development of the self*. Other Press.

Forgas, J. P. (1995). Mood and judgment: The affect infusion model (AIM). *Psychological Bulletin, 117*(1), 39–66. https://doi.org/10.1037/0033-2909.117.1.39

Fosha, D. (2000). *The transforming power of affect: A model for accelerated change*. Basic Books.

Fosha, D. (2004). "Nothing that feels bad is ever the last step": The role of positive emotion in experiential work with difficult emotional experiences. *Clinical Psychology & Psychotherapy, 11*(1), 30–43. https://doi.org/10.1002/cpp.390

Frank, J. (1973). *Persuasion and healing: A comparative study of psychotherapy* (2nd ed.). Johns Hopkins University Press.

Frankl, V. E. (1959). *Man's search for meaning: An introduction to logotherapy*. Simon & Schuster.

Fredrickson, B. L. (1998). What good are positive emotions? *Review of General Psychology, 2*(3), 300–319. https://doi.org/10.1037/1089-2680.2.3.300

Fredrickson, B. L. (2001). The role of positive emotions in positive psychology. The broaden-and-build theory of positive emotions. *American Psychologist, 56*(3), 218–226. https://doi.org/10.1037/0003-066X.56.3.218

Fredrickson, B. L. (2009). *Positivity: Groundbreaking research reveals how to embrace the hidden strength of positive emotions, overcome negativity, and thrive*. Crown Publishers.

Fredrickson, B. L., & Levenson, R. W. (1998). Positive emotions speed recovery from the cardiovascular sequelae of negative emotions. *Cognition and Emotion, 12*(2), 191–220. https://doi.org/10.1080/026999398379718

Fredrickson, B. L., Mancuso, R. A., Branigan, C., & Tugade, M. M. (2000). The undoing effect of positive emotions. *Motivation and Emotion, 24*, 237–258. https://doi.org/10.1023/A:1010796329158

Freud, S. (1955). Repression. In J. Strachey (Ed. & Trans.), *The standard edition of the complete psychological works of Sigmund Freud* (Vol. 14; pp. 141–158). Hogarth Press. (Original work published 1915)

Freud, S. (1976). Introductory lectures on psycho-analysis. In J. Strachey (Ed.), *The complete psychological works* (Vol. 15). W. W. Norton & Company. (Original work published 1917)

Fried, E. I., & Nesse, R. M. (2015). Depression is not a consistent syndrome: An investigation of unique symptom patterns in the STAR*D study. *Journal of Affective Disorders, 172,* 96–102. https://doi.org/10.1016/j.jad.2014.10.010

Frijda, N. H. (1986). *The emotions.* Cambridge University Press.

Frijda, N. H. (2016). The evolutionary emergence of what we call "emotions." *Cognition and Emotion, 30*(4), 609–620. https://doi.org/10.1080/02699931.2016.1145106

Gallese, V. (2009). Mirror neurons, embodied simulation, and the neural basis of social identification. *Psychoanalytic Dialogues, 19*(5), 519–536. https://doi.org/10.1080/10481880903231910

Gard, M. G., & Kring, A. M. (2007). Sex differences in the time course of emotion. *Emotion, 7*(2), 429–437. https://doi.org/10.1037/1528-3542.7.2.429

Gazzaniga, M. S. (1998). *The mind's past.* University of California Press.

Geller, S. M., & Greenberg, L. S. (2002). Therapeutic presence: Therapists' experience of presence in the psychotherapy encounter. *Person-Centered & Experiential Psychotherapies, 1*(1–2), 71–86. https://doi.org/10.1080/14779757.2002.9688279

Geller, S. M., & Greenberg, L. S. (2012). *Therapeutic presence: A mindful approach to effective therapy.* American Psychological Association. https://doi.org/10.1037/13485-000

Gendlin, E. T. (1969). Focusing. *Psychotherapy, 6*(1), 4–15. https://doi.org/10.1037/h0088716

Gendlin, E. T. (1981). *Focusing.* Bantam Books.

Gendlin, E. T. (1991). On emotion in therapy. In J. D. Safran & L. S. Greenberg (Eds.), *Emotion, psychotherapy, and change* (pp. 255–279). Guilford Press.

Gendlin, E. T. (1996). *Focusing-oriented psychotherapy: A manual of the experiential method.* Guilford Press.

Gilbert, P. (1992). *Depression: The evolution of powerlessness.* Lawrence Erlbaum.

Gilbert, P. (2010). *The compassionate mind: A new approach to life's challenges.* New Harbinger Publications.

Gilboa-Schechtman, E., & Foa, E. B. (2001). Patterns of recovery from trauma: The use of intraindividual analysis. *Journal of Abnormal Psychology, 110*(3), 392–400. https://doi.org/10.1037/0021-843X.110.3.392

Glaser, B. G., & Strauss, A. (1967). *Discovery of grounded theory. Strategies for qualitative research.* California Sociology Press.

Goldfried, M. R. (1980). Toward the delineation of therapeutic change principles. *American Psychologist, 35*(11), 991–999. https://doi.org/10.1037/0003-066X.35.11.991

Goldfried, M. R. (2012). The corrective experience: A core principle for therapeutic change. In L. G. Castonguay & C. E. Hill (Eds.), *Transformation in psychotherapy: Corrective experiences across cognitive behavioral, humanistic, and psychodynamic approaches* (pp. 13–29). American Psychological Association. https://doi.org/10.1037/13747-002

Goldfried, M. R., & Davison, G. C. (1976). *Clinical behavior therapy*. Holt, Rinehart and Winston.

Goldman, R. N., & Fox-Zurawic, A. (2012, July 10–14). *Self-soothing in emotion-focused therapy: Findings from a task analysis* [Paper presentation]. Conference of World Association for Person-Centred and Experiential Psychotherapy & Counselling, Antwerp, Belgium.

Goldman, R. N., & Greenberg, L. S. (2015). *Case formulation in emotion-focused therapy: Co-creating clinical maps for change*. American Psychological Association. https://doi.org/10.1037/14523-000

Goldman, R. N., Greenberg, L. S., & Angus, L. (2006). The effects of adding emotion-focused interventions to the client-centered relationship conditions in the treatment of depression. *Psychotherapy Research, 16*(5), 537–549. https://doi.org/10.1080/10503300600589456

Goldman, R. N., Greenberg, L. S., & Pos, A. E. (2005). Depth of emotional experience and outcome. *Psychotherapy Research, 15*(3), 248–260. https://doi.org/10.1080/10503300512331385188

Greenberg, L. S. (1984). A task analysis of intrapersonal conflict resolution. In L. N. Rice & L. S. Greenberg (Eds.), *Patterns of change: Intensive analysis of psychotherapy process* (pp. 67–123). Guilford Press.

Greenberg, L. S. (2002). *Emotion-focused therapy: Coaching clients to work through their feelings*. American Psychological Association. https://doi.org/10.1037/10447-000

Greenberg, L. S. (2007). A guide to conducting a task analysis of psychotherapeutic change. *Psychotherapy Research, 17*(1), 15–30. https://doi.org/10.1080/10503300600720390

Greenberg, L. S. (2011). *Emotion-focused therapy*. American Psychological Association.

Greenberg, L. S. (2015). *Emotion-focused therapy: Coaching clients to work through their feelings* (2nd ed.). American Psychological Association. https://doi.org/10.1037/14692-000

Greenberg, L. S. (2017). *Emotion-focused therapy* (Rev. ed.). American Psychological Association.

Greenberg, L. S. (2019). Theory of functioning in emotion-focused therapy. In L. S. Greenberg & R. N. Goldman (Eds.), *Clinical handbook of emotion-focused therapy* (pp. 37–59). American Psychological Association. https://doi.org/10.1037/0000112-002

Greenberg, L. S., & Angus, L. E. (2004). The contributions of emotion processes to narrative change in psychotherapy: A dialectical constructivist approach.

In L. E. Angus & J. McLeod (Eds.), *The handbook of narrative and psychotherapy: Practice, theory, and research* (pp. 330–349). SAGE Publishing. https://doi.org/10.4135/9781412973496.d25

Greenberg, L. S., Auszra, L., & Herrmann, I. R. (2007). The relationship among emotional productivity, emotional arousal, and outcome in experiential therapy of depression. *Psychotherapy Research, 17*(4), 482–493. https://doi.org/10.1080/10503300600977800

Greenberg, L. S., & Bolger, E. (2001). An emotion-focused approach to the overregulation of emotion and emotional pain. *Journal of Clinical Psychology, 57*(2), 197–211. https://doi.org/10.1002/1097-4679(200102)57:2<197::AID-JCLP6>3.0.CO;2-O

Greenberg, L. S., & Elliott, R. (1997). Varieties of empathic responding. In A. C. Bohart & L. S. Greenberg (Eds.), *Empathy reconsidered: New directions in psychotherapy* (pp. 167–186). American Psychological Association. https://doi.org/10.1037/10226-007

Greenberg, L. S., Ford, C. L., Alden, L. S., & Johnson, S. M. (1993). In-session change in emotionally focused therapy. *Journal of Consulting and Clinical Psychology, 61*(1), 78–84. https://doi.org/10.1037/0022-006X.61.1.78

Greenberg, L. S., & Geller, S. M. (2001). Congruence and therapeutic presence. In G. Wyatt (Eds), *Rogers' therapeutic conditions: Evolution, theory and practice: Vol 1. Congruence* (pp. 131–149). PCCS Books.

Greenberg, L. S., & Goldman, R. N. (2008). *Emotion-focused couples therapy: The dynamics of emotion, love and power*. American Psychological Association. https://doi.org/10.1037/11750-000

Greenberg, L. S., & Goldman, R. N. (2019). *Theory of practice of emotion-focused therapy*. In L. S. Greenberg & R. N. Goldman (Eds.), *Clinical handbook of emotion-focused therapy* (pp. 61–89). American Psychological Association. https://doi.org/10.1037/0000112-003

Greenberg, L. S., & Iwakabe, S. (2013). Emotion-focused therapy and shame. In R. L. Dearing & J. Tangney (Eds.), *Shame in the therapy hour* (pp. 69–90). American Psychological Association. https://doi.org/10.1037/12326-003

Greenberg, L. S., & Johnson, S. M. (1988). *Emotionally focused therapy for couples*. Guilford Press.

Greenberg, L. S., Malberg, N. T., & Tompkins, M. A. (2019). *Working with emotion in psychodynamic, cognitive behavior, and emotion-focused psychotherapy*. American Psychological Association. https://doi.org/10.1037/0000130-000

Greenberg, L. S., & Malcolm, W. (2002). Resolving unfinished business: Relating process to outcome. *Journal of Consulting and Clinical Psychology, 70*(2), 406–416. https://doi.org/10.1037/0022-006X.70.2.406

Greenberg, L. S., & Paivio, S. C. (1997). *Working with emotions in psychotherapy*. Guilford Press.

Greenberg, L. S., & Pascual-Leone, J. (1995). A dialectical constructivist approach to experiential change. In R. A. Neimeyer & M. J. Mahoney (Eds.), *Constructivism in psychotherapy* (pp. 169–191). American Psychological Association. https://doi.org/10.1037/10170-008

Greenberg, L. S., & Pascual-Leone, J. (2001). A dialectical constructivist view of the creation of personal meaning. *Journal of Constructivist Psychology, 14*(3), 165–186. https://doi.org/10.1080/10720530125970

Greenberg, L. S., & Pascual-Leone, A. (2006). Emotion in psychotherapy: A practice-friendly research review. *Journal of Clinical Psychology, 62*(5), 611–630. https://doi.org/10.1002/jclp.20252

Greenberg, L. S., Rice, L. N., & Elliott, R. K. (1993). *Facilitating emotional change: The moment-by-moment process.* Guilford Press.

Greenberg, L. S., & Ruchanski-Rosenberg, R. (2002). Therapists' experience of empathy. In J. C. Watson, R. N. Goldman, & M. S. Warner (Eds.), *Client-centered and experiential psychotherapy in the 21st century: Advances in theory, research and practice* (pp. 204–220). PCCS Books.

Greenberg, L. S., & Safran, J. D. (1987). *Emotion in psychotherapy: Affect, cognition, and the process of change.* Guilford Press.

Greenberg, L. J., Warwar, S. H., & Malcolm, W. M. (2008). Differential effects of emotion-focused therapy and psychoeducation in facilitating forgiveness and letting go of emotional injuries. *Journal of Counseling Psychology, 55*(2), 185–196. https://doi.org/10.1037/0022-0167.55.2.185

Greenberg, L. S., & Watson, J. (1998). Experiential therapy of depression: Differential effects of client-centered relationship conditions and process experiential interventions. *Psychotherapy Research, 8*(2), 210–224. https://doi.org/10.1080/10503309812331332317

Greenberg, L. S., & Watson, J. C. (2006). *Emotion-focused therapy for depression.* American Psychological Association. https://doi.org/10.1037/11286-000

Gross, J. J. (1998). The emerging field of emotion regulation: An integrative review. *Review of General Psychology, 2*(3), 271–299. https://doi.org/10.1037/1089-2680.2.3.271

Gross, J. J. (1999). Emotion and emotion regulation. In L. A. Pervin & O. P. John (Eds.), *Handbook of personality: Theory and research* (2nd ed., pp. 525–552). Guilford Press.

Gross, J. J. (2002). Emotion regulation: Affective, cognitive, and social consequences. *Psychophysiology, 39*(3), 281–291. https://doi.org/10.1017/S0048577201393198

Gross, J. J. (2013). Emotion regulation: Taking stock and moving forward. *Emotion, 13*(3), 359–365. https://doi.org/10.1037/a0032135

Gross, J. J., & John, O. P. (2003). Individual differences in two emotion regulation processes: Implications for affect, relationships, and well-being. *Journal of Personality and Social Psychology, 85*(2), 348–362. https://doi.org/10.1037/0022-3514.85.2.348

Gross, J. J., & Levenson, R. W. (1997). Hiding feelings: The acute effects of inhibiting negative and positive emotion. *Journal of Abnormal Psychology, 106*(1), 95–103. https://doi.org/10.1037/0021-843X.106.1.95

Hareli, S., Kafetsios, K., & Hess, U. (2015). A cross-cultural study on emotion expression and the learning of social norms. *Frontiers in Psychology, 6*, Article 1501. https://doi.org/10.3389/fpsyg.2015.01501

Harlow, H. F. (1960). Primary affectional patterns in primates. *American Journal of Orthopsychiatry, 30*(4), 676–684. https://doi.org/10.1111/j.1939-0025. 1960.tb02085.x

Harvey, A., Watkins, E., Mansell, W., & Shafran, R. (2004). *Cognitive behavioural processes across psychological disorders: a transdiagnostic approach to research and treatment.* Oxford University Press. https://doi.org/10.1093/med:psych/ 9780198528883.001.0001

Hayes, S. C., & Hofmann, S. G. (Eds.). (2018). *Process-based CBT: The science and core clinical competencies of cognitive behavioral therapy.* New Harbinger Publications.

Hayes, S. C., Strosahl, K. D., & Wilson, K. G. (2008). *Acceptance and commitment therapy: The process and practice of mindful change* (2nd ed.). Guilford Press.

Hebb, D. O. (1949). *The organization of behavior.* Wiley.

Heidegger, M. (2000). *Introduction to metaphysics* (G. Fried & R. Polt, Trans.; rev. ed.). Yale University Press. (Original work published 1953)

Hendricks, M. N. (2002). Focusing-oriented/experiential psychotherapy. In D. J. Cain (Ed.), *Humanistic psychotherapies: Handbook of research and practice* (pp. 221–251). American Psychological Association. https://doi.org/10.1037/ 10439-007

Herrmann, I. R., Greenberg, L. S., & Auszra, L. (2016). Emotion categories and patterns of change in experiential therapy for depression. *Psychotherapy Research, 26*(2), 178–195. https://doi.org/10.1080/10503307.2014.958597

His Holiness the Dalai Lama. (2001). *Ethics for the new millennium.* Riverhead Books.

Hofmann, S. G., & Doan, S. N. (2018). *The social foundations of emotion: Developmental, cultural, and clinical dimensions.* American Psychological Association. https://doi.org/10.1037/0000098-000

Hupbach, A., Hardt, O., Gomez, R., & Nadel, L. (2008). The dynamics of memory: Context-dependent updating. *Learning & Memory, 15*(8), 574–579. https:// doi.org/10.1101/lm.1022308

Hwang, J. (2006). *A processing model of emotion regulation: Insights from the attachment system* [Doctoral dissertation, Georgia State University]. ScholarWorks. *Dissertation Abstracts International: Section B. The Sciences and Engineering, 67*(4-B), 2280.

Iberg, J. R. (1991). Applying statistical control theory to bring together clinical supervision and psychotherapy research. *Journal of Consulting and Clinical Psychology, 59*(4), 575–586. https://doi.org/10.1037/0022-006X.59.4.575

Inda, M. C., Muravieva, E. V., & Alberini, C. M. (2011). Memory retrieval and the passage of time: From reconsolidation and strengthening to extinction. *The Journal of Neuroscience, 31*(5), 1635–1643. https://doi.org/10.1523/ JNEUROSCI.4736-10.2011

Ingram, B. L. (2006). *Clinical case formulations: Matching the integrative treatment plan to the client.* Wiley.

Ito, M., Greenberg, L. S., Iwakabe, S., & Pascual-Leone, A. (2010, June 2–5). *Compassionate emotion regulation: A task analytic approach to studying the process of self-soothing in therapy session* [Paper presentation]. World Congress of Behavioral and Cognitive Therapies, Boston, MA, United States.

James, W. (1890). *The principles of psychology*. Henry Holt and Company.

Jaycox, L. H., Foa, E. B., & Morral, A. R. (1998). Influence of emotional engagement and habituation on exposure therapy for PTSD. *Journal of Consulting and Clinical Psychology, 66*(1), 185–192. https://doi.org/10.1037/0022-006X.66.1.185

Johnson, S. M., & Greenberg, L. S. (1988). Relating process to outcome in marital therapy. *Journal of Marital and Family Therapy, 14*(2), 175–183. https://doi.org/10.1111/j.1752-0606.1988.tb00733.x

Jones, E. E., & Pulos, S. M. (1993). Comparing the process in psychodynamic and cognitive–behavioral therapies. *Journal of Consulting & Clinical Psychology, 61*(2), 306–316. https://doi.org/10.1037/0022-006X.61.2.306

Jurist, E. (2019). *Minding emotions: Cultivating mentalization in psychotherapy*. The Guilford Press.

Kashdan, T. B., Barrios, V., Forsyth, J. P., & Steger, M. F. (2006). Experiential avoidance as a generalized psychological vulnerability: Comparisons with coping and emotion regulation strategies. *Behaviour Research and Therapy, 44*(9), 1301–1320. https://doi.org/10.1016/j.brat.2005.10.003

Kendi, I. X. (2019). *How to be an antiracist*. One World.

Kendler, K. S. (1996). Major depression and generalised anxiety disorder: Same genes, (partly) different environments—Revisited. *The British Journal of Psychiatry, 168*(S30), 68–75. https://doi.org/10.1192/S0007125000298437

Kennedy-Moore, E., & Watson, J. C. (1999). *Expressing emotion: Myths, realities, and therapeutic strategies*. Guilford Press.

Kernberg, O. (1967). Borderline personality organization. *Journal of the American Psychoanalytic Association, 15*(3), 641–685. https://doi.org/10.1177/000306516701500309

Kernberg, O. F. (1984). *Object relations theory and clinical psychoanalysis*. Jason Aronson.

Kerr, T., Walsh, J., & Marshall, A. (2001). Emotional change processes in music-assisted reframing. *Journal of Music Therapy, 38*(3), 193–211. https://doi.org/10.1093/jmt/38.3.193

Kessler, R. C., Berglund, P., Demler, O., Jin, R., Merikangas, K. R., & Walters, E. E. (2005). Lifetime prevalence and age-of-onset distributions of *DSM-IV* disorders in the National Comorbidity Survey Replication. *Archives of General Psychiatry, 62*(6), 593–602. https://doi.org/10.1001/archpsyc.62.6.593

Kircanski, K., Lieberman, M. D., & Craske, M. G. (2012). Feelings into words: Contributions of language to exposure therapy. *Psychological Science, 23*(10), 1086–1091. https://doi.org/10.1177/0956797612443830

Kitayama, S., Markus, H. R., & Kurokawa, M. (2000). Culture, emotion, and well-being: Good feelings in Japan and the United States. *Cognition and Emotion, 14*(1), 93–124. https://doi.org/10.1080/026999300379003

Klein, M. H., Mathieu, P. L., Gendlin, E. T., & Kiesler, D. J. (1969). *The Experiencing Scale: A research and training manual: Volume 1.* Wisconsin Psychiatric Institute.

Klein, M. H., Mathieu-Coughlan, P., & Kiesler, D. J. (1986). The experiencing scales. In L. S. Greenberg & W. Pinsof (Eds.), *The psychotherapeutic process: A research handbook* (pp. 21–71). Guilford Press.

Kramer, U., & Pascual-Leone, A. (2016). The role of maladaptive anger in self-criticism: A quasi-experimental study on emotional processes. *Counselling Psychology Quarterly, 29*(3), 311–333. https://doi.org/10.1080/09515070.2015.1090395

Kramer, U., Pascual-Leone, A., Berthoud, L., de Roten, Y., Marquet, P., Kolly, S., Despland, J. N., & Page, D. (2016). Assertive anger mediates effects of dialectical behavior-informed skills training for borderline personality disorder: A randomized controlled trial. *Clinical Psychology & Psychotherapy, 23*(3), 189–202. https://doi.org/10.1002/cpp.1956

Kramer, U., Pascual-Leone, A., Despland, J.-N., & de Roten, Y. (2015). One minute of grief: Emotional processing in short-term dynamic psychotherapy for adjustment disorder. *Journal of Consulting and Clinical Psychology, 83*(1), 187–198. https://doi.org/10.1037/a0037979

Lane, R. D., Ryan, L., Nadel, L., & Greenberg, L. (2015). Memory reconsolidation, emotional arousal, and the process of change in psychotherapy: New insights from brain science. *Behavioral and Brain Sciences, 38*, Article E1. Advance online publication. https://doi.org/10.1017/S0140525X14000041

LeDoux, J. E. (1996). *The emotional brain: The mysterious underpinnings of emotional life.* Simon & Schuster.

LeDoux, J. E. (2012). Rethinking the emotional brain. *Neuron, 73*(4), 653–676. https://doi.org/10.1016/j.neuron.2012.02.004

Le Grange, D., Swanson, S. A., Crow, S. J., & Merikangas, K. R. (2012). Eating disorder not otherwise specified presentation in the U.S. population. *International Journal of Eating Disorders, 45*(5), 711–718. https://doi.org/10.1002/eat.22006

Leijssen, M. (1998). Focusing microprocesses. In L. S. Greenberg, J. C. Watson, & G. Lietaer (Eds.), *Handbook of experiential psychotherapy* (pp. 121–154). Guilford Press.

Leijssen, M. (1996–1997). Focusing processes in client-centered/experiential psychotherapy. An overview of my research findings. *The Folio: A Journal for Focusing and Experiential Therapy, 15*(2), 1–6.

Leijssen, M., Lietaer, G., Stevens, I., & Wels, G. (2000). Focusing training for stagnating clients: An analysis of four cases. In J. Marques-Teixeira & S. Antunes (Eds.), *Client-centered and experiential psychotherapy* (pp. 207–224). Vale & Vale.

Levinas, E. (1969). *Totality and infinity: An essay on exteriority* (A. Lingis, Trans.). Duquesne University Press.

Levinas, E. (2000). *Entre nous: On thinking-of-the-other* (B. Harshav & M. B. Smith, Trans.). Columbia University Press.

Levine, P. (2010). *In an unspoken voice: How the body releases trauma and restores goodness*. North Atlantic Books.

Levy Berg, A., Sandell, R., & Sandahl, C. (2009). Affect-focused body psychotherapy in patients with generalized anxiety disorder: Evaluation of an integrative method. *Journal of Psychotherapy Integration, 19*(1), 67–85. https://doi.org/10.1037/a0015324

Lewin, J. K. (2001). *Both sides of the coin: Comparative analyses of narrative process patterns in poor and good outcome dyads engaged in brief experiential psychotherapy for depression* [Unpublished master's thesis]. York University.

Lieberman, M. D., Eisenberger, N. I., Crockett, M. J., Tom, S. M., Pfeifer, J. H., & Way, B. M. (2007). Putting feelings into words: Affect labeling disrupts amygdala activity in response to affective stimuli. *Psychological Science, 18*(5), 421–428. https://doi.org/10.1111/j.1467-9280.2007.01916.x

Lin, K. M. (1983). Hwa-Byung: A Korean culture-bound syndrome? *The American Journal of Psychiatry, 140*(1), 105–107. https://doi.org/10.1176/ajp.140.1.105

Linehan, M. M. (1993). *Cognitive–behavioral treatment of borderline personality disorder*. Guilford Press.

Luedke, A. J., Peluso, P. R., Diaz, P., Freund, R., & Baker, A. (2017). Predicting dropout in counseling using affect coding of the therapeutic relationship: An empirical analysis. *Journal of Counseling and Development, 95*(2), 125–134. https://doi.org/10.1002/jcad.12125

MacLeod, R., Elliott, R., & Rodgers, B. (2012). Process-experiential/emotion-focused therapy for social anxiety: A hermeneutic single-case efficacy design study. *Psychotherapy Research, 22*(1), 67–81. https://doi.org/10.1080/10503307.2011.626805

Magnavita, J. J. (2008). Toward unification of clinical science: The next wave in the evolution of psychotherapy? *Journal of Psychotherapy Integration, 18*(3), 264–291. https://doi.org/10.1037/a0013490

Magnavita, J. J., & Anchin, J. C. (2014). *Unifying psychotherapy: Principles, methods, and evidence from clinical science*. Springer Publishing Company.

Makinen, J. A., & Johnson, S. M. (2006). Resolving attachment injuries in couples using emotionally focused therapy: Steps toward forgiveness and reconciliation. *Journal of Consulting and Clinical Psychology, 74*(6), 1055–1064. https://doi.org/10.1037/0022-006X.74.6.1055

Maren, S. (2011). Seeking a spotless mind: Extinction, deconsolidation, and erasure of fear memory. *Neuron, 70*(5), 830–845. https://doi.org/10.1016/j.neuron.2011.04.023

Markowitsch, H. J. (1998). Differential contribution of right and left amygdala to affective information processing. *Behavioural Neurology, 11*(4), 233–244.

Markus, H. R., & Kitayama, S. (1991). Culture and the self: Implications for cognition, emotion, and motivation. *Psychological Review, 98*(2), 224–253. https://doi.org/10.1037/0033-295X.98.2.224

Markus, H. R., & Kitayama, S. (2001). The cultural construction of self and emotion: Implications for social behavior. In W. G. Parrott (Ed.), *Emotions in social psychology: Essential reading* (pp. 119–137). Psychology Press.

Maslow, A. H. (1954). *Motivation and personality*. Harper and Row.

Maslow, A. H. (1968). *Toward a psychology of being* (2nd ed.). D. Van Nostrand.

McCullough, L. (1999). Short-term psychodynamic therapy as a form of desensitization: Treating affect phobias. *In Session: Psychotherapy in Practice*, 4(4), 35–53. https://doi.org/10.1002/(SICI)1520-6572(199924)4:4<35::AID-SESS4>3.0.CO;2-G

McCullough, L., Kuhn, N., Andrews, S., Kaplan, A., Wolf, J., & Hurley, C. L. (2003). *Treating affect phobia: A manual for short term dynamic psychotherapy*. Guilford Press.

McGaugh, J. L. (2002). Memory consolidation and the amygdala: A systems perspective. *Trends in Neurosciences*, 25(9), 456–461. https://doi.org/10.1016/S0166-2236(02)02211-7

McGilchrist, I. (2009). *The master and his emissary: The divided brain and the making of the Western world*. Yale University Press.

McKinnon, J. M., & Greenberg, L. S. (2013). Revealing underlying vulnerable emotion in couple therapy: Impact on session and final outcome. *Journal of Family Therapy*, 35(3), 303–319. https://doi.org/10.1111/1467-6427.12015

McWilliams, N. (1994). *Psychoanalytic diagnosis: Understanding personality structure in the clinical process*. Guilford Press.

Merleau-Ponty, M. (1962). *Phenomenology of perception* (C. Smith, Trans.). Routledge and Kegan Paul. (Original work published 1945)

Merleau-Ponty, M. (1964). *Sense and nonsense* (H. L. Dreyfus & P. A. Dreyfus, Trans.). Northwestern University Press. (Original work published 1948)

Merleau-Ponty, M. (1968). *The visible and the invisible* (C. Lefort, Ed., & A. Lingis, Trans.). Northwestern University Press.

Merrill, C. (2008). Carl Rogers and Martin Buber in dialogue: The meeting of divergent paths. *The Person-Centred Journal*, 15(1–2), 4–12.

Mesquita, B., & Albert, D. (2007). The cultural regulation of emotions. In J. J. Gross (Ed.), *Handbook of emotion regulation* (pp. 486–503). Guilford Press.

Miller, W. R., & Rollnick, S. (2013). *Motivational interviewing: Helping people change* (3rd ed.). Guilford Press.

Min, S. K., Suh, S.-Y., & Song, K.-J. (2009). Symptoms to use for diagnostic criteria of Hwa-Byung, an anger syndrome. *Psychiatry Investigation*, 6(1), 7–12. https://doi.org/10.4306/pi.2009.6.1.7

Missirlian, T. M., Toukmanian, S. G., Warwar, S. H., & Greenberg, L. S. (2005). Emotional arousal, client perceptual processing, and the working alliance in experiential psychotherapy for depression. *Journal of Consulting and Clinical Psychology*, 73(5), 861–871. https://doi.org/10.1037/0022-006X.73.5.861

Morikawa, Y. (1997). Making practical the focusing manner of experiencing in everyday life: A consideration of factor analysis. *The Journal of Japanese Clinical Psychology*, 15(1), 58–65.

Morin, A. (2020, September 20). *7 strategies to help you on your anti-racism journey.* Verywell Mind. https://www.verywellmind.com/anti-racism-strategies-5069386

Munder, T., Brütsch, O., Leonhart, R., Gerger, H., & Barth, J. (2013). Researcher allegiance in psychotherapy outcome research: An overview of reviews. *Clinical Psychology Review, 33*(4), 501–511. https://doi.org/10.1016/j.cpr.2013.02.002

Murray, H. A. (1938). *Explorations in personality.* Oxford University Press.

Myers, D. G. (1996). *Exploring psychology* (3rd ed.). Worth Publishers.

Nadel, L., & Bohbot, V. (2001). Consolidation of memory. *Hippocampus, 11*, 56–60. https://doi.org/10.1002/1098-1063(2001)11:1<56::AID-HIPO1020>3.0.CO;2-O

Nadel, L., Hupbach, A., Gomez, R., & Newman-Smith, K. (2012). Memory formation, consolidation and transformation. *Neuroscience and Biobehavioral Reviews, 36*(7), 1640–1645. https://doi.org/10.1016/j.neubiorev.2012.03.001

Nadel, L., & Moscovitch, M. (1997). Memory consolidation, retrograde amnesia and the hippocampal complex. *Current Opinion in Neurobiology, 7*(2), 217–227. https://doi.org/10.1016/S0959-4388(97)80010-4

Nader, K. (2003). Memory traces unbound. *Trends in Neuroscience, 26*(2), 65–72. https://doi.org/10.1016/S0166-2236(02)00042-5

Nader, K., & Hardt, O. (2009). A single standard for memory: The case for reconsolidation. *Nature Reviews Neuroscience, 10*, 224–234. https://doi.org/10.1038/nrn2590

Nader, K., Schafe, G. E., & LeDoux, J. E. (2000). Fear memories require protein synthesis in the amygdala for reconsolidation after retrieval. *Nature, 406*(6797), 722–726. https://doi.org/10.1038/35021052

Nichols, M. P., & Efran, J. S. (1985). Catharsis in psychotherapy: A new perspective. *Psychotherapy, 22*(1), 46–58. https://doi.org/10.1037/h0088525

Nichols, M. P., & Zax, M. (1977). *Catharsis in psychotherapy.* Gardner Press.

Norcross, J. C., & Goldfried, M. R. (Eds.). (1992). *Handbook of psychotherapy integration.* Basic Books.

Oatley, K., Keltner, D., & Jenkins, J. M. (2006). *Understanding emotions* (2nd ed.). Blackwell Publishing.

Ogden, P. (2015). *Sensorimotor psychotherapy: Interventions for trauma and attachment.* W. W. Norton.

Ogrodniczuk, J. S., Piper, W. E., & Joyce, A. S. (2008). Alexithymia and therapist reactions to the patient: Expression of positive emotion as a mediator. *Psychiatry, 71*(3), 257–265. https://doi.org/10.1521/psyc.2008.71.3.257

Orlinsky, D. E., & Howard, K. I. (1986). Process and outcome in psychotherapy. In S. L. Garfield & A. E. Bergin (Eds.), *Handbook of psychotherapy and behavior change* (3rd ed.; pp. 311–384). John Wiley & Sons.

Paivio, S. C., & Greenberg, L. S. (1995). Resolving "unfinished business": Efficacy of experiential therapy using empty-chair dialogue. *Journal of Consulting and Clinical Psychology, 63*(3), 419–425. https://doi.org/10.1037/0022-006X.63.3.419

Paivio, S. C., Hall, I. E., Holowaty, K. A. M., Jellis, J. B., & Tran, N. (2001). Imaginal confrontation for resolving child abuse issues. *Psychotherapy Research, 11*(4), 433–453. https://doi.org/10.1093/ptr/11.4.433

Paivio, S. C., & Nieuwenhuis, J. A. (2001). Efficacy of emotion focused therapy for adult survivors of child abuse: A preliminary study. *Journal of Traumatic Stress, 14*, 115–133. https://doi.org/10.1023/A:1007891716593

Paivio, S. C., & Pascual-Leone, A. (2010). *Emotion-focused therapy for complex trauma: An integrative approach.* American Psychological Association. https://doi.org/10.1037/12077-000

Panksepp, J. (1998). *Affective neuroscience: The foundations of human and animal emotions.* Oxford University Press.

Panksepp, J., & Biven, L. (2012). *The archeology of mind.* W. W. Norton & Company.

Parrott, W. G., & Sabini, J. (1990). Mood and memory under natural conditions: Evidence for mood incongruent recall. *Journal of Personality and Social Psychology, 59*(2), 321–336. https://doi.org/10.1037/0022-3514.59.2.321

Pascual-Leone, A. (2018). How clients "change emotion with emotion": A programme of research on emotional processing. *Psychotherapy Research, 28*(2), 165–182. https://doi.org/10.1080/10503307.2017.1349350

Pascual-Leone, A., & Greenberg, L. S. (2007). Emotional processing in experiential therapy: Why "the only way out is through." *Journal of Consulting and Clinical Psychology, 75*(6), 875–887. https://doi.org/10.1037/0022-006X.75.6.875

Pascual-Leone, A., & Yeryomenko, N. (2016). The client "experiencing" scale as a predictor of treatment outcomes: A meta-analysis on psychotherapy process. *Psychotherapy Research, 27*(6), 653–665. https://doi.org/10.1080/10503307.2016.1152409

Pascual-Leone, J. (1987). Organismic processes for neo-Piagetian theories: A dialectical causal account of cognitive development. *International Journal of Psychology, 22*(5–6), 531–569. https://doi.org/10.1080/00207598708246795

Pascual-Leone, J. (1991). Emotions, development, and psychotherapy: A dialectical-constructivist perspective. In J. D. Safran & L. S. Greenberg (Eds.), *Emotion, psychotherapy, and change* (pp. 302–335). Guilford Press.

Pascual-Leone, J., & Johnson, J. (1991). The psychological unit and its role in task analysis. A reinterpretation of object permanence. In M. Chandler & M. Chapman (Eds.), *Criteria for competence: Controversies in the assessment of children's abilities* (pp. 153–187). Lawrence Erlbaum Associates.

Pascual-Leone, J., & Johnson, J. (2011). A developmental theory of mental attention: Its applications to measurement and task analysis. In P. Barrouillet & V. Gaillard (Eds.), *Cognitive development and working memory: A dialogue between neo-Piagetian and cognitive approaches* (pp. 13–46). Psychology Press.

Paul, G. L. (1967). Strategy of outcome research in psychotherapy. *Journal of Consulting Psychology, 31*(2), 109–118. https://doi.org/10.1037/h0024436

Peluso, P. R., & Freund, R. R. (2018). Therapist and client emotional expression and psychotherapy outcomes: A meta-analysis. *Psychotherapy, 55*(4), 461–472. https://doi.org/10.1037/pst0000165

Peluso, P. R., Liebovitch, L. S., Gottman, J. M., Norman, M. D., & Su, J. (2012). A mathematical model of psychotherapy: An investigation using dynamic non-linear equations to model the therapeutic relationship. *Psychotherapy Research, 22*(1), 40–55. https://doi.org/10.1080/10503307.2011.622314

Pennebaker, J. W. (1990). *Opening up: The healing power of confiding in others.* William Morrow.

Perls, F. S. (1969). *Gestalt therapy verbatim.* Real People Press.

Perls, F. S. (1973). *The Gestalt approach & eye witness to therapy.* Bantam Books.

Perls, F. S., Hefferline, R. F., & Goodman, P. (1951). *Gestalt therapy.* Julian Press.

Piliero, S. (2004). *Patients reflect on their affect-focused experiential psychotherapy: A retrospective study* [Doctoral dissertation, Adelphi University]. *Dissertation Abstracts International: Section B. The Sciences and Engineering, 65*(4-B), 2108.

Pine, F. (1986). On the development of the "borderline-child-to-be." *American Journal of Orthopsychiatry, 56*(3), 450–457. https://doi.org/10.1111/j.1939-0025.1986.tb03476.x

Porges, S. W. (2004). Neuroception: A subconscious system for detecting threats and safety. *Zero to Three, 24*(5), 19–24.

Porges, S. W. (2007). The polyvagal perspective. *Biological Psychology, 74*(2), 116–143. https://doi.org/10.1016/j.biopsycho.2006.06.009

Porges, S. W. (2011). *The polyvagal theory: Neuro-physiological foundations of emotions, attachment, communication, self-regulation.* W. W. Norton & Company.

Pos, A. E., & Greenberg, L. S. (2012). Organizing awareness and increasing emotion regulation: Revising chair work in emotion-focused therapy for borderline personality disorder. *Journal of Personality Disorders, 26*(1), 84–107. https://doi.org/10.1521/pedi.2012.26.1.84

Pos, A. E., Greenberg, L. S., Goldman, R. N., & Korman, L. M. (2003). Emotional processing during experiential treatment of depression. *Journal of Consulting and Clinical Psychology, 71*(6), 1007–1016. https://doi.org/10.1037/0022-006X.71.6.1007

Pos, A. E., Greenberg, L. S., & Warwar, S. H. (2009). Testing a model of change in the experiential treatment of depression. *Journal of Consulting and Clinical Psychology, 77*(6), 1055–1066. https://doi.org/10.1037/a0017059

Pos, A. E., & Paolone, D. A. (2019). *Emotion-focused therapy for personality disorders.* In L. S. Greenberg & R. N. Goldman (Eds.), *Clinical handbook of emotion-focused therapy* (pp. 381–402). American Psychological Association. https://doi.org/10.1037/0000112-017

Prochaska, J. O., & DiClemente, C. C. (1983). Stages and processes of self-change of smoking: Toward an integrative model of change. *Journal of Consulting and Clinical Psychology, 51*(3), 390–395. https://doi.org/10.1037/0022-006X.51.3.390

Purton, C. (2004). *Person-centred therapy: The focusing-oriented approach.* Palgrave Macmillan.

Rice, L. N., & Kerr, G. P. (1986). Measures of client and therapist vocal quality. In L. S. Greenberg & W. M. Pinsof (Eds.), *The psychotherapeutic process: A research handbook* (pp. 73–105). Guilford Press.

Rice, L. N., Koke, C., Greenberg, L. S., & Wagstaff, A. (1979). *Manual for client vocal quality.* York University Counselling and Development Centre.

Rice, L. N., & Wagstaff, A. K. (1967). Client voice quality and expressive style as indexes of productive psychotherapy. *Journal of Consulting Psychology, 31*(6), 557–563. https://doi.org/10.1037/h0025164

Richman, L. S., & Leary, M. R. (2009). Reactions to discrimination, stigmatization, ostracism, and other forms of interpersonal rejection. *Psychological Review, 116*(2), 365–383.

Roemer, L., Salters, K., Raffa, S. D., & Orsillo, S. M. (2005). Fear and avoidance of internal experiences in GAD: Preliminary tests of a conceptual model. *Cognitive Therapy and Research, 29,* 71–88. https://doi.org/10.1007/s10608-005-1650-2

Rogers, C. R. (1957). The necessary and sufficient conditions of therapeutic personality change. *Journal of Consulting Psychology, 21*(2), 95–103. https://doi.org/10.1037/h0045357

Rogers, C. R. (1959). A theory of therapy, personality and interpersonal relationships, as developed in the client-centered framework. In S. Koch (Ed.), *Psychology: A study of a science* (Vol. 3, pp. 184–256). McGraw Hill.

Rogers, C. R. (1980). *A way of being.* Houghton Mifflin.

Ruby, M. B., Falk, C. F., Heine, S. J., Villa, C., & Silberstein, O. (2012). Not all collectivisms are equal: Opposing preferences for ideal affect between East Asians and Mexicans. *Emotion, 12*(6), 1206–1209. https://doi.org/10.1037/a0029118

Russell, J. A. (2003). Core affect and the psychological construction of emotion. *Psychological Review, 110*(1), 145–172. https://doi.org/10.1037/0033-295X.110.1.145

Sachse, R. (2019). Case conceptualization in clarification-oriented psychotherapy. In U. Kramer (Ed.), *Case formulation for personality disorders: Tailoring psychotherapy to the individual client* (pp. 113–135). Elsevier Academic Press. https://doi.org/10.1016/B978-0-12-813521-1.00007-2

Safdar, S., Friedlmeier, W., Matsumoto, D., Yoo, S. H., Dwantes, C. T., Kakai, H., & Shigemasu, E. (2009). Variations of emotional display rules within and across cultures: A comparison between Canada, USA, and Japan. *Canadian Journal of Behavioural Science, 41*(1), 1–10. https://doi.org/10.1037/a0014387

Safran, J. D., & Muran, J. C. (2000). *Negotiating the therapeutic alliance: A relational treatment guide.* Guilford Press.

Sarbin, T. R. (Ed.). (1986). *Narrative psychology: The storied nature of human conduct.* Praeger.

Schank, R. C. (2000). *Tell me a story: Narrative and intelligence.* Northwestern University Press.

Scherer, A., Boecker, M., Pawelzik, M., Gauggel, S., & Forkmann, T. (2017). Emotion suppression, not reappraisal, predicts psychotherapy outcome. *Psychotherapy Research, 27*(2), 143–153. https://doi.org/10.1080/10503307.2015.1080875

Schore, A. N. (1994). *Affect regulation and the origin of the self: The neurobiology of emotional development*. Lawrence Erlbaum Associates.

Schore, A. N. (2003). *Affect dysregulation and disorders of the self*. W. W. Norton & Company.

Shahar, B. (2014). Emotion-focused therapy for the treatment of social anxiety: An overview of the model and a case description. *Clinical Psychology & Psychotherapy, 21*(6), 536–547. https://doi.org/10.1002/cpp.1853

Shahar, B., Bar-Kalifa, E., & Alon, E. (2017). Emotion-focused therapy for social anxiety disorder: Results from a multiple-baseline study. *Journal of Consulting and Clinical Psychology, 85*(3), 238–249. https://doi.org/10.1037/ccp0000166

Shahar, B., Doron, G., & Szepsenwol, O. (2015). Childhood maltreatment, shame-proneness and self-criticism in social anxiety disorder: A sequential mediational model. *Clinical Psychology & Psychotherapy, 22*(6), 570–579. https://doi.org/10.1002/cpp.1918

Sicoli, L. A. (2005). *Development and verification of a model of resolving hopelessness in process-experiential therapy of depression* (Publication No. 2006-99014-142) [Doctoral dissertation, York University]. ProQuest Dissertations and Theses Global.

Silberschatz, G., Fretter, P. B., & Curtis, J. T. (1986). How do interpretations influence the process of psychotherapy? *Journal of Consulting and Clinical Psychology, 54*(5), 646–652. https://doi.org/10.1037/0022-006X.54.5.646

Sloan, E., Hall, K., Moulding, R., Bryce, S., Mildred, H., & Staiger, P. K. (2017). Emotion regulation as a transdiagnostic treatment construct across anxiety, depression, substance, eating and borderline personality disorders: A systematic review. *Clinical Psychology Review, 57*, 141–163. https://doi.org/10.1016/j.cpr.2017.09.002

Spinoza, B. (1967). *Ethics (part IV)*. Hafner Publishing Company.

Sroufe, A. L. (1996). *Emotional development: The organization of emotional life in the early years*. Cambridge University Press.

Staunton, H. (Ed.). (1898). *The plays of Shakespeare* (Vol. 1). George Routledge.

Stern, D. N. (1985). *The interpersonal world of the infant: A view from psychoanalysis and developmental psychology*. Basic Books.

Stricker, G., & Gold, J. R. (Eds.). (1993). *Comprehensive handbook of psychotherapy integration*. Plenum Press.

Tamietto, M., & de Gelder, B. (2010). Neural bases of the non-conscious perception of emotional signals. *Nature Reviews Neuroscience, 11*, 697–709. https://doi.org/10.1038/nrn2889

Taylor, C. (1990). *Human agency and language*. Cambridge University Press.

Timulak, L. (2015). *Transforming emotional pain in psychotherapy: An emotion-focused approach*. Routledge.

Timulak, L., & McElvaney, J. (2016). Emotion-focused therapy for generalized anxiety disorder: An overview of the model. *Journal of Contemporary Psychotherapy, 46*(1), 41–52. https://doi.org/10.1007/s10879-015-9310-7

Totton, N. (2003). *Body psychotherapy: An introduction*. Open University Press.

Tugade, M. M., & Fredrickson, B. L. (2004). Resilient individuals use positive emotions to bounce back from negative emotional experiences. *Journal of Personality and Social Psychology, 86*(2), 320–333. https://doi.org/10.1037/0022-3514.86.2.320

Vrana, G. (2020). *A task analysis of the resolution of aversion to emotion and self-interruption in emotion-focused therapy* [Unpublished doctoral dissertation]. York University.

Warwar, S. H. (2005). Relating emotional processing to outcome in experiential psychotherapy of depression. *Dissertation Abstracts International: B. The Sciences and Engineering, 66*, 581.

Warwar, S. H., & Greenberg, L. S. (1999). *Client Emotional Arousal Scale–III–R* [Unpublished manuscript]. York Psychotherapy Research Clinic, York University.

Warwar, S. H., Greenberg, L. S., & Perepeluk, D. (2003, June). *Reported in-session emotional experience in therapy* [Paper presentation]. 34th International Annual Meeting of the Society for Psychotherapy Research, Weimar, Germany.

Warwar, S. H., Links, P. S., Greenberg, L., & Bergmans, Y. (2008). Emotion-focused principles for working with borderline personality disorder. *Journal of Psychiatric Practice, 14*(2), 94–104. https://doi.org/10.1097/01.pra.0000314316.02416.3e

Watson, J. C. (2019). Role of the therapeutic relationship in emotion-focused therapy. In L. S. Greenberg & R.N. Goldman (Eds.), *Clinical handbook of emotion-focused therapy* (pp. 111–128). American Psychological Association. https://doi.org/10.1037/0000112-005

Watson, J. C., Timulak, L., & Greenberg, L. S. (2019). Emotion-focused therapy for generalized anxiety disorder. In L. S. Greenberg & R. N. Goldman (Eds.), *Clinical handbook of emotion-focused therapy* (pp. 315–336). American Psychological Association. https://doi.org/10.1037/0000112-014

Watson, J. C. (2002). *Re-visioning empathy*. In D. J. Cain (Ed.), *Humanistic psychotherapies: Handbook of research and practice* (pp. 445–471). American Psychological Association. https://doi.org/10.1037/10439-014

Watson, J. C. (2016). The role of empathy in psychotherapy: Theory, research and practice. In D. J. Cain, K. Keenan, & S. Rubin (Eds.), *Humanistic psychotherapies: Handbook of research and practice* (2nd ed., pp. 115–145). American Psychological Association.

Watson, J. C., & Bedard, D. L. (2006). Clients' emotional processing in psychotherapy: A comparison between cognitive-behavioral and process-experiential therapies. *Journal of Consulting and Clinical Psychology, 74*(1), 152–159. https://doi.org/10.1037/0022-006X.74.1.152

Watson, J. C., Chekan, S. S., & McMullen, E. (2017). Emotion-focused psychotherapy for GAD: Individual case comparison of a good and poor outcome case. *Person-Centered and Experiential Psychotherapies, 16*(2), 118–139. https://doi.org/10.1080/14779757.2017.1330707

Watson, J. C., Goldman, R. N., & Greenberg, L. S. (2007). *Case studies in emotion-focused treatment of depression: A comparison of good and poor outcome.* American Psychological Association. https://doi.org/10.1037/11586-000

Watson, J. C., Gordon, L. B., Stermac, L., Kalogerakos, F., & Steckley, P. (2003). Comparing the effectiveness of process-experiential with cognitive-behavioral psychotherapy in the treatment of depression. *Journal of Consulting and Clinical Psychology, 71*(4), 773–781. https://doi.org/10.1037/0022-006X.71.4.773

Watson, J. C., & Greenberg, L. S. (1996). Pathways to change in the psychotherapy of depression: Relating process to session change and outcome. *Psychotherapy, 33*(2), 262–274. https://doi.org/10.1037/0033-3204.33.2.262

Watson, J. C., & Greenberg, L. S. (2017). *Emotion-focused therapy for generalized anxiety.* American Psychological Association. https://doi.org/10.1037/0000018-000

Watson, J. C., & McMullen, E. J. (2005). An examination of therapist and client behavior in high- and low-alliance sessions in cognitive-behavioral therapy and process experiential therapy. *Psychotherapy, 42*(3), 297–310. https://doi.org/10.1037/0033-3204.42.3.297

Watson, J. C., & Prosser, M. (2002). Development of an observer-related measure of therapist empathy. In J. Watson, R. Goldman, & M. Warner (Eds.), *Client-centered and experiential psychotherapy in the 21st century: Advances in theory, research, and practice* (pp. 3030–314). PCCS Books.

Watson, J. C., Steckley, P. L., & McMullen, E. J. (2014). The role of empathy in promoting change. *Psychotherapy Research, 24*(3), 286–298. https://doi.org/10.1080/10503307.2013.802823

Webb, T. L., Miles, E., & Sheeran, P. (2012). Dealing with feeling: A meta-analysis of the effectiveness of strategies derived from the process model of emotion regulation. *Psychological Bulletin, 138*(4), 775–808. https://doi.org/10.1037/a0027600

Webster, M. (2019). *Emotion-focused psychotherapy: A practitioner's guide.* The Annandale Institute.

Weiss, J., Sampson, H., & Mt. Zion Psychotherapy Research Group. (1986). *The psychoanalytic process: Theory, clinical observations, and empirical research.* Guilford Press.

Weston, J. L. (2018). *Protection from dangerous emotions: interruption of emotional experience in psychotherapy* [Unpublished doctoral dissertation]. York University. https://yorkspace.library.yorku.ca/xmlui/bitstream/handle/10315/34982/Weston_Janice_L_2018_PhD.pdf?sequence=2&isAllowed=y

Whelton, W. J. (2004). Emotional processing in psychotherapy: Evidence across therapeutic modalities. *Clinical Psychology & Psychotherapy, 11*(1), 58–71. https://doi.org/10.1002/cpp.392

Whelton, W. J., & Greenberg, L. S. (2000). The self as a singular multiplicity: A process-experiential perspective. In J. C. Muran (Ed.), *Self-relations in the psychotherapy process* (pp. 87–110). American Psychological Association. https://doi.org/10.1037/10391-004

White, R. W. (1959). Motivation reconsidered: The concept of competence. *Psychological Review, 66*(5), 297–333. https://doi.org/10.1037/h0040934

Wile, D. B. (1992). *Couples therapy: A nontraditional approach.* John Wiley & Sons.

Williams, J. M. G., Barnhofer, T., Crane, C., Herman, D., Raes, F., Watkins, E., & Dalgleish, T. (2007). Autobiographical memory specificity and emotional disorder. *Psychological Bulletin, 133*(1), 122–148. https://doi.org/10.1037/0033-2909.133.1.122

Wingfield, A. H. (2010). Are some emotions marked "whites only"? Racialized feeling rules in professional workplaces. *Social Problems, 57*(2), 251–268. https://doi.org/10.1525/sp.2010.57.2.251

Winnicott, D. W. (1965). *The maturational processes and the facilitating environment.* International Universities Press.

Wong, C. F., Schrager, S. M., Holloway, I. W., Meyer, I. H., & Kipke, M. D. (2014). Minority stress experiences and psychological well-being: The impact of support from and connection to social networks within the Los Angeles House and Ball communities. *Prevention Science, 15*, 44–55. https://doi.org/10.1007/s11121-012-0348-4

Ye, Z. (2002). Different modes of describing emotions in Chinese: Bodily changes, sensations, and bodily images. *Pragmatics & Cognition, 10*(1–2), 307–339. https://doi.org/10.1075/pc.10.12.13ye

Yeomans, F. E., Clarkin, J. F., & Kernberg, O. F. (2015). *Transference-focused psychotherapy for borderline personality disorder: A clinical guide.* American Psychiatric Publishing. https://doi.org/10.1176/appi.books.9781615371006

Zimbardo, P. G., Ebbesen, E. B., & Maslach, C. (1977). *Influencing attitudes and changing behavior: An introduction to method, theory, and applications of social control and personal power* (2nd ed.). Addison-Wesley Publishing Company.

Index

About the Author

Leslie S. Greenberg, PhD, is Distinguished Research Professor Emeritus of Psychology at York University in Toronto, Canada, and the primary developer of emotion-focused therapy. He authored two of the first clinical titles in the field: *Emotion in Psychotherapy: Affect, Cognition, and the Process of Change* (with Jeremy D. Safran; 1987) and *Emotionally Focused Therapy for Couples* (with Susan M. Johnson; 1988). More recent books include *Emotion-Focused Couples Therapy: The Dynamics of Emotion, Love and Power* (with Rhonda N. Goldman; 2008), *Therapeutic Presence: A Mindful Approach to Effective Therapy* (with Shari M. Geller; 2012), the second edition of *Emotion-Focused Therapy: Coaching Clients to Work Through Their Feelings* (2015), *Emotion-Focused Therapy for Generalized Anxiety* (with Jeanne C. Watson; 2017), and *Forgiveness and Letting Go in Emotion-Focused Therapy* (with Catalina Woldarsky Meneses; 2019). Dr. Greenberg currently conducts international trainings on emotion-focused approaches. He has received the Distinguished Career (Senior) Award of the Society for Psychotherapy Research as well as the Carl Rogers Award and the Award for Distinguished Professional Contributions to Applied Research of the American Psychological Association. He also has received the Canadian Psychological Association Award for Distinguished Contributions to Psychology as a Profession. He is a past president of the Society for Psychotherapy Research.